COLORECTAL SURGERY

Seventh Edition

A Companion to Specialist Surgical Practice

Series Editors
O. James Garden
Simon Paterson-Brown

Seventh Edition

COLORECTAL SURGERY

Edited by

Sue Clark, MA, MD, FRCS(Gen Surg), EBSQ(Coloproctology)

Consultant Colorectal Surgeon, St Mark's, The National Bowel Hospital;
Professor of Practice (Colorectal Surgery), Department of Surgery and Cancer,
Imperial College, London, UK

Phil Tozer, MBBS, FRCS, MD(Res)

Consultant Colorectal Surgeon, St Mark's, The National Bowel Hospital;
Honorary Senior Lecturer, Department of Surgery and Cancer,
Imperial College, London, UK

For additional online content visit eBooks+

ELSEVIER

First edition 1997
Second edition 2001
Third edition 2005
Fourth edition 2009
Fifth edition 2014
Sixth edition 2019
Seventh edition 2024

Notices

Practitioners and researchers must always rely on their own experience and knowledge in evaluating and
using any information, methods, compounds or experiments described herein. Because of rapid advances in
the medical sciences, in particular, independent verification of diagnoses and drug dosages should be made.
To the fullest extent of the law, no responsibility is assumed by Elsevier, authors, editors or contributors for
any injury and/or damage to persons or property as a matter of products liability, negligence or otherwise, or
from any use or operation of any methods, products, instructions, or ideas contained in the material herein.

ISBN: 978-0-7020-8501-7

Content Strategist: Alexandra Mortimer
Content Project Manager: Arindam Banerjee
Design: Ryan Cook
Art Buyer: Muthukumaran Thangaraj
Marketing Manager: Deborah Watkins

Printed in India

Last digit is the print number: 9   8   7   6   5   4   3   2   1

Contents

Series Editors' preface

The *Companion to Specialist Surgical Practice* series has now reached its Seventh Edition and continues to remain popular for both surgeons in training as well as consultant surgeons in independent practice. The strength of this series has always been founded on contemporary, evidence-based information on the subspecialist areas relevant to their general surgical practice and this Seventh Edition has followed this plan.

This Edition continues to keep abreast of increasing subspecialisation in general surgery. The ongoing developments in minimal access and increasingly robotic surgery are discussed, along with the desire of some subspecialities, such as breast and vascular surgery, to separate away from 'general surgery' in some countries. However, all volumes also underline the importance for all surgeons of being aware of current developments in their surgical field. The importance of evidence-based practice and in particular the management of emergency conditions remains throughout, and authors have provided recommendations and highlighted key resources within each chapter. The ebook version of the textbook has also enabled improved access to the reference abstracts and links to video content relevant to many of the chapters.

As in all the previous editions, we are greatly indebted to the volume editors, and contributors, who have all put so much hard work into delivering such a high quality piece of work. We remain grateful for the support and encouragement of the team at Elsevier and we trust that our original vision of delivering an up-to-date, affordable text has been met and that readers, whether in training or independent practice, will find this Seventh Edition an invaluable resource.

We are grateful to Kathryn Rigby and Jonathan Michaels who wrote the guidelines on Evidence-based Practice in Surgery for previous editions of the series. These have been well received and have been retained again for this new edition in order to help guide readers in their assessment of the various levels of evidence discussed in each chapter.

O. James Garden, CBE, BSc, MBChB, MD, DSc(Hon), FRCS (Glas), FRCS(Ed), FRCP(Ed), FRACS(Hon), FRCSC (Hon), FACS(Hon), FCSHK(Hon), FRCSI(Hon), FRCS(Engl)(Hon), FRSE, MAMSE, FFST(RCSEd)

Professor Emeritus, Clinical Surgery, University of Edinburgh, UK.

Simon Paterson-Brown, MBBS, MPhil, MS, FRCS(Ed), FRCS (Engl), FCSHK, FFST(RCSEd)

Honorary Senior Lecturer, Clinical Surgery, University of Edinburgh, UK.

Series Editors' preface

Editors' preface

In this Seventh Edition we have incorporated material from the previous separate chapter on 'investigation' into the relevant topic chapters and updated it. A number of authors have joined the team, and as a result we have fresh chapters on rectal cancer, chemotherapy and radiotherapy for colorectal cancer, Crohn's disease and anal fistula. The presentation of anal neoplasia has been revamped, with an entirely new chapter covering HPV, AIN and anal cancer.

There are links to videos, which will complement the written descriptions and diagrams. Multiple choice questions to enable readers to test their knowledge have been introduced in this edition.

The aim has been to be clear, concise, authoritative and contemporary, and to emphasise the underlying evidence-base. This is achieved using clearly signposted 'expert opinion' (one tick) and 'strong recommendation' (two tick) panels, together with brief descriptions of the key papers.

This volume provides more than enough information for those preparing for general and colorectal surgical examinations, and to support those in consultant practice. Each print volume gives access to the accompanying ebook version, which should enhance the overall experience and ensure that it is enjoyable to read and to use.

ACKNOWLEDGEMENTS

The editors would like to acknowledge and offer grateful thanks for the input of all previous editions' contributors, without whom this new edition would not have been possible.

Sue Clark
Phil Tozer
London

Evidence-based practice in surgery

Critical appraisal for developing evidence-based practice can be obtained from a number of sources, the most reliable being randomised controlled clinical trials, systematic literature reviews, meta-analyses and observational studies. For practical purposes three grades of evidence can be used, analogous to the levels of 'proof' required in a court of law:

1. **Beyond all reasonable doubt**. Such evidence is likely to have arisen from high-quality randomised controlled trials, systematic reviews or high-quality synthesised evidence such as decision analysis, cost-effectiveness analysis or large observational datasets. The studies need to be directly applicable to the population of concern and have clear results. The grade is analogous to burden of proof within a criminal court and may be thought of as corresponding to the usual standard of 'proof' within the medical literature (i.e. $P < 0.05$).

2. **On the balance of probabilities**. In many cases a high-quality review of literature may fail to reach firm conclusions due to conflicting or inconclusive results, trials of poor methodological quality or the lack of evidence in the population to which the guidelines apply. In such cases it may still be possible to make a statement as to the best treatment on the 'balance of probabilities'. This is analogous to the decision in a civil court where all the available evidence will be weighed up and the verdict will depend upon the balance of probabilities.

3. **Not proven**. Insufficient evidence upon which to base a decision, or contradictory evidence.

Depending on the information available, three grades of recommendation can be used:

Strong recommendation, which should be followed unless there are compelling reasons to act otherwise.

    a. A recommendation based on evidence of effectiveness, but where there may be other factors to take into account in decision-making, for example the user of the guidelines may be expected to take into account patient preferences, local facilities, local audit results or available resources.

    b. A recommendation made where there is no adequate evidence as to the most effective practice, although there may be reasons for making a recommendation in order to minimise cost or reduce the chance of error through a locally agreed protocol.

✓✓ Evidence where a conclusion can be reached 'beyond all reasonable doubt' and therefore where a **strong recommendation** can be given.

This will normally be based on evidence levels:

- Ia. Meta-analysis of randomised controlled trials
- Ib. Evidence from at least one randomised controlled trial
- IIa. Evidence from at least one controlled study without randomisation
- IIb. Evidence from at least one other type of quasi-experimental study.

✓ Evidence where a conclusion might be reached 'on the balance of probabilities' and where there may be other factors involved which influence the recommendation given. This will normally be based on less conclusive evidence than that represented by the double tick icons:

- III. Evidence from non-experimental descriptive studies, such as comparative studies and case–control studies
- IV. Evidence from expert committee reports or opinions or clinical experience of respected authorities, or both.

Evidence that is associated with either a **strong recommendation** or **expert opinion** is highlighted in the text in panels such as those shown above, and is distinguished by either a double or single tick icon, respectively. The references associated with double-tick evidence are listed as Key References at the end of each chapter, along with a short summary of the paper's conclusions where applicable. The full reference list for each chapter is available in the ebook.

The reader is referred to Chapter 1, 'Evaluation of surgical evidence' in the volume *Core Topics in General and Emergency Surgery* of this series, for a more detailed description of this topic.

Contributors

Beshar Allos, BMedSci, MBChB, MRCP, PgDip, FRCR
Consultant Clinical Oncology
Cancer Centre
University Hospitals Birmingham NHS Foundation Trust
Birmingham, United Kingdom

Omer Aziz, MBBS, BSc(Hons), DIC, PhD, FRCS
Manchester Academic Health Science Centre Chair in
   Surgery
Division of Cancer Sciences
University of Manchester
Manchester, United Kingdom

Ayan Banerjea, MA, PhD, FRCS
Consultant Colorectal Surgeon
Nottingham Colorectal Service
Nottingham University Hospitals NHS Trust
Nottingham, United Kingdom

Steven R. Brown, MBChB, FRCS, MD, BMedSci
Professor
Department of Surgery
Sheffield Teaching Hospitals
Yorkshire, United Kingdom

**Tamzin Cuming, MA(Cantab), MBBS, FRCS(Eng),
FRCS(Gen Surg), MEd**
Consultant Surgeon
Chair, Women in Surgery Forum
Royal College of Surgeons of England
London, United Kingdom

Eric J. Dozois, MD, FACS, FACRS
Chair
Division of Colon and Rectal Surgery
Mayo Clinic
Rochester, Minnesota, United States

Anton V. Emmanuel, MD, FRCP
Professor
GI Physiology
University College London Hospitals NHS Foundation
   Trust
London, United Kingdom

Ian Geh, MB BS, MRCP, FRCR
Consultant Clinical Oncologist
Cancer Centre
University Hospitals Birmingham NHS Foundation Trust
Birmingham, United Kingdom

Pasquale Giordano, MD, FRCS, FRCSEd
Consultant General and Colorectal Surgeon
Department of Colorectal Surgery
Pelvic Floor Service Clinical Lead
Complex Benign Abdominal & Pelvic Service Clinical Lead
Barts Health NHS Trust;
Honorary Senior Lecturer
Queen Mary University of London
London, United Kingdom

Gaetano Gallo, MD, PhD
Assistant Professor of Surgery
Department of Surgery
Sapienza University of Rome
Rome, Italy

Alison J. Hainsworth, MBBS, BSc, FRCS
Consultant Colorectal Surgeon
Colorectal and Pelvic Floor Unit
Guy's and St Thomas' Hospital
London, United Kingdom

Adam Haycock, MBBS, MRCP, BSc, MD
Consultant Gastroenterologist and Endoscopist
Wolfson Unit for Endoscopy
St Mark's Hospital;
Honorary Senior Lecturer
Imperial College
London, United Kingdom

**Alexander Heriot, MB BChir, MA, MD, MBA, FRACS,
FRCS(Gen), FRCSEd, FACS, FASCRS, GAICD**
Consultant Colorectal Surgeon
Director of Surgery
Division of Cancer Surgery
Peter MacCallum Cancer Centre
Melbourne, Australia

Nicola Hodges, FRACS
Clinical Research Fellow
St Mark's Hospital
Imperial College London
London, United Kingdom

Scott R. Kelley, MD, FACS, FASCRS
Consultant
Colon and Rectal Surgery
Mayo Clinic
Rochester, Minnesota, United States

Andrew Latchford, MBBS, BSc(Hons), MRCP, MD
Consultant Gastroenterologist
Centre for Familial Intestinal Cancer
St Mark's Hospital;
Department of Surgery and Cancer
Imperial College
London, United Kingdom

Paul-Antoine Lehur, MD, PhD
Professor
Coloproctology Unit
EOC Lugano
Lugano, Switzerland

Alan J. Lobo, MB, BS, MD, FRCP, FAoP
Professor of Gastroenterology
Inflammatory Bowel Disease Centre
Sheffield Teaching Hospitals and University of Sheffield
Sheffield, United Kingdom

Akash Mehta, MD
Consultant Colorectal and Intestinal Failure Surgeon
Department of Colorectal Surgery and The Lennard-Jones
    Intestinal Rehabilitation Unit
St Mark's Hospital
Harrow, United Kingdom

Danilo Miskovic, PhD, FRCS
Consultant Surgeon
Department of Surgery
St Mark's Hospital;
Honorary Senior Lecturer
Department of Surgery
Imperial College
London, United Kingdom

Katy Newton, MBChB, FRCS, MD, MA
Consultant Colorectal Surgeon
Department of Surgery
Manchester Royal Infirmary
Manchester, United Kingdom

Gregory P. Thomas, MBBS, BSc, MD, FRCS
Consultant Colorectal Surgeon
The Sir Alan Parks Department of Physiology
St Mark's Hospital, The National Bowel Hospital, London
    Northwest University Healthcare NHS Trust;
Honorary Senior Clinical Lecturer
Imperial College
London, United Kingdom

Siwan Thomas-Gibson, MD, FRCP
Consultant Gastroenterologist
Wolfson Unit for Endoscopy
St Mark's Hospital;
Professor of Practice
Imperial College
London, United Kingdom

Phil Tozer, MBBS, FRCS, MD(Res)
Consultant Colorectal Surgeon
St Mark's, The National Bowel Hospital;
Honorary Senior Lecturer
Department of Surgery and Cancer
Imperial College
London, United Kingdom

Carolynne Vaizey, MBChB, MD, FRCS(Gen), FCS(SA)
Consultant Colorectal and Intestinal Failure Surgeon
Department of Colorectal Surgery and The Lennard-Jones
    Intestinal Rehabilitation Unit
St Mark's, The National Bowel Hospital
London, United Kingdom

Andrew B. Williams, MBBS, BSc, MS, FRCS
Consultant Colorectal and Pelvic Floor Surgeon
London, United Kingdom

Des Winter, MD, FRCSI, FRCS(Gen)
Consultant Surgeon
St Vincent's University Hospital;
Professor
National University of Ireland
Dublin, Ireland

Lower gastrointestinal endoscopy

Siwan Thomas-Gibson | Adam Haycock

INTRODUCTION

Since flexible endoscopy of the colon was introduced in 1963, it has become the gold-standard diagnostic test for evaluation of colonic disease. Improvements in technique and technology have also led to advances in therapeutic procedures, and the boundary between endoscopic and surgical procedures is becoming increasingly blurred. A good understanding of both the technique and technology is essential for an endoscopist to perform high-quality, safe endoscopy. This chapter gives an insight into how lower gastrointestinal (GI) endoscopy is influencing the practice of colorectal surgery.

INDICATIONS AND CONTRAINDICATIONS

FLEXIBLE SIGMOIDOSCOPY OR COLONOSCOPY?

Indications for colonoscopy or flexible sigmoidoscopy must be weighed against the risk/benefit profile. Diagnostic colonoscopy has a higher risk of complications relating to sedation and bowel preparation than diagnostic flexible sigmoidoscopy. Flexible sigmoidoscopy is also quicker, cheaper and easier to perform, and detection of distal pathology can be considered as a marker for possible proximal pathology, prompting full colonoscopy.

CONTRAINDICATIONS

The only absolute contraindications are a competent patient who is unwilling to give consent or a known free colonic perforation. Relative contraindications include: acute diverticulitis, immediately post-operative patients, a recent myocardial infarction (within 30 days), acute pulmonary embolism, severe coagulopathy (particularly for therapeutic procedures) or haemodynamic instability. In fulminant colitis, a limited examination to ascertain extent of disease and acquire confirmatory biopsies is often helpful. In general, colonoscopy or flexible sigmoidoscopy is considered to be safe in pregnancy but should only be performed for strong indications and after careful consent and liaison with an obstetrician.[1]

CHECKLIST

Checklists prevent errors, have a positive impact on patient morbidity and mortality in surgical settings and are now commonplace, or mandatory, in many endoscopy units.

SEDATION

Sedation during colonoscopy is the subject of much debate and research. A large multicentre European audit showed that most colonoscopies were done using moderate (conscious) sedation and that although deep sedation was associated with shorter procedure times and fewer technical difficulties, it was also more resource-intensive and required more hospitalisations for complications. American Society of Gastrointestinal Endoscopy recommendations are that routine use of deep sedation in average-risk patients cannot be endorsed. A recent British position statement noted that the need for deep sedation and anaesthesia is increasing because of the growing complexity of GI endoscopy.[2] Flexible sigmoidoscopy is most often performed unsedated, as the use of intravenous sedation would negate many of the potential benefits of the procedure. Unsedated colonoscopy is certainly possible with few complications and good acceptability.[3] Nitrous oxide (Entonox) can be a useful adjunct in unsedated patients as it is short acting and reversible, but does have a cost implication and is implicated in climate change, as it is 300 times more potent as a greenhouse gas than carbon dioxide.

✔ Research and audit have identified continued avoidable morbidity and mortality from sedation. Recommendations are for competency-based formal training for all healthcare professionals involved in sedation.[4]

INSERTION TECHNIQUE

Insertion technique varies even amongst expert colonoscopists. Technique depends on local circumstances, sedation practice, endoscopist preference and equipment available. However, there are some basic principles that are recognised to contribute to safe, efficient colonoscopy.

HANDLING AND SCOPE CONTROL

Most skilled colonoscopists now adopt the one-person, single-handed approach, where the right hand is used to manipulate the shaft and the left hand operates the angulation controls. Tip control is gained by a combination of up/down angulation with the large wheel and clockwise/anti-clockwise torque applied with the right hand. Left/right angulation using the small wheel is used for maintaining the luminal view while torque is being applied with the right hand.

1

INSERTION AND STEERING

A digital rectal examination should be performed to lubricate the anal canal and detect any anal and distal rectal pathology before insertion. Intubation of the anus should be under direct visualisation. The initial view is often a 'redout' because of the lens pressing against the rectal mucosa. Gentle insufflation, slow withdrawal and small amounts of tip angulation are used to gain a view of the lumen. Rectal retroflexion is best performed at the start of the procedure to identify any distal pathology.

TIPS FOR INSERTION AND STEERING

- **Pull back more, push in less.** The first rule of good colonoscopy is to keep the shaft straight. This allows accurate tip control, prevents stretching of the mesentery, minimises discomfort and shortens the colon by a 'concertina' effect, telescoping the bowel wall over the shaft. Pulling back often reduces acute angles of bends, disimpacts the tip of the scope and improves the view. In contrast, excessive pushing of the scope often results in formation of large loops, excessive pain, loss of one-to-one tip control and increases the risk of iatrogenic perforation.[5]
- **Use torque frequently.** Twisting clockwise or anticlockwise with the right hand applies torque to the shaft of the scope. With a straight shaft and bent tip, use of torque will provide lateral movement at the tip and help to stiffen the scope to prevent looping during advancement. Application of torque is also essential for loop resolution. Without the use of an image guidance device, the application of torque will be determined both by frequency of loop type and 'feel' of the instrument. The majority of sigmoid loops (N-loops, 80%; alpha loops, 10%) require clockwise torque and pull-back to resolve; atypical loops (reverse sigmoid N-spiral, 1%; reverse-alpha, 5%) require anti-clockwise torque.
- **Minimise insufflation.** Pain or discomfort during colonoscopy is often caused by stretching of the bowel wall by excessive gas insufflation. Pneumatic perforation of the right colon from over-insufflation has been reported. Frequent suctioning of gas prevents this and may often allow progression of the tip through the colon by the concertina effect. The use of carbon dioxide rather than air has been shown to cause less discomfort and is widely recommended.[6] The use of water-aided (either water-immersion or water-exchange) colonoscopy is also now advocated to improve comfort scores and may improve adenoma detection rate.[7]

PATIENT POSITION CHANGE

Moving the patient's position from the left lateral position during both insertion and withdrawal can shift both fluids away from, and air into, the uppermost segment of bowel, preventing unnecessary suctioning of fluid and insufflation of gas. It can provide mechanical advantage by opening up acute bends, especially at the rectosigmoid junction, splenic and hepatic flexures. The effective use of gravity to assist the passage of the endoscope is a simple, technique that is easily learnt. It has been shown to be effective in promoting endoscope tip advancement in two-thirds of cases,[8] but it

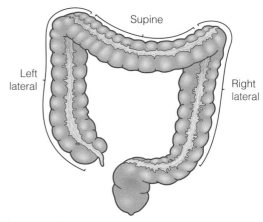

Figure 1.1 Schema for optimal patient position change.

does require cooperation from the patient and can be difficult if heavy sedation or general anaesthesia is used (Fig. 1.1). If water immersion or exchange is used, the patient should remain in the left lateral position while negotiating the left colon, as the water helps weigh down the sigmoid, minimising loop formation by reducing acute bends and tight angulations.

ABDOMINAL HAND PRESSURE

The use of abdominal hand pressure aims to prevent the shaft of the endoscope looping by opposing pressure close to the anterior abdominal wall. Pressure is best used to prevent a loop forming rather than applying it to an already formed loop, which is unlikely to be successful and may increase the discomfort felt by the patient. Specific pressure on anterior-protruding loops is more likely to be helpful than non-specific pressure.[9] Magnetic imaging devices can help with guided pressure, although efficacy in promoting tip advancement is less than for patient position change,[8] as many loops do not protrude anteriorly. The use of deep inspiration can also be used to splint the diaphragm and provide pressure on the splenic and hepatic flexures if external pressure is unsuccessful.

THREE-DIMENSIONAL IMAGER

Magnetic imaging systems (ScopeGuide, Olympus Optical Company; ScopePilot, Pentax Medical) use low-voltage magnetic fields to produce a real-time, three-dimensional image of the entire colonoscope shaft in both anteroposterior and lateral views, allowing the colonoscopist to visualise the configuration of the scope within the patient (Fig. 1.2). This can help determine if there is an anterior component to a loop and so assist with loop resolution, as well as aiding accurate tip location. A sensor can assist with accurate hand-pressure placement.

✔ Meta-analysis of eight randomised controlled trials has shown real-time magnetic imaging to be of benefit in training and educating inexperienced endoscopists and improves the caecal intubation rate for experienced and inexperienced endoscopists.[10]

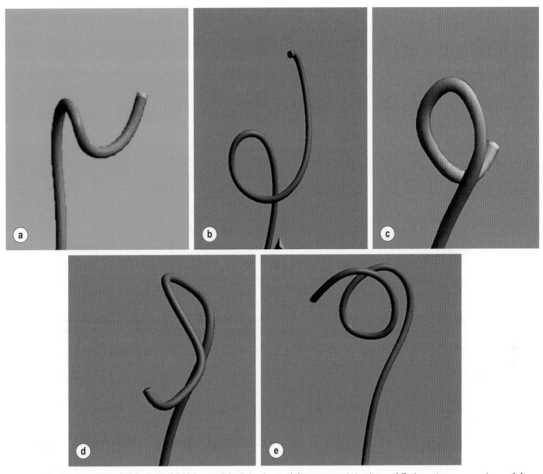

Figure 1.2 ScopeGuide images of: **(a)** sigmoid N-loop; **(b)** alpha loop; **(c)** reverse alpha loop; **(d)** deep transverse loop; **(e)** gamma loop.

WITHDRAWAL AND EXAMINATION TECHNIQUE

It should be remembered that the aim of colonoscopy is to visualise the whole of the colonic mucosa to identify pathology. A systematic review of back-to-back studies[11] has shown a polyp miss rate at colonoscopy of 22%, even in expert hands, although most missed polyps were small (<1 cm). All studies investigating miss rates have shown a variation in performance between endoscopists, and this can be wide even with expert examiners (>10 000 procedures), with sensitivities ranging from 17–48% in one large study.[12] This implies that there is a link between individual technical skill and outcome measures. Studies looking at the causes of post-colonoscopy colorectal cancers have shown that up to 89% may be avoidable,[13] although tumour biology may be more important than endoscopist factors.[14]

WITHDRAWAL TIME

Recent publications have stressed the importance of spending sufficient time inspecting the colonic mucosa on withdrawal as a key marker for the adequacy of the examination.

The current recommendation is that colonoscopists should spend more than 6 minutes during withdrawal inspecting the colonic mucosa in colonoscopies with normal results.[15] A landmark study[16] looking specifically at withdrawal time found that endoscopists who spent longer than 6 minutes on withdrawal in a negative colonoscopy had significantly higher adenoma detection rates (ADR) than quicker examinations, but there was no advantage in taking over 10 minutes.

OPTIMAL EXAMINATION TECHNIQUE

It seems logical that those colonoscopists who take longer to withdraw also use techniques that increase visualisation of abnormalities. In one study looking at differences in technique between two colonoscopists with different polyp miss rates,[17] a lower miss rate was associated with superior withdrawal technique for each of the following examination criteria: (1) examining the proximal sides of flexures, folds and valves; (2) cleaning and suctioning; (3) adequacy of distension; and (4) adequacy of time spent viewing. A study looking at the quality of inspection at flexible sigmoidoscopy[18] has included similar criteria: (1) time spent viewing the mucosa; (2) re-examination of poorly viewed areas; (3) suctioning of fluid pools; (4) distension of the lumen; and (5) lower rectal examination.

The following continuous quality improvement targets regarding withdrawal (adapted from Rex et al.[17]) aim to standardise withdrawal technique to maximise detection rates:

1. Mean examination times during withdrawal should average at least 6–10 minutes.
2. Adenoma prevalence rates detected during colonoscopy in persons over 50 years of age undergoing first-time examination should be ≥25% in men and ≥15% in women.
3. Documentation of quality of bowel preparation in all cases.

The implementation of systematic monitoring of withdrawal time and other quality indicators may, in itself, increase the performance of endoscopists.[19]

BOWEL PREPARATION

It is self-evident that pools of fluid or faeces will obscure good visualisation of the mucosa, and many studies have examined the effectiveness of various bowel preparations for clearing the colon before colonoscopy.

✓✓ Evidence-based recommendations on bowel preparation for colonoscopy are available from many national and international societies.[20,21]

It has been shown that better quality preparation at flexible sigmoidoscopy results in a higher ADR,[22] and that endoscopists with a higher ADR are more likely to be critical of the quality of bowel preparation.

POSITION CHANGE

The use of position change has been shown in a randomised controlled trial to improve luminal distension between the hepatic flexure and sigmoid-descending junction during colonoscope withdrawal.[23] The same schema can be used for each segment as previously illustrated for insertion (see Fig. 1.1). Although four cross-over trials have shown that the improved visualisation that results can also improve polyp and adenoma detection rates, three parallel trials did not, and a meta-analysis concluded that the effectiveness is uncertain.[24]

ANTISPASMODICS

Pre-medication with an antispasmodic such as hyoscine *N*-butyl bromide (Buscopan) has been used for colonoscopy to decrease the amount of muscular spasm caused by peristalsis. There is insufficient evidence to conclude whether antispasmodics improve caecal intubation rate, predominantly because the baseline rates were already high. Antispasmodics probably have efficacy in reducing caecal intubation time, especially in those with marked colonic spasm, but do not offer significant benefit in polyp detection or improving patient comfort during diagnostic colonoscopy.[25] Caution must be exercised in patients with known cardiac history as there is a risk of sinus tachycardia.

RECTAL AND RIGHT-SIDED RETROFLEXION

Colorectal cancer is most common distally, and most experts routinely perform retroflexion in the rectum. Although the evidence that this significantly improves detection rates is still being debated,[26] it probably allows clearer views of the proximal sides of rectal valves and the top of the anal canal. There is a risk of iatrogenic perforation if the rectal lumen is narrow, in which case a paediatric colonoscope or thin upper GI endoscope can be used. A recent meta-analysis of publications looking at the value of retroflexion in the proximal colon concluded there is a benefit in terms of adenoma detection and small risk of adverse events.[27] A quality improvement study has shown that a training bundle consisting of routine use of hyoscine, rectal retroflexion and minimum withdrawal time can improve global ADR, driven by improvements among the poorest performing colonoscopists.[28] Some adjuncts such as distal attachments on the scope may reduce the need to retroflex by improving the view in these positions.

NEW TECHNIQUES IN ENDOSCOPIC MUCOSAL VISUALISATION

There are many new developments in colonoscopic technique and technology that may improve polyp detection and identification of pathology.

ASSISTED-VIEWING DEVICES

Cuffs, caps and rings have been developed that attach to the tip of the colonoscope and improve the view by flattening the folds of the colon during withdrawal, allowing for improved visibility behind folds. They have all been shown to increase ADR, particularly for small proximal polyps, and there may also be additional benefit of rings and cuffs in improved caecal intubation rates and decreased pain scores.[29] Retrograde (Third-Eye RetroScope) and 360-degree viewing endoscopes (Third-Eye Panoramic, Fuse FullSpectrum Endoscopy, Ewave) have shown some efficacy in improving ADR but have not shown benefit when incorporated into routine practice.[30]

CHROMOENDOSCOPY

Chromoendoscopy is a technique that uses a surface dye such as indigo carmine to make irregularities in the colonic mucosa more readily apparent to the endoscopist (Fig. 1.3).

✓✓ The use of chromoendoscopy has been shown to significantly improve adenoma detection during surveillance of high-risk groups such as ulcerative colitis[31–33] and familial colorectal cancer syndromes.[34]

It has also been shown to aid identification of flat or depressed adenomas, which are much more prevalent than was previously thought and have a high risk of malignant transformation. It can, however, be time-consuming and currently, there is no evidence for its use during routine colonoscopy.

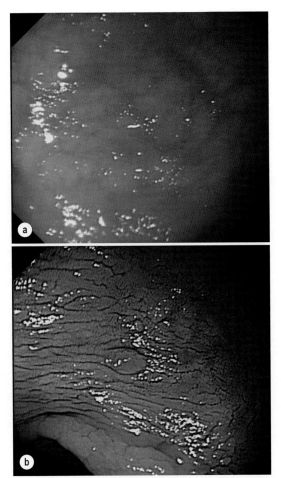

Figure 1.3 **(a)** Polyp in white light. **(b)** With indigo carmine dye-spray.

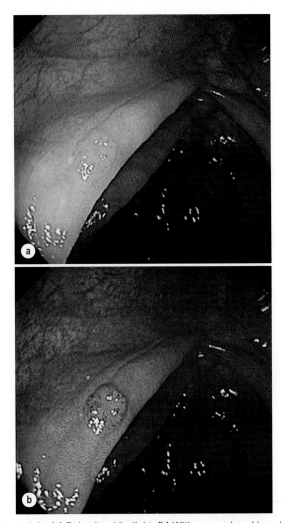

Figure 1.4 **(a)** Polyp in white light. **(b)** With narrow band imaging.

Optical enhancement (or electronic chromoendoscopy) uses optical filters to narrow the bandwidth of white light (narrow-band imaging, NBI), or spectral emission processing of white light (I-scan, Flexible Spectrum Imaging Colour Enhancement, FICE) to enhance the visualisation of the capillary network or microsurface pattern of colonic adenomas (Fig. 1.4).[35] These technologies are activated by the push of a button on enabled scopes, which has clear advantages over the use of dye-spray. They are recommended for use in high-risk groups such as Lynch syndrome patients where spotting even diminutive adenomas is crucial, but randomised trials have not shown significant benefit in routine endoscopy.[36,37] Confocal laser endomicroscopy combines a standard video endoscope with a miniaturised laser microscope. Using intravenous sodium fluorescein as a contrast agent, 'virtual histology' can be created, allowing visualisation of both the surface epithelium and some of the lamina propria, including the microvasculature. This can potentially provide accurate identification of colonic intra-epithelial neoplasia and carcinoma, although many barriers have so far prevented uptake in routine use.[38]

HIGH-MAGNIFICATION ENDOSCOPY

High-magnification endoscopes can magnify the image up to 100 times, and newer high-definition scopes have a much greater pixel density and ability to improve detail discrimination. In conjunction with dye-spray or electronic chromoendoscopy, their use permits identification of a polyp's surface 'pit pattern' to assist in distinguishing between cancerous, adenomatous and non-adenomatous polyps. A classification system devised by Kudo has been shown to have a reasonable diagnostic accuracy (overall 86.1%, sensitivity 90.8%, specificity 72.7%) when compared to histological findings[39] (Fig. 1.5). There is a learning curve in identification of the patterns, however, so for inexperienced endoscopists, it does not significantly reduce the number of histological samples taken. Further work has resulted in a simple classification system, the Narrow-band Imaging International Colorectal Endoscopic (NICE) Classification,[40] but studies have yet to confirm its real-world utility, and current evidence does not support a 'resect-and-discard' approach.[41]

ARTIFICIAL INTELLIGENCE AND COMPUTER-AIDED DIAGNOSIS

In lower GI endoscopy, Artificial Intelligence (AI) and deep-learning algorithms have the potential to assist with both computer-aided polyp detection (CADe) and polyp characterisation (CADx). Initial studies demonstrated the ability of AI in real-time recognition and identification for colonic

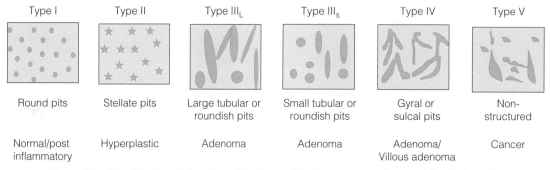

Figure 1.5   Classification of pit pattern at high-magnification chromoendoscopy (after Kudo et al.).

adenomas of >90%.[42] One AI system (GI Genius, Medtronic) has shown initial promise in a randomised controlled trial, increasing ADR by 9% compared to standard withdrawal without significantly impacting withdrawal time.[43]

QUALITY ASSURANCE

There are now detailed guidelines for quality standards in colonoscopy, which include key performance indicators, measurable outcomes and minimum standards.[15,44,45] These aim to ensure a high-quality, effective and patient-centred service by setting benchmarks for both individual endoscopists and unit performance. Development of these guidelines has been driven by the implementation of bowel cancer screening programmes, which involve asymptomatic individuals choosing to undergo invasive investigations. It is imperative to minimise risk for this group by provision of a safe, high-quality service. This has had the benefit of improving quality assurance standards for the whole of endoscopy.[46]

The COVID-19 pandemic has reinforced the need for high quality safety practices within all hospital and procedural disciplines. A toolkit of cognitive aids, based on human factors principles, has been developed to help teams adapt to working safely in the era of COVID-19.[47]

SUSTAINABLE ENDOSCOPY

Given the recognition of the impact of climate change, many healthcare organisations (e.g., NHS Net Zero) are seeking practical ideas to attain net carbon zero targets. Endoscopy is a major contributor to the environmental footprint of health care, generating about 3.09 kg of waste per bed per day. There is a growing interest in sustainability and minimising the environmental impact by targeted interventions such as improved waste segregation, increased recycling, or the avoidance of single-use items where possible. Detailed analyses of the sustainability of each step in endoscopy activities may allow the identification of small but cumulative beneficial changes.[48]

ENDOSCOPY TRAINING

Guidelines on training have been published both in the UK and US to improve access to and quality of endoscopy training.[49,50] Accredited national courses in endoscopy have

been developed to provide more readily available and structured training, and have now become essential components of gastroenterology training. Focus has also been placed on ensuring that those endoscopists responsible for training or performing screening procedures on healthy populations are themselves competent to do so. 'Training the Trainers' courses teach experienced endoscopists adult education theory and its application to skills training in endoscopy.

Accreditation for colonoscopists wishing to undertake colorectal cancer screening is now mandatory in England and Wales. Both initiatives are aimed at maximising the provision of high-quality endoscopy and training on a national basis and not just in teaching centres. A national audit in 2011 of all colonoscopies done in England demonstrated improvements in virtually all aspects of colonoscopy,[46] including training, validating the rigorous quality assurance process undertaken in recent years.

The use of both computer and animal endoscopic simulation has now been shown to be of value in the early phase of colonoscopy training,[51] with transfer of skills to live patients. The importance of non-technical skills and teamwork is vital to the performance of high-quality endoscopy. Training can improve safety-related knowledge and attitudes,[52] and observation of behavioural markers relating to these non-technical skills now forms part of the UK assessment and credentialing process.[53]

✔ Current European recommendations are that endoscopy simulators, where available, should be used to allow training to occur in a safe, controlled environment.[54]

ENDOSCOPIC THERAPY

One of the exciting benefits of improving endoscopic skills and technology is the increasingly successful application of novel therapeutic techniques. Therapy that previously required open surgical procedures can now be performed with minimally invasive techniques.

BASIC THERAPY

POLYPECTOMY
The ability to remove neoplastic lesions endoscopically forms the basis of all cancer prevention and surveillance programmes. The resectability of a polyp depends on its site, morphology, size and accessibility.[55] Polyps that are unlikely to be endoscopically resectable are those with submucosal

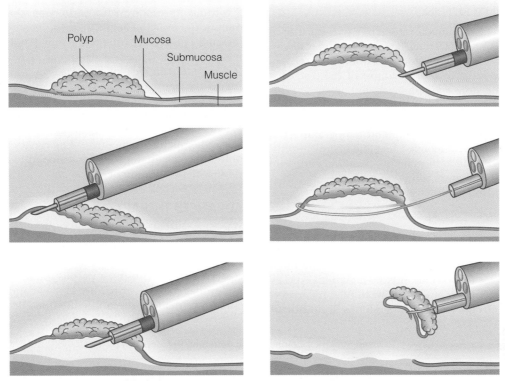

Figure 1.6 Technique for endoscopic mucosal resection.

invasion, large sessile polyps extending beyond 50% of the bowel circumference, low rectal polyps extending beyond the dentate line, or lesions encircling the appendix orifice.[56] It is recognised that serrated lesions are also more difficult to resect as they have indistinct edges.[57]

Very tiny polyps 2 mm or less in size can be removed by cold forceps but are more commonly now removed using cold snare. Hot biopsy is no longer recommended by either the American or European endoscopy societies. Polyps up to 10 mm are now routinely resected using cold snare, and cold-snare endoscopic mucosal resection (EMR) is safe and effective up to 20 mm, with higher complete resection rates than conventional EMR.[58] The risk of significant bleeding is very low, even in patients on anticoagulation, and the practice of bridging with heparin does now seem to have a higher risk than remaining on single agent anticoagulants or antiplatelet agents.[59]

Larger stalked polyps are best removed using a conventional hot snare. The stalk should be transected approximately halfway between the polyp and the bowel wall. This ensures a clear resection margin whilst leaving sufficient stalk in place to facilitate endoscopic treatment should post-polypectomy bleeding occur. Diathermy settings should be chosen to ensure enough coagulating current is applied to allow adequate haemostasis of the blood vessels within the polyp stalk. A validated Direct Observation of Polypectomy Skills assessment tool has been developed to assist with the training and evaluation of polypectomy technique,[60] and is now in clinical use for competency assessment of trainees and in the Bowel Cancer Screening accreditation processes in England and for trainees in the United States.

Retrieval of the polyp is important to determine the histology and grade of dysplasia. Small polyps can be sucked through the scope into a polyp trap, while larger polyps can be grasped or snared and withdrawn with the scope. Retrieval baskets or nets are particularly useful for retrieving more than one piece of tissue or multiple polyps.

ENDOSCOPIC MUCOSAL RESECTION

EMR involves injection of fluid into the submucosal space to lift the mucosa (and the polyp) away from the muscle layer of the bowel wall (Fig. 1.6). This facilitates removal of sessile or flat lesions, reducing the risk of thermal injury to the bowel wall. The authors find the addition of dilute adrenaline (1:200 000) to improve haemostasis and a few drops of contrast dye (e.g., indigocarmine or methylene blue) to differentiate the submucosal plane helpful. Large lesions (>2 cm) can be removed in a piecemeal fashion safely using a submucosal lift. Polyp recurrence may be reduced following piecemeal resection by the judicious use of thermal coagulation to destroy small areas of residual polyp around the resection margin, although the evidence for this is weak.

The 'non-lifting' sign, when a polyp fails to lift with a submucosal injection, should raise the suspicion of malignant invasion of the submucosa, assuming it is a de novo lesion. Lesions that do not lift should be biopsied, tattooed (Fig. 1.7) and referred for expert assessment and consideration of advanced techniques such as endoscopic submucosal dissection (ESD) or surgical resection. Underwater EMR[61] may be therapeutically successful for non-lifting recurrent lesions but should be performed by very experienced endoscopists.

INVESTIGATION OF ACUTE LOWER GASTROINTESTINAL BLEEDING

The lower GI tract accounts for a quarter to a third of all hospitalised cases of GI bleeding,[62] with diverticular disease being by far the most common cause. Colitis, cancer, polyps and angiodysplasia account for most of the rest. Most lower GI bleeding stops spontaneously and, in those cases, an elective colonoscopy with standard bowel preparation is appropriate. In the uncommon case of continued bleeding requiring hospitalisation, computed tomography (CT) angiography is the recommended first-line investigation to localise the source of blood loss before planning endoscopic or radiological therapy.[63] Surgery is reserved for cases of recurrent, uncontrolled or massive bleeding.

COLONIC DECOMPRESSION

The three main causes of bowel obstruction are cancer, diverticular disease and sigmoid volvulus. Flexible sigmoidoscopy with placement of a decompression tube is the initial treatment of choice for volvulus. It has a high initial success rate (78%) but is only a temporising measure as recurrence is common and elective surgery is therefore still considered

the definitive treatment. Emergency surgery is reserved for a volvulus unresponsive to endoscopic therapy or for patients with bowel ischaemia or peritonitis.

Acute colonic pseudo-obstruction (Ogilvie's syndrome) may mimic the signs and symptoms of bowel obstruction. It may be initially treated conservatively with removal of any triggering factors, mobilisation and the use of a parasympathomimetic agent such as neostigmine (if not contraindicated). If this approach fails, then endoscopic placement of a decompression tube is generally accepted as the first invasive therapeutic manoeuvre. Emergency surgery is again only indicated in resistant or complicated cases, such as those with perforation or ischaemia.

ADVANCED THERAPY

ENDOSCOPIC SUBMUCOSAL DISSECTION
ESD is a technique that has been developed for 'en bloc' resection of large lesions in the GI tract. A deep, submucosal lift is created using a viscous solution such as sodium hyaluronate or 10% glycerine. Mucosal and submucosal incisions are made using a modified needle knife to dissect

Revised St Mark's Colonoscopic Tattooing Protocol 2011

Indications	Equipment	Procedure
• Prior to surgery to localise pathology • To mark lesions for endoscopic surveillance • **Do not tattoo rectal lesions** as they disrupt surgical planes • There is no need to tattoo lesions in the caecum; however, **if in doubt, then place a tattoo**	• Primed variceal injection needle with 10mL syringe filled with normal saline • 5mL syringe filled with Spot® (or 0.9mL sterilised Black (Indian) Ink made up to 5mL with normal saline)	• Direct needle at an angle to mucosa • Raise a bleb using 1-2mL of saline • Swap to syringe filled with Spot® or Indian Ink • Inject 1mL into the bleb to create tattoo • Swap to syringe filled with saline and flush ink out with 1mL saline before removing needle • Repeat process for 3 tattoos

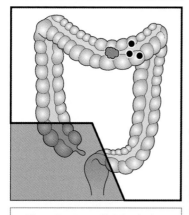

Place 3 tattoos **distal** to lesion

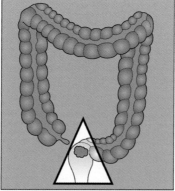

Do not place tattoo below 20cm but clearly record distance of LESION from anal verge

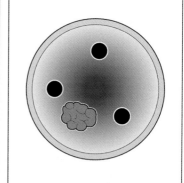

Place tattoos 120° apart **as close to lesion as possible** but separate from it

Remember: To document **how many** tattoos were placed and **the position relative to the lesion**

Figure 1.7 St Mark's colonoscopic tattooing protocol.

the mucosa from the submucosa. A transparent hood is attached to the endoscope tip to help retract tissue and maintain the submucosal field of view. The benefit of this technique is that it produces en bloc specimens for complete histological analysis, but the technique itself is difficult with a long learning curve, and success depends on excellent endoscopic and haemostatic skills. As a time-consuming procedure, usually taking between 2 and 3 hours in expert hands, ESD should be performed only when carefully planned with appropriate consent and nursing team and where surgical backup is available. It does achieve a higher rate of en bloc and R0 resection compared to EMR, at the cost of a higher risk of complications.[64]

STRICTURE DILATATION AND STENTING

The dilatation of colonic strictures is generally reserved for benign disease, whereas the use of self-expandable metal stents (SEMS) is usually indicated for malignant disease.[65]

Through-the-scope balloon dilators have been used in the management of strictures associated with inflammatory bowel disease, non-steroidal anti-inflammatory drug–induced colonic strictures and anastomotic strictures. Success rates vary, with recent studies suggesting short-term relief in 70–100%, but with frequent recurrence. Complication rates are significant, with a risk of perforation of 2% and bleeding between 4% and 11%.

SEMS are usually inserted through the scope and can be deployed as far as the proximal ascending colon. Preoperative stenting of malignant strictures can, in carefully selected cases, allow for one-stage surgical procedures, but are mostly used for palliation, with patency established up to a year. SEMS can also be considered as a potential therapy for selected benign strictures and has been reported for anastomotic strictures unresponsive to dilatation, Crohn's disease, diverticular disease and radiation-induced strictures.

NOVEL THERAPIES

As technology and endoscopic skill evolve, the lines between what is possible endoscopically, laparoscopically and traditionally have become increasingly blurred. Although initial interest in natural orifice transluminal endoscopic surgery was high, most studies have concluded that the standard laparoscopic techniques are quicker and safer. However, enthusiasts continue to innovate. A novel trans-anal endo-surgical approach to large, complex rectal polyps may allow for minimally invasive management of polyps that were previously destined for surgery.[66] Endoscopic full-thickness resection techniques may allow for wider local oncological resection, although new platforms and prospective clinical trials are required before they are taken up in routine clinical practice.[67] Balloon-assisted colonoscopy can be used to provide a stable platform for advanced endoscopic therapy and may enable access in cases that were previously incomplete because of technical difficulties.

COMPETING TECHNOLOGIES

Currently, optical colonoscopy remains the gold-standard test for examination of the colon because of its relatively high pathology detection rate and the ability to perform therapy. However, newer techniques are emerging that may be considered as 'disruptive technologies' that will undoubtedly change the current position.

COMPUTED TOMOGRAPHY COLONOGRAPHY

Computed tomography colonography (CTC), also known as *virtual colonoscopy* (VC; or 'CT pneumocolon'), is now an established technique for detecting colon cancer and colonic polyps. It comprises two low-dose CT scans of the abdomen and pelvis, and is less invasive than optical colonoscopy, requires no conscious sedation and may be better tolerated by patients. The diagnostic performance characteristics can be comparable to expert optical colonoscopy with sensitivity for detecting large polyps (>10 mm in maximal diameter) exceeding 90% and 96% for cancer,[68] but it lacks the facility for mucosal biopsy or polyp removal. It has, however, now superseded barium enema as the radiological test of choice for the colon.

SELF-PROPELLING COLONOSCOPES

One disadvantage of traditional optical colonoscopy is the prolonged training required for expertise. There would be significant advantages to providing the same examination and potential for therapy without the need for an experienced operator. A number of self-propelling or self-navigating colonoscopes have been developed, but these have not been widely adopted despite initial tests showing them to be safe and effective. The current trend is clearly towards greater quality and accuracy of traditional colonoscopy performance, rather than widespread adoption of new technology.

COLON CAPSULE

Wireless capsule endoscopy is a safe, minimally invasive, nonsedation requiring, patient-friendly modality to visualise the bowel, and is now considered first line for investigation of small bowel disease in appropriate patients without contraindications such as stricturing disease. The development of the PillCam colon capsule (Given Imaging Ltd, Yoqneam, Israel) aims to widen the application to investigation of colonic disease so that pan-endoscopy can be achieved. It is attractive for similar reasons and, unlike optical colonoscopy, only requires expertise in image interpretation. The second-generation PillCam Colon Capsule 2 has a wider field of view and adaptive frame rate than the first-generation, and a meta-analysis has demonstrated high specificity for polyps over 10 mm in a screening setting. European guidelines now consider it as an option following incomplete colonoscopy or in patients with no alarm-symptoms, although the evidence base is low.[68]

CONCLUSIONS

This chapter has given an overview of the role of lower GI endoscopy in the diagnosis, treatment and prevention of colorectal disease. Traditional optical endoscopy is becoming more refined and new technologies are emerging that will impact on its diagnostic and therapeutic capability. The current focus is on quality assurance and improvements in training with continual skill development essential for all those endoscopists wishing to perform high-quality, safe endoscopy. Future developments include incorporation of AI/CAD to improve performance outcomes and the provision of more environmentally sustainable endoscopy.

Key points

- Good technique is vital for high-quality safe endoscopy.
- Sedation should be standardised, tailored to patient needs and administered by clinicians with formal training.
- Withdrawal times should be a minimum of 6 minutes in normal colonoscopies.
- Advanced imaging techniques are now becoming more widely available and may impact on diagnostic capabilities.
- All endoscopists should be familiar with basic therapeutic techniques (polypectomy, diathermy, decompression) and indications for referral for advanced therapy (EMR, ESD, stenting).
- Adjunctive and competing technologies are evolving and need to be evaluated for their utility in clinical practice.
- Performance in technical skills should be considered in conjunction with non-technical skills and team working.

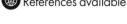 References available at http://ebooks.health.elsevier.com/

▶ RECOMMENDED VIDEOS

- http://www.stmarksacademicinstitute.org.uk/resources/colonoscopy-insertion-steering-and-examination/.
- http://www.stmarksacademicinstitute.org.uk/resources/colonoscopy-experts-in-action-part-1/.
- http://www.stmarksacademicinstitute.org.uk/resources/colonoscopy-experts-in-action-part-2/.
- http://www.stmarksacademicinstitute.org.uk/resources/colonoscopy-equipment-and-accessories/.
- http://www.stmarksacademicinstitute.org.uk/resources/olympus-scopeguide-3d-imager/.
- http://www.stmarksacademicinstitute.org.uk/resources/polypectomy-training-polypectomy-in-detail/.

KEY REFERENCES

[15] Rizk MK, Sawhney MS, Cohen J, et al. Quality indicators common to all GI endoscopic procedures. Gastrointest Endosc 2015;81(1):3–16. PMID: 25480102.

[16] Barclay RL, Vicari JJ, Doughty AS, et al. Colonoscopic withdrawal times and adenoma detection during screening colonoscopy. N Engl J Med 2006;355(24):2533–41. PMID: 17167136.

Observational study of 12 experienced colonoscopists over 7882 colonoscopies showing a 10-fold difference in ADR between endoscopists and a significant difference in those who spent more or less than 6 minutes during withdrawal in normal colonoscopies.

[20] ASGE Standards of Practice Committee. Bowel preparation before colonoscopy. Gastrointest Endosc 2015;81(4):781–94. PMID: 25595062.

[21] Hassan C, East J, Radaelli F, et al. Bowel preparation for colonoscopy: European Society for Gastrointestinal Endoscopy (ESGE) guideline – update 2019. Endoscopy 2019;51(8):775–94. PMID: 31295746.

[31] Hurlstone DP, Sanders DS, McAlindon ME, et al. High-magnification chromoscopic colonoscopy in ulcerative colitis: a valid tool for in vivo optical biopsy and assessment of disease extent. Endoscopy 2006;38(12):1213–7. PMID: 17163321.

Biphasic examination with 1800 images from 300 patients obtained via conventional or magnification imaging. Magnification imaging was significantly better than conventional colonoscopy for predicting disease extent in vivo (P < 0.0001).

[32] Kiesslich R, Fritsch J, Holtmann M, et al. Methylene blue-aided chromoendoscopy for the detection of intraepithelial neoplasia and colon cancer in ulcerative colitis. Gastroenterology 2003;124(4):880–8. PMID: 12671882.

Randomised controlled trial of 165 patients showing a significantly better correlation between the endoscopic assessment of degree (P = 0.0002) and extent (89% vs. 52%; P <0.0001) of colonic inflammation and the histopathological findings in the chromoendoscopy group compared with the conventional colonoscopy group. More targeted biopsies were possible and significantly more neoplasias were detected (32 vs. 10; P = 0.003).

[33] Rutter MD, Saunders BP, Schofield G, et al. Pancolonic indigo carmine dye spraying for the detection of dysplasia in ulcerative colitis. Gut 2004;53(2):256–60. PMID: 14724160.

Back-to-back colonoscopies in 100 patients showing significantly more dysplasia detection with chromoendoscopy and targeted biopsies (P = 0.02). Chromoendoscopy required fewer biopsies (157 vs. 2904) yet detected nine dysplastic lesions, seven of which were only visible after indigo carmine application.

[34] Hurlstone DP, Karajeh M, Cross SS, et al. The role of high-magnification-chromoscopic colonoscopy in hereditary nonpolyposis colorectal cancer screening: a prospective 'back-to-back' endoscopic study. Am J Gastroenterol 2005;100(10):2167–73. PMID: 16181364.

Back-to-back colonoscopies in 25 asymptomatic HNPCC patients. Panchromoscopy identified significantly more adenomas than conventional colonoscopy (P = 0.001) and a significantly higher number of flat adenomas (P = 0.004).

Colorectal cancer

2

Ayan Banerjea

INTRODUCTION

Colorectal cancer is a significant healthcare issue in terms of prevention, timely diagnosis, treatment and survivorship. Improving outcomes remains a key healthcare challenge in the UK, where bowel cancer is the second most common cause of cancer death, accounting for over 16 000 deaths annually.[1] Over 42 000 new cases are diagnosed each year, the majority arising in the elderly, although increasing incidence in younger patients has been recorded worldwide. Overall numbers are higher in men, especially in the rectum, but right colon cancer incidence is higher in women. The overall 5-year survival rate is around 58%, with 'early' disease yielding 5-year survival over 90%, compared to only 10% in those with metastases at diagnosis.[1]

New National Institute for Health and Care Excellence (NICE) guidance[2] focuses on information for patients and shared decision making, reflecting changes in UK societal expectations around valid consent; quality of life considerations also feature, as do minimum numbers for rectal cancer major resections. Accurate outcome data are key to quality improvement and the National Bowel Cancer Audit Project underpins this process in England and Wales.[3]

Distinguishing the colon and rectum is important – treatment regimens differ and comparisons between treatments, or minimum numbers for site-specific treatments, cannot be measured without uniform definitions. The colon comprises the large bowel proximal to the rectum but, historically, the definition of the rectum has been variable. Anatomical texts describe the top of the rectum as the point where the sigmoid mesocolon ends or that part of the large bowel level with the third sacral vertebra, whilst some surgeons think of the rectum as the large bowel segment lying within the true pelvis. Another intra-operative definition is the fusion of the two anti-mesenteric taenia into an amorphous area where the true rectum begins. In the UK, a rectal cancer is a tumour within 15 cm of the anal verge,[3] whereas US authorities have preferred 11 or 12 cm. Standardised use of cross-sectional radiology for staging and expanding non-operative options for rectal cancer mean a radiological definition may be most appropriate. The 'sigmoid take-off' is the point where the fixed mesorectum ends and no longer tethers the rectum to the sacrum, whilst the mesocolon elongates, and consensus around this reproducible radiological definition may grow over time.[4]

NATURAL HISTORY

Approximately 50% of cancers arise in the rectum and left colon, 25% in the right, with synchronous lesions in around 5% of cases (Fig. 2.1). Most colorectal cancers arise from pre-existing polyps (Box 2.1).[5] The majority of adenomas diagnosed in the West are polypoid or exophytic, but the flat adenoma, where the depth of the dysplastic tissue is no more than twice that of the mucosa, may account for up to 40% of all adenomas. In addition, the serrated lesion, which is histologically distinct and related to the hyperplastic polyp, is now a recognised pre-malignant condition.[6] These characteristically right-sided lesions, are easily missed and may represent pre-malignant lesions in an 'accelerated' cancer pathway, perhaps explaining some interval cancers that arise between endoscopies. Reliable diagnosis requires a skilful, experienced endoscopist, using dye spray on the colonic mucosa and narrow band imaging (NBI) to aid detection. Newer techniques, including mechanical adjuncts that improve luminal views and digital software that highlights irregular mucosa for closer inspection, are discussed in Chapter 1.

When invasion has taken place, colorectal cancer can spread directly and by the lymphatic, blood and transcoelomic routes.

DIRECT SPREAD

Direct spread occurs longitudinally, transversely and radially, but as adequate proximal and distal clearance is technically feasible in most colorectal cancers, radial spread is a key surgical consideration. A retroperitoneal colonic cancer may involve the ureter, duodenum or posterior abdominal wall muscles; intra-peritoneal tumours may involve small intestine, stomach, pelvic organs or the anterior abdominal wall. Rectal tumours may involve the pelvic organs or side walls.

LYMPHATIC SPREAD

Lymphatic spread progresses from the paracolic nodes along the main colonic vessels to the nodes associated with either cephalad or caudal vessels, eventually reaching the para-aortic glands in advanced disease. However, this orderly process may be inconsistent, and in about 30% of cases nodal involvement can skip a tier of glands.[7] In contrast to rectal disease, where drainage is via the mesorectal nodes, it is unusual for a colonic cancer that has not breached the muscle wall to exhibit lymph node metastases.

BLOOD-BORNE SPREAD

The most common site for blood-borne spread of colorectal cancer is the liver, presumably arriving by the portal venous system. Up to 37% of patients may have occult liver metastases at the time of operation, and approximately 50% of

Bowel cancer cases:
percentage distribution by anatomical site

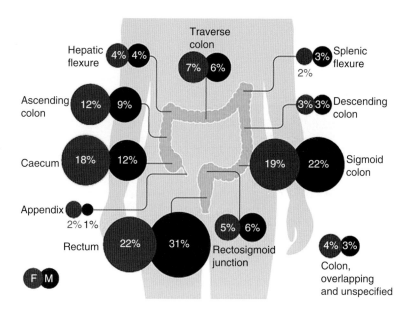

Figure 2.1 Frequency of anatomical locations of colorectal cancer for men and women in the UK (2010–2012). (Credit: Cancer Research UK[1])

cruk.org/cancerstats
Together we will beat cancer

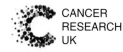
CANCER
RESEARCH
UK

Box 2.1 Evidence for the polyp-cancer (adenoma-carcinoma) sequence that underlies most colorectal cancers

1. Adenoma prevalence correlates well with that of carcinomas, the average age of adenoma patients being around 5 years younger than patients with carcinomas.
2. Adenomatous tissue often accompanies cancer, and it is unusual to find small cancers with no contiguous adenomatous tissue.
3. Most sporadic adenomas are identical histologically to the adenomas of familial adenomatous polyposis (FAP), and this condition is unequivocally premalignant.
4. Large adenomas are more likely to display cellular atypia and genetic abnormalities than smaller lesions.
5. The distribution of adenomas and carcinomas is similar throughout the large bowel.
6. Adenomas are found in up to one-third of all surgical specimens resected for colorectal cancer.
7. The incidence of colorectal cancer falls with a long-term screening programme involving colonoscopy and polypectomy.

---

patients develop overt disease at some time. The lung is the next most common site, with around 10% of patients developing lung metastases at some stage; other reported sites include ovary, adrenal, bone, brain and kidney.

TRANSCOELOMIC SPREAD

Colonic cancer may spread throughout the peritoneum, either via the subperitoneal lymphatics or by virtue of viable cells being shed from the serosal surface of a tumour, giving rise to malignant ascites, which is relatively rare.

AETIOLOGY

Colorectal cancers arise as a result of a combination of environmental and inherited risk factors. In most, environmental factors are the main cause, with only 5% of cancer patients having a high-risk inherited genetic predisposition, although lower risk genetic variants probably play a part in many more. Cancers arise due to a complex interplay between the intraluminal environment, host-tumour immune responses and the colonic mucosa, wherein genetic alterations drive neoplasia. Knowledge of the molecular genetics of colorectal cancer has increased rapidly and it is now evident that numerous pathways exist, layers of redundancy allowing cancers to escape host responses and progress. The gut microbiome may act as a mediator of environmental factors.[8] The microbiomes of colorectal cancer patients display distinct properties, although it is not clear whether this is a 'cause or effect' of disease. Certain bacterial species demonstrate altered profiles in bowel cancer patients and perhaps some ability to modulate disease progression and response to treatment (Fig. 2.2). Further studies in this area might drive improvements in prevention, diagnosis, individualised treatment and quality of life – the use of pre-operative antibiotics with mechanical bowel preparation demonstrates these concepts influencing current practice.

GENETIC PATHWAYS

The predisposing genetic factors and molecular changes underlying familial colorectal cancer have been widely studied (Chapter 3). In summary, the two most commonly inherited forms of colorectal cancer are Lynch syndrome, caused by deoxyribonucleic acid (DNA) mismatch repair gene mutation, and familial adenomatous polyposis (FAP), caused by *APC*

Microorganisms may drive colorectal cancer

Three examples of the possible mechanisms by which bacteria might influence colorectal cancer. It remains unclear whether they have a causative role in colorectal carcinogenesis and the potential mechanisms involved.

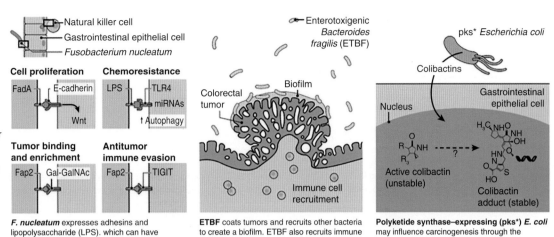

Gal-GalNAc, galactose N-acetyl-D-galactosamine: miRNA, microRNA: TIGIT, T cell immunoreceptor with Ig and ITIM domains: TLR4, Toll-like receptor 4.

Figure 2.2 Possible mechanisms of interactions between microbiomes and colorectal carcinogenesis. (Reproduced with permission from Garrett WS. The gut microbiota and colon cancer. Science 2019.[8] Illustratorr: V. ALTOUNIAN/*SCIENCE*.)

gene mutation. However, family history in the absence of these mutations does confer increased risk, reflecting a combination of shared environmental factors and lower penetrance inherited genetic polymorphisms. Sporadic colorectal cancer mirrors inherited pathways in two of four groups, now defined as Consensus Molecular Subtypes (CMS).[9] Around 14% demonstrate microsatellite instability (MSI), arising from acquired dysfunction in mismatch repair (CMS1), and associations with serrated adenomas, the right colon, older female patients and smoking. Another 37% demonstrate chromosomal instability associated with more traditional adenomas and genetic changes (CMS2). Two further groups are described although some cancers sit across these four categories.

Immunohistochemical staining for mismatch repair genes in resection specimens is now recommended for improved Lynch kindred identification, but also promotes identification of sporadic MSI colorectal cancer. This is clinically relevant as this subset has altered response to standard chemotherapeutic agents. Molecular testing for certain gene mutations is now considered routine practice to guide adjuvant chemotherapy.

DIET AND LIFESTYLE

The World Cancer Research Fund (WCRF) updates a systematic review of the world literature on Food, Nutrition, Physical Activity and the Prevention of Cancer every 10 years.[10]

✔✔ Physical activity reduces the risk of colorectal cancer, whilst processed meat intake, obesity, adult attained height and alcohol consumption increase risk.[10] Probable associations include reduced risk with dietary fibre, wholegrains, dairy and calcium, and increased risk with red meat consumption. The increased risk reported with diabetes is intertwined with obesity. Obesity and physical activity are recognised areas for preventive action. Long-term smoking is associated with colorectal cancer (particularly with sporadic CMS 1 subtype), and quitting reduces this risk.[11]

PREDISPOSING CONDITIONS

Long-standing inflammatory bowel disease, both ulcerative colitis and Crohn's disease, increases the risk of colorectal cancer. Previous gastric surgery (gastrectomy and vagotomy) has also been implicated, and although the association is controversial, the risk may be about twofold – altered bile acid metabolism may play a role in this process. The risk after ureterosigmoidostomy is well established, although this operation has now been superseded by ileal conduit formation for urinary diversion.

PRESENTATION

Around 20% of colorectal cancers present as emergencies, despite established pathways that encourage urgent referral for recognised chronic symptoms. This highlights that patients with colorectal cancer at all stages may be asymptomatic, fail to consult for symptoms, or only report vague symptoms. The commonest emergency presentations are bowel obstruction and rectal bleeding. Occasionally, emergency presentation may relate to a palpable mass, more rarely a sigmoid cancer causes pneumaturia or urinary infection by fistulation into the bladder, or a gastrocolic fistula may cause faecal vomiting or severe diarrhoea.

Most diagnoses are made after primary care referral and since 2000, pathways to investigate 'high risk' patients urgently, based on age and symptoms, have been implemented in the UK (Table 2.1). However, notwithstanding an initial decrease in emergency presentations, these pathways and sustained public awareness campaigns have increased the number of patients being investigated without positive effect on the stage at diagnosis,[12] and similar numbers of diagnoses are made on routine pathways. Updated guidelines broadened referral criteria in 2015, reducing the threshold for urgent referral criteria to a positive predictive value of 3%, aiming to increase diagnosis at early stage and improve clinical outcomes.[13] This further exacerbated demand for diagnostics without any demonstrable benefit, but also reintroduced the concept of testing for occult blood in faeces. There is now significant interest in the use of quantitative faecal immunochemical testing (FIT) for detection of faecal haemoglobin (fHb) in symptomatic patients, although initial guidance recommended use specifically in 'low-risk' patients that do not qualify for urgent referral.[14]

Table 2.1   Comparison of referral guidelines before and after NICE guideline NG12,[13] which aimed to increase the proportion of cancers diagnosed at early stage by defining the predictive value of referral criteria to 3% or above

Urgent referral guidelines for colorectal cancer – England and Wales		
	Pre 2015	**NICE guideline NG12 (2015)**
All ages	Definite palpable right sided abdominal mass	Consider referral for abdominal mass
	Definite palpable rectal (not pelvic) mass	Consider referral for rectal mass
	Unexplained Iron deficiency anaemia **and** Hb <11.0 males Hb <10 non-menstruating females	*See later*
Over 40 years	Rectal bleeding WITH a change of bowel habit to looser stools and/or increased frequency >6 weeks	Aged under 50 years with rectal bleeding **and** any of the following unexplained symptoms or findings: <ul><li>abdominal pain</li><li>change in bowel habit</li><li>weight loss</li><li>Iron-deficiency anaemia.</li></ul> Unexplained weight loss and abdominal pain Aged under 60 years **and** positive for occult blood in faeces **without** rectal bleeding with: <ul><li>changes in their bowel habit **or**</li><li>iron-deficiency anaemia</li></ul>
Over 50 years		Unexplained rectal bleeding Aged over 50 years and positive for occult blood in faeces **without** rectal bleeding and unexplained: <ul><li>abdominal pain or</li><li>weight loss, or</li></ul> Aged under 60 years **and** positive for occult blood in faeces **without** rectal bleeding with: <ul><li>changes in their bowel habit or</li><li>iron-deficiency anaemia.</li></ul>
Over 60 years	Rectal bleeding >6 weeks without a change in bowel habit or anal symptoms	Unexplained rectal bleeding
		Iron-deficiency anaemia Any anaemia **and** positive for occult blood in faeces
	Change of bowel habit to looser stools and/or increased frequency >6 weeks without rectal bleeding	Changes in bowel habit

Hb, Haemoglobin; *NICE*, National Institute for Health and Care Excellence.
NICE. Suspected cancer: recognition and referral. NICE guidelines[NG12] 2015 (updated July 2017) Available from: https://www.nice.org.uk/guidance/ng12/chapter/Introduction accessed March 2021.

FIT is a risk stratification tool and effectively segments the symptomatic population into a majority with very low risk (around 0.5%), and groups with higher risk.

The NICE FIT study, a large multi-centre double-blinded study of 9822 'high-risk' patients undergoing colonoscopy, demonstrated that the risk of bowel cancer was around 0.2% in those with undetectable levels of fHb and 0.4% using a cut-off of 10 μg Hb/g faeces.[15] Fifty-six percent of 3143 patients referred with rectal bleeding had undetectable fHb, and the risk of bowel cancer remained very low.[16]

These data broadly concur with other research studies and three large service evaluations where FIT was used to stratify symptomatic patients in Primary Care. In Northern Spain[17] and Tayside,[18] all symptoms were included, and in Nottingham rectal mass and bleeding were excluded;[19] the cancer diagnosis rate after reassurance without investigation based on low fHb results in primary care was

consistently 0.3% or less at follow-up. FIT misses a small number of colorectal cancers, but far fewer than referral criteria based on symptoms and age and identifies a population with low risk in whom investigation might be deferred or undertaken routinely. Anaemia,[20] iron deficiency and thrombocytosis[21] may all have added value in defining optimal thresholds, or may yet combine with FIT and demographics to improve on existing scoring systems. Patients with very high fHb readings harbour increased risk of bowel cancer, or significant bowel pathology, and should be prioritised for urgent investigation and 'one-stop' services. Point-of-care testing platforms are emerging but clear guidelines around current uncertainties are awaited (Box 2.2).

Newer technologies may in future combine with, or supersede FIT ; these include 'liquid biopsy' concepts.[22] Blood tests for cell-free circulating tumour DNA (ctDNA) or circulating tumour cells have mainly been considered for surveillance, but diagnostic uses may emerge as the

Box 2.2 Considerations in the use of FIT in symptomatic patients

Sampling, storage and analysers

- User error: Patients usually collect their own samples. Storage over 14 days or in heated areas increases 'false negatives'. Different 'pickers' and different platforms may yield different results, particularly at low levels of fHb.

Thresholds

- A threshold of 10 µg Hb/g faeces misses marginally more cancers than the limit of detection – this varies between platforms. Most studies demonstrate colorectal cancer risk is around 0.5–1% in 'high-risk symptom' populations with fHb less than 10 µg Hb/g faeces.
- Anaemia, iron deficiency and thrombocytosis are recognised markers of risk that may prompt lower thresholds and improve cut-off selection.
- 10 µg Hb/g faeces may be too low for younger patients with vague symptoms and normal bloods. Opportunistic testing in Primary Care is likely.

Primary care or secondary care

- FIT improves selection of patients for urgent referral, but access in primary care prompts referral of some patients previously managed by routine referral or without referral. It is not clear that access in primary care reduces demand on urgent diagnostic capacity.
- Use in secondary care may guide resource allocation and test selection but may cause delay in timed pathways. Point of care platforms may address this concern.

Palpable rectal mass

- A well-performed digital rectal examination remains the most cost-effective way to detect a palpable rectal cancer. FIT negative palpable rectal cancer has been documented. Bleeding rectal cancers would be expected to demonstrate overt bleeding.

Rectal bleeding

- FIT may be used in rectal bleeding – undetectable fHb identifies a lower risk cohort, potentially allowing reassurance or selection between colonoscopy and flexible sigmoidoscopy. Highest fHb results are seen in left-sided tumours, perhaps because blood is closer to the surface of stools. It is unclear whether FIT is better at predicting pathology beyond the splenic flexure than anaemia, abdominal mass and thrombocytosis.

Iron-deficiency anaemia

- Right-sided cancers yield lower fHb results (haemoglobin degradation may explain this) and commonly present with anaemia and/or iron deficiency – the liquid nature of the faeces and wider colon lumen make obstructive symptoms unusual. Blood from tumours might be distributed more evenly in the eventual solid stool and hence, easier to miss at sampling.

Imminent obstruction

- In left-sided tumours change of bowel habit, colicky abdominal pain and rectal bleeding are the commonest symptoms. Watery diarrhoea caused by obstruction represents a sampling challenge and is another cause of 'FIT negative' cancers.

Repeat testing

- There is no clarity on the value or recommended interval for repeat FIT testing, but some pathways are exploring a second negative test for reassurance.

FIT, Faecal immunochemical testing; *fHb*, faecal haemoglobin.

---

technique advances. Multi-target stool DNA testing detects DNA shed from adenomas and cancers, as well as fHb, and is approved in the United States, where one screening study demonstrated increased sensitivity but lower specificity than fHb alone.[23] It remains expensive and data on use in symptomatic patients is limited. Utility of volatile organic compounds in blood, urine, stool and breath, requires further evaluation and the value of microbiome profiles is speculative.

INVESTIGATION

Currently, the main investigative techniques are sigmoidoscopy, colonoscopy and computed tomography colonography (CTC) – barium enema has fallen out of favour. Colonoscopy remains the 'gold standard' for whole colon investigation but even in the best hands carries a small risk of perforation, with significant consequences for the patient, may be incomplete in around 5% of cases and misses some lesions. One UK study demonstrated that 7.4% of individuals having negative colonoscopy were diagnosed with colorectal cancer within 3 years, with lower rates in those examined by accredited screening colonoscopists.[24]

Precise tumour localisation at colonoscopy is challenging as the only reliable landmarks are the anus and the terminal ileum, although the use of magnetic scope guides allows more accurate estimation of the site of a lesion. In the era of laparoscopic surgery, a tattoo should be placed 'anal' to any colonic cancer.

✓ CT colonography or 'virtual colonoscopy' is effective in detecting polypoid lesions down to 6 mm in diameter and superior to barium enema for the detection of cancers and significant polyps.[25]

CT colonography is particularly useful in older, frail or co-morbid patients, or when cessation of anticoagulants or antiplatelets is undesirable. It offers increased capacity for whole colon investigation and might be preferred in patients with low or undetectable fHb, in whom weight loss, abdominal mass or altered bowel habit may be caused by extra-colonic pathology. Capsule endoscopy has now been modified to allow examination of the large bowel and may become an important tool in colorectal investigation. Rigid sigmoidoscopy has been largely superseded by flexible sigmoidoscopy for examination of the rectum and distal colon. The majority of cancers are within reach of a flexible

Table 2.2   Clinicopathological staging of colorectal cancer[26]

TNM staging

T[†]	Primary tumour
TX	Primary tumour cannot be assessed
T0	No evidence of primary tumour
Tis	Carcinoma in situ
T1	Tumour invades submucosa
T2	Tumour invades muscularis propria
T3	Tumour invades through muscularis propria into subserosa or into non-peritonealised pericolic or perirectal tissues
T4a	Tumour perforates the visceral peritoneum
T4b	Tumour directly invades other organs or structures[‡]
N	Regional lymph nodes
NX	Regional lymph nodes cannot be assessed
N0	No regional lymph node metastasis
N1	Metastasis in 1–3 pericolic or perirectal lymph nodes
N1a	1 nearby node involved
N1b	2 or 3 nearby nodes involved
N1c	Tumour deposits (satellites) – discrete mesenteric cancer nodules that are discontinuous from the primary, without histological evidence of residual lymph node (lymphatic invasion) or identifiable vascular (vascular invasion) or neural (perineural invasion) structures.
N2	Metastasis in 4 or more pericolic or perirectal lymph nodes
N2a	4 to 6 nearby nodes involved
N2b	7 or more nodes involved
M	Distant metastasis
M0	No distant metastases
M1	Distant metastases
M1a	Single distant organ or set of nodes involved, without distant peritoneal involvement
M1b	More than one distant organ or set of nodes involved, without distant peritoneum involved
	Distant peritoneum involved

Stage	Estimated 5-year UK survival	TNM
I	93%	T1-2, N0, M0
IIA	84%	T3, N0, M0
IIB		T4a, N0, M0
IIC		T4b, N0, M0
IIIA	65%	T1-2, N1/1c, M0 OR T1, N2a, M0
IIIB		T3/4a, N1/1c OR T2-3, N2a, M0 OR T1-2, N2b, M0
IIIC		T4a, N2a, M0 OR T3-4a, N2b, M0 OR T4b, N1-2, M0
IVA-C	10%	Any T, Any N, M1 (further divided a-c)

[†]Additional letters used include UT, ultrasound depth; yT, following neoadjuvant therapy; pT, following pathological examination. [‡]Direct invasion in T4 includes invasion of other segments of the colorectum by way of the serosa, e.g., invasion of the sigmoid colon by a carcinoma of the caecum.
Brierley JD GM, Wittekind C. The TNM Classification of Malignant Tumours. 8th ed 2016.

sigmoidoscopy, and more proximal disease is uncommon in the absence of anaemia, iron deficiency or abdominal mass.[20] Detection of a sentinel left-sided adenoma should prompt completion colonoscopy if feasible. However, the extent to which the colon can be visualised is highly variable when enema preparation is used.

After diagnosis, radiological staging of the primary tumour, liver and lungs aims to predict the pathological stage and is crucial to choosing the appropriate sequence of treatments. Dukes' staging is simple, reproducible and widely recognised, but TNM staging is now the international standard (Table 2.2).[26] Classical markers of poor prognosis – metastatic disease and lymph node involvement – remain important, but poorer outcomes are also reported with T4 status, local mesenteric tumour deposits (termed *N1c*) and lymphovascular invasion. In rectal cancer, involvement of the circumferential resection margin determines the choice between surgery and chemoradiotherapy in the first instance.

✔ CT of the chest, abdomen and pelvis is the staging modality of choice. In rectal cancer, magnetic resonance imaging (MRI) allows accurate pre-operative staging, assessing key prognostic markers that guide treatment planning. Endorectal ultrasound may help to discriminate T1 from T2 tumours but is highly operator dependent. Positron emission tomography–CT helps to exclude occult disease when surgical resection of metastases or advanced primary cancer is being considered.[27]

SCREENING

Colorectal cancer is suitable for population screening. Prognosis is much better when treating early-stage disease and the polyp–cancer sequence offers opportunities to prevent cancer by treating pre-malignant disease. The ideal screening test detects relevant pathology, with high sensitivity and specificity, and should be safe and acceptable to the population offered screening. Screen-detected tumours are much more likely to be at an early stage than symptomatic disease, but this does not prove that screening is beneficial. Even improved survival in patients whose tumours are detected by screening is not conclusive because of selection bias, length bias and lead-time bias:

- Selection bias arises as people who accept screening tend to be more health conscious than the general population.
- Length bias reflects the disproportionate diagnosis of cancers that are slow growing, thereby having good prognosis.
- Lead-time bias is the interval between detection by screening and the date that cancer would have been diagnosed otherwise. As survival is measured from the time of diagnosis, screening advances the diagnosis date, thus lengthening the survival time, without necessarily affecting the date of death.

✅✅ Effectiveness should be assessed by comparing disease-specific mortality in a population offered screening with that in an identical population not offered screening. In colorectal cancer, testing for occult blood in faeces (FOB) was evaluated in three randomised controlled trials. Annual FOB testing in Minnesota yielded 33% reduction in colorectal cancer-specific mortality and a 21% reduction with biennial screening.[28] In Nottingham, biennial FOB testing demonstrated a 15% reduction in cumulative mortality[29] and a similar study from Funen, Denmark, showed an 18% reduction in mortality.[30]

The UK Bowel Cancer Screening Programme (BCSP) was introduced using Haemoccult, a guaiac-based FOB test that detects the peroxidase-like activity of haematin in faeces, accepting recognised disadvantages with uptake, sensitivity and specificity. Quantitative FIT is now the preferred test and uses antibody to detect globin, conferring better specificity and sensitivity for occult blood. FIT is associated with higher uptake, as, unlike the guaiac test, only one sample is required, and the collection device is more hygienic. Automated and objective quantification avoids the human observational error of its predecessor, and thresholds and performance characteristics can be set to suit the screening programme. Interestingly, concerns around diagnostic capacity, specifically colonoscopy, have yielded different cut-offs across the UK – England adopting 120 µg Hb/g faeces, Wales 150 µg Hb/g faeces and Scotland 80 µg Hb/g faeces – at roll-out.

Endoscopy may be used as a primary screening test. Colonoscopy is used in some countries but as 70% of cancers and large adenomas are found in the distal 60 cm of the large bowel, flexible sigmoidoscopy has also been evaluated. Once-only flexible sigmoidoscopy, between the ages of 55 and 64 years, reduced colorectal cancer mortality *and* incidence, particularly in the rectum and left colon, in a multi-centre randomised study.[31] The incidence reduction is undoubtedly because of adenoma removal at the time of flexible sigmoidoscopy. In the UK, flexible sigmoidoscopy screening was introduced in this younger age group but is due to be replaced by FIT in 2021.

SURVEILLANCE AFTER ADENOMA DETECTION

Surveillance of patients diagnosed with adenomatous polyps creates a significant demand on colonoscopy resources, particularly with the introduction of population screening. In the UK, the adoption of lower thresholds of FIT or lower age cut-offs in BCSP have been constrained by endoscopy capacity. New guidelines aim to reduce the frequency and longevity of polyp surveillance, restricting follow-up to those under the age of 75 years, and/or life expectancy of at least 10 years, with large non-pedunculated lesions and other high-risk findings.[32] This significant shift represents a pragmatic approach, as the evidence for these guideline changes is not very strong, and aims to create capacity for a more inclusive and more sensitive screening programme, with younger cohorts and lower fHb thresholds in time.

THE SUSPICIOUS OR MALIGNANT POLYP

Improved access to colonoscopy and screening have increased the detection of polyps that harbour a focus of invasive cancer. In the UK, the Suspicious Polyp Early Colorectal Cancer (SPECC) programme[33] promotes:

i. Increased awareness of malignant potential in polyps of 2cm or more, or those with adverse features.
ii. Enhanced endoscopic assessment (Fig. 2.3).[34]
iii. Separate consideration of confirmed cancers up to 3cm in size.
iv. Pre-intervention radiological staging where appropriate.
v. Multi-disciplinary discussion of these polyps and small rectal cancers.

Approximately 15% of suspicious polyps harbour malignancy and a considered approach allows planned endoscopic removal by an appropriately trained endoscopist, transanal endoscopic surgery for some rectal lesions, or formal surgical resection where appropriate. Increased awareness of the potential for malignancy might in practice deter some endoscopists from removing simpler polyps at the index procedure and hence add to the demand for colonoscopy. The concept of organ preservation is well-established in the rectum where partial and full-thickness transanal excision has been used for some years; in future endoscopic techniques may supersede partial-thickness transanal excision. In the colon, combining laparoscopic surgery with endoscopic approaches allows partial-thickness excision of more challenging lesions. Full-thickness endoscopic lesion excision has been described but is yet to be used widely. The site of a SPECC lesion should be flagged with an appropriately placed injection of submucosal ink (tattoo) to guide future interventions.

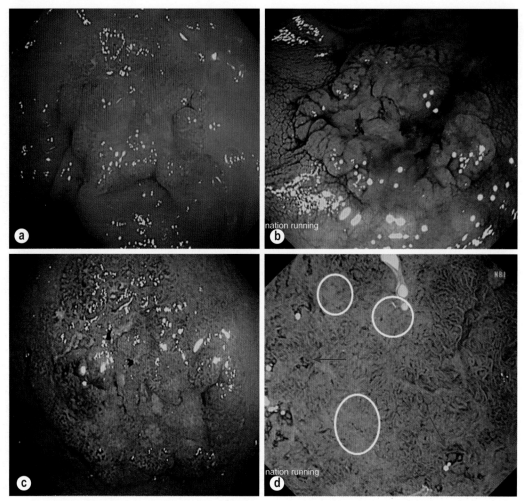

Figure 2.3 Enhanced endoscopic assessment of suspicious polyps (a) White light picture shows a laterally spreading tumour with a central nodule. (b) Indigo dye spray allows better visualisation of the margins of the lesion – a central well-demarcated depressed area appears evident too. (c) NBI assessment reveals irregular vascular pattern. The peripheral area shows a brown colour given by the vascular network – typical of adenoma. The central depressed area appears lighter in colour, suggesting loose vessels areas. (d) Magnified view of the central depressed area: the vascular pattern appears highly irregular, with some loose vessel areas (see *yellow circles*) and interrupted thick vessels (*red arrows*). This is classified as JNET type 3 and is suggestive of deep submucosal invasive cancer. In this case, surgical treatment is indicated.[34] (With thanks to Dr Stefano Sansone and Dr Adolfo Parra-Blanco, Nottingham University Hospitals NHS Trust, UK).

After planned or inadvertent local excision of a malignant polyp, formal resection is considered if there is a risk of residual tumour in the bowel wall or regional lymph nodes, but quantifying this risk is challenging. The pathologist's assessment of the resected lesion is crucial. Haggitt and colleagues reported that cancer infiltrating the head, neck or stalk of a pedunculated polyp yields residual disease risk of less than 1%.[35] In contrast, if cancer involves submucosa at the base of the stalk (Haggitt level 4), the risk is far greater (Fig. 2.4). Sessile adenomas have similar risks to Haggitt level 4 lesions. Kikuchi and colleagues categorised these risks in full-thickness rectal biopsies taken at transanal surgery by subdividing the depth of invasion into thirds of the submucosa. The most superficial invasion is termed *sm1*, and the deepest *sm3*: risks of nodal metastasis have been quoted as 2, 8 and 23% for these respective levels.[36]

Clear tumour margins on histology reduce the risk of recurrent disease – less than 1 mm clearance yields the same clinical significance as a positive margin, where the risk of residual disease is quoted as 21–33%.[37] In one study, this translated to a 5-year survival of 81% with a margin less than 1 mm, compared to 95% with a clear margin.[38] Even with clear margins, other 'adverse' features may worsen prognosis, and in one multivariate analysis lymphatic invasion, submucosal invasion depth of 1 mm or more, tumour budding and poor differentiation appeared most significant (Table 2.3).[39] Combinations of these may amplify risk and piecemeal specimens make predictions unreliable. However, when these 'adverse' features are absent, there is little evidence to recommend resection.[2] In discussions with the patient, it is important to present the predicted risk of residual disease, and all its consequences, whilst acknowledging that the highest risk malignant polyps yield no cancer in 60% of subsequent resection specimens. The patient should also be aware of the sequelae of surgery, with or without complications.

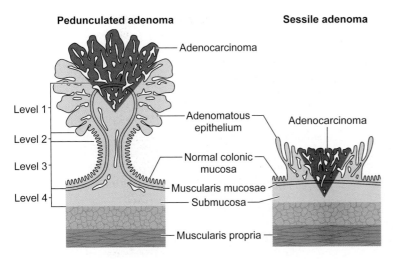

Pedunculated adenoma

- Adenocarcinoma
- Level 1
- Level 2
- Level 3
- Level 4
- Adenomatous epithelium
- Normal colonic mucosa
- Muscularis mucosae
- Submucosa
- Muscularis propria

Sessile adenoma

- Adenocarcinoma

Figure 2.4 Haggitt classification describing invasion depth of pedunculated and sessile malignant polyps.[35] The focus of invasive cancer is represented by dark shading as having penetrated through the muscularis mucosae to level 1 (carcinoma limited to the head of the polyp). Level 2 is where carcinoma invades to the level of the neck (the junction of the head and stalk) of the adenoma. Level 3 is carcinoma invading any part of the stalk. Level 4 is where carcinoma invades into the submucosa of the bowel wall below the level of the stalk. In the sessile adenoma, a stalk is absent and so, by definition, the lesion is defined as being level 4. (Adapted from Williams JG, Pullan RD, Hill J, et al. Management of the malignant colorectal polyp: ACPGBI position statement. Colorectal Dis. 2013;15(Suppl.2):1-38.[50])

Table 2.3 The risk of lymph node involvement in pT1 colorectal cancer in a systematic review of studies including 3621 patients. Background adenoma not included

Dichotomous histological feature	Risk of lymph node involvement (feature present:absent [%])	Relative risk of lymph node involvement (95% CI) if feature present
Lymphatic invasion alone	26.7:5.4	5.2 (4.0–6.8)
Submucosal invasion depth 1 mm or more	12.3:1.5	5.2 (1.8–15.4)
Positive tumour budding	21.3:5.0	5.1 (3.6–7.3)
High grade	24.5:8.9	4.8 (3.3–6.9)
Lymphovascular invasion	22.0:7.1	3.9 (2.7–5.6)
Submucosal invasion width 5 mm or more	16.9:5.6	2.7 (1.4–5.4)
Poor differentiation at invasive front	19.2:10.2	2.5 (1.8–3.5)
Submucosal invasion depth 2 mm or more	13.3:5.4	2.4 (1.6–3.7)
Vascular invasion alone	20.8:9.9	2.2 (1.4–3.2)
Located in Rectum	13.8:9.9	1.4 (1.1–1.7)

Adapted from Bosch et al.[39]

SURGERY

Surgical resection is the cornerstone of curative treatment for colorectal cancer and gives the greatest level of oncological security (see Chapters 4 and 5). Resection aims to remove the affected bowel and adjacent draining lymph nodes. A laparoscopic approach is increasing, with attendant improvements in short-term outcomes when conversion is avoided, but there is still a definite role for open surgery in more challenging cases. Robotic surgery is also growing, with new platforms driving uptake and in future, competition might improve cost-effectiveness. Single incision laparoscopic surgery (SILS), where all minimally invasive instruments are passed through a single port, usually at the umbilicus, is feasible, may reduce post-operative pain and expedite return to function. SILS has not been adopted widely, perhaps because of concerns around consistency of such benefits and added operative time, especially early in learning curves. Advances in robotic technology might yield lightweight technology that enables synergy between these two approaches. Improved survival after complete mesocolic excision for colon cancer has been reported,[40] but concerns regarding operative morbidity and patient selection have slowed widespread adoption.

In rectal cancer, the choice is usually between anterior resection where intestinal continuity is preserved and abdomino-perineal excision (APER), which results in a permanent colostomy. In both operations, the principle of mesorectal excision to ensure disease clearance is established, and in APER, there is increasing emphasis on pelvic floor excision (often referred to as *extra-levator abdomino-perineal* or *ELAP excision*) for adequate clearance of very low cancers. Transanal total mesorectal excision (TaTME) incorporates a transanal approach to address the visualisation challenges of the lower rectum. Cohort data from one national database has raised concerns around the risk of aberrant pelvic side wall recurrence. These findings have not been widely reproduced and may highlight the importance of appropriate training when introducing new techniques. Further evaluation should determine whether these observations mirror the concerns raised around port-site recurrence in the early era of laparoscopic surgery, or whether TaTME is genuinely compromised by this risk.

Quality of surgery is paramount, both in terms of avoiding post-operative morbidity and obtaining good long-term outcomes. There is now unequivocal evidence that both volume and specialisation are associated with better short-term outcomes in a range of cancer operations, and in the UK, it is recognised that colorectal cancer surgery should only be performed by appropriately trained surgeons whose work is audited.[3]

ADJUVANT THERAPY

Adjuvant radiotherapy is not recommended for primary colon cancer, as the risk of radiation enteritis affecting adjacent small bowel is high. Thus, adjuvant therapy for colon cancer is restricted to systemic treatment, commonly based on fluoropyrimidines (5-fluorouracil and the orally available derivative, capecitabine). More recently, combinations with oxaliplatin have proved to be more effective, but these are most appropriate for fitter patients. The more targeted agents, bevacizumab (an antibody against vascular endothelial growth factor [VEGF] receptor) and cetuximab (an antibody against epidermal growth factor [EGF] receptor), have not been found to be effective in the adjuvant setting in randomised trials. Traditionally, the indication for adjuvant chemotherapy has been stage III disease, but now a more personalised approach considers other histological 'adverse' features; the presence of microsatellite instability, *BRAF* and *KRAS* mutations, are used as predictors of risk and response, and guide chemotherapy choices. The FOx-TROT trial demonstrated that pre-operative chemotherapy in patients with radiologically-staged T3/4 colon cancer may improve outcomes, particularly in microsatellite stable cancer.[41] Further iterations of this trial platform may demonstrate effective regimes for MSI cancer. This marks a potential paradigm shift in the management of colon cancer with locally advanced radiological features. A comparison of neoadjuvant chemotherapy and complete mesocolic excision in an appropriately conducted trial seems warranted.

Pre-operative or neoadjuvant treatment is now standard for selected rectal cancers, but there is still wide variation in the use of neoadjuvant strategies. In patients at moderate risk of local recurrence after mesorectal excision, in whom the circumferential margin is not involved on MRI, short-course pre-operative radiotherapy (25 Gy in five fractions over 1 week) followed by immediate surgery may be appropriate. Those where MRI demonstrates margin involvement, or extra-mural vascular invasion, long-course combination chemotherapy and radiotherapy is indicated, followed by a period of 3 months to allow for cytoreduction before surgery.[42] Pre-operative radiotherapy produces better disease control and less morbidity than post-operative treatment, and with appropriate pre-operative MRI staging of the primary tumour, the latter should no longer be necessary.

In some cases, particularly early-stage tumours, pre-operative treatment may result in a complete clinical response, and there is debate around managing such patients, with a strategy of 'watch and wait' gaining traction.[43] Evaluation in clinical practice suggests that regrowth of disease is seen in a quarter to a third of complete clinical responders but over 80% can be salvaged with surgery. Thus, intensive follow-up is recommended in those who pursue a 'watch and wait' strategy, and for some patients this causes anxiety. Three-year survival appears comparable and stoma avoidance more likely in those who 'watch and wait'. Time intervals to surgery are now under question, as the response to long-course radiotherapy clearly continues beyond traditional timeframes, and immediate clinical outcomes appear unchanged up to 1 year after short-course.[44]

Organ preservation is also considered in patients staged with early rectal cancer (T1, and perhaps T2), particularly when the patient has co-morbidities or declines resection. The optimal strategy is unclear; primary local excision is established but the STAR TREC trial is evaluating pre-operative radiotherapy followed by local excision of any residual disease after 6 weeks or so. Some centres use (chemo)radiotherapy after local excision with best results in pT1 cancer.[45] Contact radiotherapy, or Papillon technique, allows high-dose radiotherapy to be applied directly using a rigid transanal probe to tumours up to 3-cm in size.[33] Access to contact radiotherapy is limited in the UK and current guidelines suggest further studies are required to evaluate the role of this technique. Combining local excision with any radiotherapy technique increases risk of bowel function disturbance, and this as well as the anxiety of follow-up, sometimes leads individuals to choose resection even when local recurrence is absent. Valid consent is challenging in individuals in whom all options are feasible, and patients are often influenced by the tone of the first consultation after diagnosis, whilst clinicians are influenced by patient factors and occasionally cognitive dissonance.

MANAGEMENT OF ADVANCED DISEASE

The surgical management of the advanced primary tumour is covered in Chapter 7. In colonic cancer, local recurrence usually occurs at the anastomosis and, in the absence of disseminated disease, re-resection should be attempted, but palliative bypass may be all that can be achieved. The patient with distant metastases poses different challenges.

OPERABLE METASTASES

Hepatic resection for colorectal cancer metastases is practised widely without randomised trial evidence. Comparative studies using retrospective data from historical controls, suggest that with careful patient selection, hepatectomy for colorectal metastases may yield 5-year survival approaching 40%.[2] Although the most widely accepted criterion for resection is one to three resectable metastases in one lobe of the liver, many services have extended their indications. There is no clear evidence to favour synchronous resection of metastases with primary tumours over staged resection, and the role of chemotherapy around liver resection remains unclear. Non-randomised evidence suggests that pre-operative chemotherapy may improve both resectability and long-term survival. In a proportion of patients with liver disease not amenable to resection, radiofrequency ablation may be used.[2]

Pulmonary metastases are also amenable to resection. The PULMICC trial addressed resection versus best alternative care, but was unable to recruit sufficient numbers, demonstrating the challenge of meaningful studies when 'hope' outweighs clinical equipoise. Although segmental lung resection may be associated with 5-year survival rates of 20–60%, PULMICC found that 29% of those fit for, but not undergoing, surgery survived 5-years without.[46] These data were excluded from a recent evidence review and metastectomy, which appears superior to other interventions, is likely to continue.

It seems unlikely that surgery for operable metastasis can be effectively assessed in randomised trials but registration and follow-up of those who decline surgery when offered it, may be one way to properly inform patients in future.

ADVANCED LOCAL DISEASE

In advanced colon cancer, defunctioning or bypass surgery may be appropriate, but multi-organ en bloc resection might be curative, and suitable patients should be given this option, with referral to tertiary centres, as appropriate. In rectal cancer, although palliative radiotherapy with or without a defunctioning stoma may produce a degree of symptom control, consideration should always be given to pelvic exenteration, particularly in younger, fitter patients. In patients with peritoneal spread alone, or with operable liver metastases, peritonectomy combined with heated intra-peritoneal chemotherapy (HIPEC) may result in long-term survival.[47] However, this has never been subjected to a randomised trial and the small number of suitable patients make this very unlikely.

INOPERABLE DISSEMINATED DISEASE

In patients with widespread disease, fluoropyrimidine chemotherapy is the established first-line option for palliative therapy. The oral 5-fluorouracil (5FU) prodrugs UFT and capecitabine are first-line single agents, yielding equivalent survival and the advantage of easier administration. Combination chemotherapy with intravenous 5FU and either irinotecan or oxaliplatin has been demonstrated to enhance survival as both first- and second-line therapy. If oxaliplatin has been used as first-line treatment, then irinotecan should be considered for second-line therapy and vice versa.

Monoclonal antibody treatments, such as bevacizumab or cetuximab, confer survival advantages in combination with conventional chemotherapy. Cetuximab, and the alternative panitumumab, are recommended for use along with 5-FU/leucovorin/oxaliplatin or FU/irinotecan as first-line treatment for patients with metastatic *KRAS* wild-type disease, as a functioning KRAS pathway is necessary for EGF-receptor signal transduction. Bevacizumab has not been recommended by NICE on the grounds that it is not cost-effective.[2]

Second-line agents include Trifluridine (nucleoside analogue) combined with Tipiracil (thymidine phosphorylase inhibitor), and Encorafenib (mitogen-activated protein kinase (MAPK) pathway inhibitor) may be used with Cetuximab. Aflibercept, an alternative VEGF inhibitor, and immune checkpoint inhibitors, such as Nivolumab and Pembrolizumab that might have benefits in mismatch repair deficient advanced cancer, are not currently approved by NICE.[2]

MULTI-DISCIPLINARY TEAM

Treatment decisions should be ratified by a multi-disciplinary team (MDT) consisting of nurse specialists, surgeons,

---

Box 2.3 Summary of key components of the minimum dataset for reporting of colorectal cancer[49]

Macroscopic description

1. Size of the tumour (greatest dimension).
2. Site of the tumour in relation to the resection margins.
3. Any abnormalities of the background bowel.

Microscopic description

1. Histological type.
2. Differentiation of the tumour, based on the predominant grade within the tumour.
3. Maximum extent of invasion into/through the bowel wall (submucosa, muscularis propria, extramural).
4. Serosal involvement by tumour, if present.
5. A statement on the completeness of excision at the cut ends (including the 'doughnuts' from stapling devices) and at any radial margin.
6. The number of lymph nodes examined, the number containing metastases, and whether the apical node is involved.
7. The number of tumour deposits, if present.
8. Deepest layer of vascular, lymphatic and perineural invasion, if present.
9. Pre-operative therapy response, if applicable.
10. Pathological staging of the tumour according to TNM classification (see Table 2.2).

---

oncologists, radiologists and pathologists with interest and expertise in the management of colorectal cancer.[48] SPECC and advanced cancer decisions benefit from the input of advanced endoscopists, liver and thoracic surgeons as appropriate, whilst urologists and gynaecologists contribute to decisions around advanced rectal cancer. Advanced peritoneal disease should be referred to reference centres that undertake peritonectomy and HIPEC. In current practice, new consent guidance determines that patients should be informed of all alternatives and progressive MDTs should list all reasonable options, perhaps ranking their recommendations. High-risk patients are also formally discussed with anaesthetic and critical care colleagues in some centres.

PATHOLOGICAL STAGING

Accurate, detailed and consistent pathology reporting for colorectal cancer is important for estimating prognosis, offering adjuvant therapy where appropriate and stratifying surveillance. Both macroscopic and histological appearances must be described in some detail (Box 2.3).[49]

SUMMARY RECOMMENDATIONS FOR BEST PRACTICE

INVESTIGATION

1. Patients with suspicious symptoms, higher levels of faecal haemoglobin or proven colorectal cancer should be investigated with complete colonoscopy or CTC.

2. Unless it cannot alter management, all patients should be staged with CT scanning, and patients with rectal cancer should have MRI of the rectum.

ELECTIVE SURGICAL TREATMENT

1. Treatment decisions should be ratified by a quorate MDT.
2. All reasonable options should be discussed with the patient. Written information, such as patient information leaflets and clinic letters to patients, are part of the consent process.
3. Colorectal cancer surgery should be performed by appropriately trained surgeons whose workload volume permits meaningful audit.

EMERGENCY TREATMENT

1. Emergency surgery should be delivered by experienced surgeons and anaesthetists, preferably during daytime.
2. In clinically obstructed patients, pseudo-obstruction should be excluded before surgery.
3. Stoma formation should be carried out in the patient's interests only, and not as a result of lack of experienced surgical staff or appropriate stenting facilities.
4. The overall mortality for emergency/urgent surgery should be 20% or less.

TREATMENT OF ADVANCED DISEASE

1. Surgical treatment should be considered in selected patients with locally advanced and metastatic disease. In particular, the patient with limited hepatic involvement should be considered for partial hepatectomy by an experienced liver surgeon.
2. Effective palliation with optimal quality of remaining life should be the main aim of therapy in others.
3. Palliative chemotherapy should be considered in patients with locally advanced and metastatic disease, with input from an oncologist when patients are well enough and agreeable.

Outcomes - Surgeons and centres should carefully audit the outcome of their colorectal cancer surgery:

1. Expected mortality of around 3% at 90 days after elective surgery.
2. Wound infection rates after colorectal cancer surgery should be less than 10%.
3. Quality of life metrics and long-term stoma rates should be monitored.
4. Surgeons and services should examine carefully their practice with a view to meeting or improving on targets set by national long-term statistics.

PATHOLOGY

All resected colorectal tumours should be submitted for histological examination. The report should comply with minimum dataset requirements.

Key points

- Most colorectal cancers arise from pre-existing adenomas or serrated polyps. Flat adenomas, which are difficult to detect without special endoscopic techniques, are significant precursor lesions.
- Obesity, lack of exercise, dietary red and processed meat, low-fibre intake, alcohol and smoking increase the risk of colorectal cancer.
- FIT helps to stratify risk in symptomatic patients.
- Colonoscopy is the gold standard investigative technique, but CT colonography is an adequate alternative. CT scanning is the optimal method of pre-operative staging.
- Screening can reduce colorectal cancer mortality – FIT is now used in the UK and many other countries.
- Treatment options for advanced disease are expanding rapidly – all patients should be considered, although many will not be suitable.
- Valid consent, for investigation and treatment, requires full discussion of all reasonable options that a patient may wish to consider.

 References available at http://ebooks.health.elsevier.com/

ACKNOWLEDGEMENT

This chapter in the sixth edition was written by Robert Steele and I am grateful to him for those parts of the chapter, which we have kept in this edition.

KEY REFERENCES

[2] NICE. Colorectal cancer NICE guideline [NG151] 2020. Available from: https://www.nice.org.uk/guidance/ng151.
Up-to-date evidence-based guideline on the management of colorectal cancer.
[10] Clinton SK, Giovannucci EL, Hursting SD. The world cancer research fund/american institute for cancer research third expert report on diet, nutrition, physical activity, and cancer: impact and future directions. J Nutr 2020;150(4):663–71.
This report lays out all the lifestyle-associated risk factors for all common cancers.
[11] Botteri E, Borroni E, Sloan EK, et al. Smoking and colorectal cancer risk, overall and by molecular subtypes: a meta-analysis. Am J Gastroenterol 2020;115(12):1940–9.
This study describes the link between smoking and molecular subtypes of colorectal cancer.
[15] D'Souza N, Georgiou Delisle T, Chen M, et al. Faecal immunochemical test is superior to symptoms in predicting pathology in patients with suspected colorectal cancer symptoms referred on a 2WW pathway: a diagnostic accuracy study. Gut 2021;70(6):1130–8. https://doi.org/10.1136/gutjnl-2020-321956.
This multicentre UK study describes clinical outcomes in patients undergoing colonoscopy on urgent symptomatic pathways stratified by faecal haemoglobin level.
[28] Mandel JS, Church TR, Ederer F, et al. Colorectal cancer mortality: effectiveness of biennial screening for fecal occult blood. J Natl Cancer Inst 1999;91:434–7. PMID: 10070942.
These three randomised trials (references 28–30) provide evidence that disease-specific mortality can be reduced by faecal occult blood screening for colorectal cancer, and form the basis for current debates regarding the introduction of national screening programmes in several countries.
[29] Hardcastle JD, Robinson MHE, Moss SM, et al. Randomised controlled trial of faecal occult blood screening for colorectal cancer. Lancet 1996;348:1472–7. PMID: 8942775.
These three randomised trials (references 28–30) provide evidence that disease-specific mortality can be reduced by faecal occult blood screening for colorectal cancer, and form the basis for current debates regarding the introduction of national screening programmes in several countries.
[30] Kronborg O, Fenger C, Olsen J, et al. A randomized study of screening for colorectal cancer with fecal occult blood test at funen in denmark. Lancet 1996;348:1467–71. PMID: 8942774.
These three randomised trials (references 28–30) provide evidence that disease-specific mortality can be reduced by faecal occult blood screening for colorectal cancer, and form the basis for current debates regarding the introduction of national screening programmes in several countries.

Colorectal cancer and genetics

3

Katy Newton | Andrew Latchford

INTRODUCTION

Individuals develop colorectal cancer (CRC) as a result of interaction between their genotype and the environment to which they are exposed. The lifetime risk of CRC in the UK population is about 5%. As it is common, many people by chance alone have at least one affected relative;[1] as the number of affected relatives increases, so does the risk of developing the disease.[2] As far as genetic factors are concerned, there is a spectrum of risk from those with no particular genetic predisposition, to very rare individuals who will inevitably develop bowel cancer. While open to error, it is possible to divide the population into four broad categories of risk for CRC: low-, moderate- and high-risk, and the highly penetrant syndromes.

In the highly penetrant syndromes group, the contribution of inheritance (genotype) is overwhelming, though environmental influences may modify disease severity (phenotype). It is this minority (accounting for less than 5% of large bowel cancer) that is traditionally described as being at risk of 'inherited bowel cancer'.

In the low-, moderate- and high-risk groups, genotype may still contribute to risk but less markedly, and is thought to account for about 30% of CRC risk.[3] This may be caused by low penetrance genes that influence dietary carcinogen metabolism, deoxyribonucleic acid (DNA) repair and a variety of other functions.

This chapter deals predominantly with those in the highly penetrant syndromes group. Although these individuals comprise a minority of those at risk overall, there is sufficient knowledge about the specific syndromes that fall within this category to provide important opportunities for cancer prevention.

ASSESSMENT OF RISK

The documentation of an accurate family history allows an empirical assessment of risk.[2] It should focus on site and age at diagnosis of all cancers in family members, as well as the presence of related features such as colorectal adenomas. This can be time-consuming, especially when the information needs to be verified. Few surgeons are able to devote the necessary time or skill to do this, and it is here that family cancer clinics or registries for inherited bowel cancer have an important role.[4]

A full personal history should also be taken, focused on:

- symptoms (e.g., rectal bleeding, change in bowel habit), which should be investigated as usual
- previous large-bowel polyps
- previous large-bowel cancers
- cancers at other sites
- other risk factors for CRC (inflammatory bowel disease, ureterosigmoidostomy, acromegaly); these conditions are not discussed further in this chapter but may warrant surveillance of the large bowel.

The family history has many limitations, particularly in small families. Other difficulties arise because of incorrect information or early death of individuals before they develop cancers. A vast range of complex pedigrees arise, and rather than try to devise guidelines to cover all of them, common sense is needed. If a family seems to fall between risk groups, it is safest to manage the family as if in the higher-risk group. Despite this, some families will appear to be at high risk simply because of chance clustering of sporadic cancer while some, particularly small families with Lynch syndrome, will be assigned to the low- or moderate-risk groups. Even in families affected with an autosomal dominant condition, 50% of family members will not have inherited the causative mutation and will therefore not be at any increased risk of developing cancer.

Family histories evolve, so that the allocation of an individual to a particular risk group may change if further family members develop tumours. It is important that patients are informed of this, particularly if they are in the low- or moderate-risk groups and therefore not undergoing regular surveillance.

LOW-RISK GROUP

Individuals in this group have:

1. no personal history of CRC; and
2. no first-degree relative (i.e., parent, sibling or child) with CRC; or
3. one first-degree relative with CRC diagnosed at age 50 years or older.

MODERATE-RISK GROUP

This group comprises:

1. those with one first-degree relative diagnosed under age 50 years; or
2. two affected first-degree relatives diagnosed at any age, of whom the patient under assessment is a first-degree relative of at least one affected individual.

HIGH-RISK GROUP

Families with a cluster of at least three affected first-degree relatives diagnosed with CRC at any age, across at least two generations, of who the individual under assessment is a first-degree relative of at least one affected individual.

HIGHLY PENETRANT SYNDROMES

This category encompasses Lynch syndrome and the various polyposis syndromes.

1. member of a family with known familial adenomatous polyposis (FAP) or other polyposis syndrome; or
2. member of a family with known Lynch syndrome; or
3. pedigree suggestive of autosomal dominantly inherited CRC (or other Lynch syndrome-associated cancer); or
4. pedigree indicative of autosomal recessive inheritance, suggestive of MYH-associated polyposis (MAP).

Diagnosis of the polyposis syndromes is comparatively straightforward as there is a recognisable phenotype in each. Lynch syndrome is more difficult as there is no such characteristic phenotype, other than the occurrence of cancers.

MANAGEMENT

Individuals with a moderate- or high-risk family history should be assessed in a specialist familial CRC. Where possible, tumour tissue from an affected family member should be tested for mismatch repair status.

LOW-RISK GROUP

The risk of CRC even in these individuals may be up to twice the average risk,[2] although this tends to be expressed after the sixth decade of life.

✅ There is no evidence to support invasive surveillance in this group.[5]

It is important to explain to these individuals that they are at only marginally increased risk of developing CRC, and that this risk is not sufficient to outweigh the disadvantages of colonoscopy. They should be aware of the symptoms of CRC, the importance of reporting if further members of the family develop tumours and be encouraged to take part in population screening.

MODERATE-RISK GROUP

✅ There is a three- to sixfold relative risk for individuals in this category,[2] but probably only a marginal benefit from surveillance.[5]

Part of the reason for this is that the incidence of CRC is very low in the young and rises markedly in the elderly. Even those aged 50 years who have a sixfold relative risk by virtue of their family history are less likely to develop CRC in the following 10 years than are 60-year-olds at average risk.[6]

✅ Current recommendations[5] are that individuals at moderate risk should be offered a one-off colonoscopy age 55 years. If normal, screening should continue in a national screening programme. If polyps are found, surveillance should continue as per national post-polypectomy guidelines.

Again, these individuals should be informed of the symptoms of CRC, the importance of reporting changes in family history and that they should take part in population screening when they reach the appropriate age.

HIGH-RISK GROUP

These are individuals who fulfil the Amsterdam family history criteria for Lynch syndrome, but have no evidence of tumour mismatch repair deficiency, and Lynch syndrome has been excluded by tumour and/or germline mutation testing. Referral to a clinical genetics service is vital for this investigation. Incidence of CRC is lower in these families than in Lynch syndrome. The term 'familial CRC type X' is now used.[5]

✅ Current recommendations are that individuals with high familial risk (familial CRC X) should be offered a colonoscopy at age 40 years, and 5 yearly thereafter until age 75 years.[5]

HIGHLY PENETRANT SYNDROMES

Referral to a clinical genetics service is essential. The polyposis syndromes are usually diagnosed from the phenotype, supplemented by genetic testing. Diagnostic confusion can arise, particularly in cases where there are adenomatous polyps insufficient to be diagnostic of FAP. This may occur, for example, in MAP, FAP with an attenuated phenotype, or Lynch syndrome. A careful search for extra-colonic features, mismatch repair immunohistochemistry or microsatellite instability assessment of tumour tissue, and germline mutation detection can sometimes help. Despite this, the diagnosis in some families remains in doubt. In these circumstances, the family members should be offered thorough surveillance.

LYNCH SYNDROME

Lynch syndrome is inherited in an autosomal dominant fashion, is responsible for about 3% of CRCs and is the commonest of the inherited bowel cancer syndromes, with current estimates that it occurs in up to 1:250–300 of the population (Table 3.1). The terminology in this area is extremely confusing and has recently been revised.[7] Labelled first as the 'cancer family syndrome', the name was changed to *hereditary non-polyposis colorectal cancer* (HNPCC) to distinguish it from the polyposis syndromes and to highlight the absence of the large numbers of colorectal adenomas found in FAP.

Table 3.1   Cancers associated with Lynch syndrome

Site	Frequency (%)
Large bowel	30–75
Endometrium	30–70 (of women)
Stomach	5–10
Ovary	5–10 (of women)
Urothelium (renal pelvis, ureter, bladder)	5
Other (small bowel, pancreas, brain)	<5

Various different diagnostic criteria have been used, including different definitions based on family history. Mutations in DNA mismatch repair (MMR) genes were identified in some, but not all, families with an apparent dominantly inherited cancer syndrome. The term Lynch syndrome should be used where there is evidence of MMR gene mutation. HNPCC is now an obsolete term. Lynch-like syndrome is a family history suggestive of Lynch with MMR deficient tumour(s), no features suggestive of sporadic MMR deficiency, and no identifiable germline mutation. These individuals and their relatives should be managed as Lynch syndrome – hence the term '*Lynch-like*'.

CLINICAL FEATURES

Lynch syndrome is characterised by early onset of CRC, the average age at diagnosis being 45 years. These tumours have certain distinguishing pathological features. There is a predilection for the proximal colon, and tumours are frequently multiple (synchronous and metachronous). They tend to be mucinous, poorly differentiated and of 'signet-ring' appearance, with marked lymphocytic infiltration and lymphoid aggregation at their margins. The associated cancers and their frequencies are continuously evolving; up to date gene and gender specific risk can be obtained from https://ehtg.org/collaborative-studies/plsd/.[8] The prognosis of these cancers tends to be better than in the same tumours arising sporadically.

GENETICS

Lynch syndrome is caused by germline mutation in MMR genes, whose role is to correct errors in base-pair matching during replication of DNA or to initiate apoptosis when DNA damage is beyond repair. The vast majority of cases are caused by mutation in the MMR genes *MLH1*, *MSH2*, *MSH6*, *PMS2*. Recently, transmissible epimutations in the non-MMR gene *EPCAM* have been identified as a cause of Lynch syndrome. Other MMR gene mutations (*MLH3*, *MSH3*, *PMS1*) have been reported in some families with Lynch syndrome but their clinical significance is not established.

The MMR genes are tumour-suppressor genes: patients with Lynch syndrome inherit a defective copy from one parent and tumorigenesis is triggered when the solitary normal gene in a cell becomes mutated or lost, so that DNA mismatches are no longer repaired in that cell. Defective MMR results in the accumulation of mutations in a host of other genes, leading to tumour formation.

A hallmark of tumours with defective MMR is microsatellite instability (MSI). Microsatellites are regions where a short DNA sequence (up to five nucleotides) is repeated. There are large numbers of such sequences in the human genome, the majority in non-coding DNA. Base-pair mismatches occurring during DNA replication are normally repaired by the MMR proteins. In tumours with a deficiency of these proteins, this mechanism fails and microsatellites become mutated, resulting in a change in the number of sequence repeats and hence the length of the microsatellite (microsatellite instability – MSI).

About 15% of sporadic CRC show MSI. Most occur in older patients, particularly right-sided cancers and are caused

Box 3.1 Amsterdam criteria II

- At least three relatives with a Lynch syndrome-associated cancer (colorectal, endometrial, small bowel, ureter, renal pelvis), one of whom should be a first-degree relative of the other two
- At least two successive generations should be affected
- At least one cancer should be diagnosed before age 50 years
- Familial adenomatous polyposis should be excluded
- Tumours should be verified by pathological examination

by inactivation of the MMR gene *MLH1* by promoter methylation, and hence will also show loss of MLH1 protein on immunohistochemistry. Promoter methylation in the vast majority of patients is not related to any inherited factor.

DIAGNOSIS

PEDIGREE

Over the years, a confusing range of 'criteria' have emerged. The International Collaborative Group on HNPCC (ICG-HNPCC) proposed the Amsterdam criteria in 1990. These were not intended as a diagnostic definition, rather to target genetic research by identifying families likely to have a dominantly inherited cancer predisposition. The Amsterdam criteria were modified by the ICG-HNPCC in 1999 (Box 3.1) to include Lynch syndrome-associated cancers other than CRC (Amsterdam II criteria).[9] Subsequent studies have shown that only around half the families that meet these criteria have Lynch syndrome (i.e., an MMR mutation is identified), and 50% of Lynch syndrome families do not meet the Amsterdam criteria.

Therefore although family history alone may be used to highlight high-risk families, it is insufficient to make a diagnosis of Lynch syndrome; genetic testing is required to make this diagnosis.

ANALYSIS OF TUMOUR TISSUE

A reference panel of five microsatellite markers is used to detect MSI; if two of the markers show instability, the tumour is designated 'MSI-high'. The value of MSI testing is that Lynch syndrome is caused by MMR mutation and therefore virtually all CRCs arising as a result of Lynch syndrome will be MSI-high. The Bethesda guidelines[10] (Box 3.2) were proposed to determine whether tumour tissue from an individual should be tested for MSI. The aim was to provide a sensitive set of guidelines that would encompass nearly all Lynch syndrome-associated CRCs but also many 'sporadic cancers', and to use MSI testing to exclude those individuals lacking MSI-high, whose cancers are extremely unlikely to be caused by Lynch syndrome. Those designated MSI-high can then be further investigated using immunohistochemistry and genetic testing.

MSI testing is expensive and requires DNA extraction. A simpler approach is to use standard immunohistochemical techniques to identify MMR protein expression.[11] However, it is not 100% sensitive, particularly in benign adenomatous colonic polyps and so care is needed in interpreting the results.

✔✔ The National Institute for Health and Care Excellence (NICE) has recently recommended universal testing of new cases of CRC to screen for evidence of Lynch syndrome (https://www.nice.org.uk/guidance/DG27). This may be done by either MSI or MMR immunohistochemistry and their analysis shows this to be cost-effective. Colonoscopic biopsy is now recommended as the source material for tumour MMR testing.

GENETIC TESTING

The decision whether to perform germline genetic testing on a blood sample from an at-risk or affected person takes the features of the patient, family and tumour into account. This cautious approach is currently justified on the grounds of cost, since genetic testing for MMR genes in the first member of the family (mutation detection) costs around £600. Once a mutation has been detected in a family, testing other at-risk family members to determine whether they too carry the abnormal gene (predictive testing) is much more straightforward, and allows those without the mutation to be discharged from further surveillance.

As with the other syndromes described in this chapter, testing should be undertaken only after the patient has been counselled and given informed consent. The consent process should include provision of written information and a frank discussion of the benefits and risks of genetic testing. A multidisciplinary clinic where counselling is available is ideal.[5] Not every individual will accept an offer of genetic testing. Significant predictors of test uptake include an increased perception of risk, greater confidence in the ability to cope with unfavourable genetic news, more frequent thoughts of cancer and having had at least one colonoscopy.[11]

Germline gene testing may have several outcomes (Box 3.3); this along with complexities of result interpretation[15] mandate that (results should be relayed via the multidisciplinary clinic, where counselling is available.[12] Failure to detect a mutation may be caused by a variety of factors: some cases may be caused by mutation in regulatory genes rather than the MMR genes themselves; there may be other as yet unidentified genes involved; there may be a technical failure to identify a mutation, which is present; or the family history may be a cluster of sporadic tumours. When this happens, the at-risk family members should continue to be screened.

SURVEILLANCE

✔✔ Colonoscopic surveillance reduces the risk of colorectal cancer in Lynch syndrome patients by 63%.[13]

Colonoscopy must be meticulous because tiny cancers may be present[14] and post-colonoscopy cancers are common. Chromoendoscopy may be helpful to increase the pick-up of flat dysplastic lesions, which are seen more commonly in Lynch syndrome. Both lifetime risk, and interval cancer risk are significantly lower in *MSH6* and *PMS2* when compared to *MLH1* and *MSH2*, such that age of onset of surveillance is now stratified according to gene.

✔ Colonoscopy every 2 years from age 25 years (or 5 years younger than the youngest affected relative, whichever is the earlier)[5] is recommended for Lynch syndrome caused by *MLH1* or *MSH2* mutation. Where the causative mutations is *MSH6 or PMS2* (or *EPCAM*) surveillance with colonoscopy can be delayed till age 35 years (or 5 years younger than the affected relative). Surveillance should continue until about 75 years or until the causative mutation in that family has been excluded in that individual.[5]

There is currently little evidence of benefit for screening for extra-colonic cancers and it is not recommended.

SURGERY

PROPHYLACTIC

The option of prophylactic colectomy rather than colonoscopic surveillance should be discussed with mutation carriers, because of the high risk of CRC. A similar situation pertains to prophylactic hysterectomy and bilateral salpingo-oophorectomy in women who have completed their families, with the exception of carriers of a *PMS2* mutation.

Colectomy might be subtotal, with an ileorectal anastomosis, or might take the form of a restorative proctocolectomy. The risk of metachronous cancer in the retained rectum after ileorectal anastomosis has been estimated to be about 12% at 12 years.[15] Regular endoscopy of residual large bowel should be carried out post-operatively, at intervals no greater than 2 years.

✔ Use of a decision analysis model indicates large gains in life expectancy for carriers of MMR mutation when offered some intervention. Benefits were quantified as 13.5 years from surveillance, 15.6 years from proctocolectomy and 15.3 years from subtotal colectomy compared with no intervention.[16] However, recognition that short intervals between high-quality colonoscopies are needed for surveillance in Lynch syndrome, and that aspirin reduces cancer risk, means that there may be no advantages of prophylactic surgery over good-quality surveillance.

Adjusting for quality of life showed that surveillance led to the greatest quality-adjusted life expectancy benefit. This study provides a mathematically based indication of benefit only: individual circumstances need to be incorporated into the decision-making process when making recommendations.

TREATMENT

For those with colon cancer, the main choice lies between segmental colectomy and colectomy with ileorectal anastomosis (IRA). Segmental resection leads to better function but an increased risk of metachronous cancers (for those with an *MLH1* or *MSH2* mutation) and need for colonoscopic surveillance. Colectomy and IRA has a prophylactic element, but without the additional morbidity of proctectomy; furthermore, ongoing surveillance is easier and more acceptable. Proctocolectomy (with or without ileoanal pouch) can be considered in patients who present with rectal cancer.

✅ There is a risk of metachronous bowel tumour of up to 16% after 10 years, and 41% after 20 years of follow-up.[17]

Total/near total colectomy should be considered in *MLH1* and *MSH2* mutation carriers who develop CRC balanced with risk of metachronous cancer, functional outcomes, age, and patient's wishes.[5]

MEDICAL MANAGEMENT

✅ The CAPP2 (Colorectal Adenoma/Carcinoma Prevention Programme 2) study[18] was a randomised controlled trial of aspirin and resistant starch as chemopreventive agents in Lynch syndrome. This study reported a significant reduction in colorectal cancer rates in those treated with 600 mg aspirin daily, and certainly draws into question the benefits of prophylactic or extended therapeutic large-bowel excision. CAPP3 is currently under way to help determine optimum dose and duration of treatment. Individuals with Lynch syndrome should be offered aspirin to reduce CRC risk.

The benefit of adjuvant cytotoxic chemotherapy (5-fluorouracil [5FU]) for cancers in the setting of Lynch syndrome has been questioned.[5] This may be because some agents act by damaging DNA, resulting in apoptosis. MMR proteins are thought to play a part in signalling the presence of irreversible DNA damage and initiating apoptosis, a pathway absent in these tumours. The current European Society for Medical Oncology guidelines suggest that the small (10–15%) subset of patients with Dukes' B (stage II) MMR deficient tumours (caused either by Lynch syndrome or by inactivation by promoter methylation) are at a very low risk of recurrence and are unlikely to benefit from chemotherapy. They do not therefore recommend the use of adjuvant 5FU in this setting. There is no evidence that deficient MMR influences the benefit from oxaliplatin, therefore the Dukes' C (stage III) disease is treated using the same chemotherapy regimens as CRC with proficient MMR. Currently, there is a great deal of interest in immunotherapy in the treatment of MMR deficient CRC. Data regarding the use of checkpoint inhibitors are emerging. The exploratory NICHE study[19] and the Keynote 177 trial[20] investigated nivolumab and pembrolizumab, in the neoadjuvant and metastatic setting respectively, in MMR deficient tumours with promising results. These checkpoint inhibitors are starting to be used in routine clinical practice.

FAMILIAL ADENOMATOUS POLYPOSIS

Less common than Lynch syndrome, the risk of CRC in patients with FAP approaches 100%.

FAP is usually characterised by:

- hundreds of colorectal adenomatous polyps at a young age (second or third decade of life) (Fig. 3.1)
- duodenal adenomatous polyps
- multiple extra-intestinal manifestations (Box 3.4)
- mutation in the tumour-suppressor adenomatous polyposis coli (*APC*) gene on chromosome 5q
- autosomal dominant inheritance (offspring of affected individuals have a 1 in 2 chance of inheriting FAP).

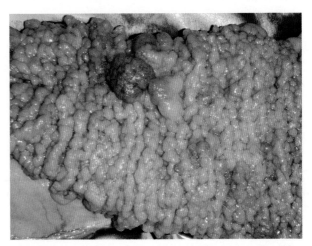

Figure 3.1 Colectomy specimen from a patient with familial adenomatous polyposis (FAP).

Box 3.4 Extracolonic manifestations in familial adenomatous polyposis

Ectodermal origin
- Epidermoid cysts
- Pilomatrixoma
- Tumours of central nervous system
- Congenital hypertrophy of the retinal pigment epithelium

Mesodermal origin
- Connective tissue: desmoid tumours, excessive adhesions
- Bone: osteoma, exostosis, sclerosis
- Dental: dentigerous cyst, odontoma, supernumerary teeth, unerupted teeth

Endodermal origin
- Adenomas and carcinomas of duodenum, stomach, small intestine, biliary tract, thyroid, adrenal cortex
- Fundic gland polyps
- Hepatoblastoma

DIAGNOSIS

FAP was originally defined by the presence of over 100 colorectal adenomas. This clinical definition is still useful, as a mutation in the *APC* gene can only be identified in up to 80% of affected individuals. The majority of new cases come from families with a known history of the disease, but approximately 20% are caused by a new mutation,[21] where there will be no relevant family history. Further potential sources of confusion are the discovery of MAP and the well-documented existence of attenuated FAP characterised by a relative paucity of polyps (10–100) and a later age of developing cCRC.[22]

Inadequate colonoscopy may lead to a false diagnosis of attenuation, an error that can be avoided by the use of dye-spray (chromoendoscopy).[23] Some individuals with Lynch syndrome have a number of adenomatous polyps. Where the diagnosis requires confirmation, the use of dye-spray and random biopsies looking for microadenomas (a hallmark of FAP but not seen in Lynch syndrome) are helpful, as are upper gastrointestinal (GI) endoscopy (up to 80% of FAP patients have gastric fundic gland polyps and the lifetime risk of duodenal adenomas is over 90%).

GENETIC TESTING

✔ The issue of genetic testing is a useful paradigm highlighting the fundamental role played by registries. Identification of at-risk family members who are offered genetic testing is critical and is usually made possible by the comprehensive collation of family pedigrees that such registries are uniquely positioned to obtain and update.

An uncontrolled approach to testing and the release of results can lead to inadequate counselling and the provision of incorrect information to patients.[24]

An affected family member should be tested first. Once the mutation has been identified, at-risk family members can be offered simple blood testing. Should the known family mutation not be found in the at-risk individual, that person can be discharged from further surveillance[25] but should be informed that they remain at the same risk of sporadic CRC as the general population. Such an approach eliminates unnecessary colonoscopy and costs less than conventional clinical screening.[26]

GENOTYPE–PHENOTYPE CORRELATION

The site of the mutation in the *APC* gene can influence the expression of FAP.[27] Genotype–phenotype correlation is seen in the association between certain mutations and severe FAP (dense colorectal polyposis with relatively early CRC), and between other mutations and attenuated FAP (AFAP).[28] However, individuals with identical mutations can display differences in phenotypic expression, suggesting that other modifier genes and the environment play a role in disease expression.[29]

Some of the multiple extra-colonic manifestations of FAP (see Box 3.4),[30] such as desmoid disease, also show correlation with the mutation site; others, notably duodenal adenomas and malignancy, do not.

These genotype–phenotype correlations have led to suggestions that the findings on molecular analysis might guide both surveillance and treatment.[28,31,32] At present, however, it is important to emphasise that management of the large bowel should be guided predominantly by an individual's phenotype and prophylactic surgery remains the management options of choice for the large bowel in nearly all patients with FAP. AFAP remains poorly defined; the diagnosis of AFAP is a phenotypic one and cannot be diagnosed by genotype.

SURVEILLANCE

If the family mutation is known, at-risk family members are usually offered predictive genetic testing in their early teens. If this is not possible, then clinical surveillance is required. It is very unusual for significant colorectal polyps to develop before the teenage years and cancers developing in children are exceptionally rare. If an individual has symptoms attributable to the large bowel (anaemia, rectal bleeding or change in bowel habit), colonoscopy should be performed, irrespective of age. Otherwise, colonoscopy starting at 12–14 years of age is recommended, with surveillance interval personalised according to polyp burden. Decision-making regarding the age at which such surveillance can be stopped depends on the specific family history.

THE LARGE BOWEL

SURGERY

Prophylactic

Once the diagnosis has been made, the aim is to offer prophylactic surgery before a cancer develops. Colonoscopy should be performed to assess the large bowel polyp burden. If the individual is symptomatic or the polyps are dense or large, surgery should be undertaken as soon as is practicable. Otherwise, it is usual to defer surgery until a time when its social and educational impact will be minimised.

As the surgical options have increased, so has the controversy surrounding the choice between them. Increasingly, laparoscopically assisted surgery is becoming the norm and has great attractions in this group, where a good cosmetic result and rapid recovery make surgery more acceptable. The available operations are:

- colectomy and IRA or ileo-distal sigmoid anastomosis (IDSA)
- restorative proctocolectomy (RPC) with an ileal pouch–anal anastomosis
- panproctocolectomy and end ileostomy (almost exclusively for those with very low rectal cancer).

Most young people facing prophylactic colectomy want to avoid a permanent ileostomy, so the choice really lies between the first two options. The biggest attraction of RPC is that the entire large bowel is removed, so that there should be no risk of polyps or cancer developing in a retained rectum. However, a cuff of rectal mucosa is retained when a stapled anastomosis is performed, and cancers at this site have been reported.[33] A mucosectomy can be done and a hand-sewn anastomosis created, but this is a more technically demanding technique, with poorer functional outcome, and does not fully protect against cancer, probably as a result of incomplete mucosectomy. Furthermore, follow-up studies have shown adenoma formation within ileoanal pouches[34] and the development of cancer has been reported.

The advantages of IRA or IDSA[35] are that it is a one-stage procedure (whereas RPC often involves a temporary defunctioning ileostomy) with better function and avoids morbidity related to pelvic dissection.

✓ The functional results in terms of defaecatory frequency and leakage are generally better after IRA (or IDSA) than after RPC.[36]

Sexual and reproductive function can both be compromised by proctectomy. There is a small but definite risk of erectile and ejaculatory dysfunction in men undergoing proctectomy. In addition, there is a pouch failure rate of about 10%, resulting in the need for a permanent ileostomy. These potential complications are particularly difficult to accept for essentially healthy young people undergoing surgery for prophylaxis.

✓ Studies have shown that RPC for both FAP[37] and ulcerative colitis adversely affects fertility in women.

The choice of surgery, is usually based on an individual's phenotype, in particular total colonic and rectal polyp burden, as well as mutation in the case of carriers of certain high-risk mutations (such as at codon 1309). Historical data show a cumulative rectal cancer risk of up to 30% by 60 years of age, but at the time most patients underwent IRA as RPC was not available. IRA was the only option to avoid a permanent ileostomy, and thus was done in circumstances when it would not now be recommended.

✓ In selected cases, the risk of rectal cancer is low and IRA is a reasonable option.[38]

Many patients will have experience of one or both operations from other family members who have undergone them, which may affect their choice. Ultimately, they need to be informed about the advantages and disadvantages of both procedures, as well as the implications of their genotype (if identified) so that their decision can be as informed as possible.

Treatment

In the presence of a colonic cancer, the surgical decision-making is essentially the same as in prophylactic surgery. In individuals with severe rectal polyposis (over 20 adenomas) or in those carrying a mutation at codon 1309 of the *APC* gene, the risk of subsequent uncontrollable rectal polyposis requiring completion proctectomy, or of rectal cancer itself, are high and outweigh the disadvantages of RPC. In those with few rectal polyps, mutations at other sites and the few patients with a genuine attenuated phenotype, IRA may represent a better option. Ultimately, it remains for the informed patient to make a choice.

When rectal cancer is present, the choice is between RPC and proctocolectomy and ileostomy. As in any case of rectal cancer, a very low tumour precludes sphincter preservation. Careful local staging and multi-disciplinary management are crucial.

Surveillance after surgery

Follow-up is required after all procedures. After IRA or RPC, per anal digital and flexible endoscopic examination

are mandatory. The non-steroidal anti-inflammatory drug (NSAID) sulindac has been used to control rectal adenomas[39] and pouch adenomas.[40] There are, however, no robust published long-term data to support the use of NSAIDs and indeed there are reports of cancer despite NSAID 'chemoprevention' and surveillance. The selective cyclo-oxygenase (COX)-2 inhibitor celecoxib showed a moderate reduction in large-bowel polyps in treated patients[41] but no longer has a licence and can no longer be recommended in FAP. More recently, the use of omega-3 fish oil supplements has been shown to have a similar 'beneficial effect' to these NSAIDs in control of colorectal polyps[42] but again this was a short-term study and there are no long-term data on cancer prevention. Aspirin has not been shown to have a significant effect.[43]

Following colectomy, the major causes of mortality and morbidity are duodenal cancers and desmoid tumours. This knowledge guides post-operative management.[44]

UPPER GASTROINTESTINAL TRACT POLYPS

Non-adenomatous gastric polyps (fundic gland polyps) occur in up to 80% of patients with FAP. It is doubted whether these lesions have malignant potential, which at most is extremely low.[45] There are emerging data regarding an increased risk of gastric adenomas and cancer in FAP and this appears to be a 'new' clinical problem that clinicians face. There are no consensus guidelines for the surveillance or management of gastric adenomas in FAP.

✓ Duodenal adenomas occur in nearly all patients with FAP but are severe in only 10%, with malignant change occurring in 5%.[46]

SURVEILLANCE OF THE UPPER GASTROINTESTINAL TRACT

Surveillance usually begins in the third decade of life (in the asymptomatic patient), with endoscopies at intervals of between 1 and 5 years depending on the severity of duodenal polyposis.[47] A staging system for duodenal polyposis has been developed (Table 3.2) to allow surveillance to be tailored to disease severity and to identify individuals at high risk of developing malignancy.[48]

✓✓ Duodenal surveillance is beneficial. Duodenal cancer detected at surveillance endoscopy has a significantly improved overall survival compared to symptomatic cancers.[49]

The ampulla and periampullary area must be examined, being at particularly high risk. If the ampulla is abnormal because of the development of an adenoma, the frequency of endoscopic surveillance may need to be altered according to the severity of the ampullary disease.[50]

MANAGEMENT OF DUODENAL POLYPOSIS

✓ Management of severe duodenal polyposis is difficult. No chemopreventive options are available. Endoscopic therapy is recommended but its impact on hard endpoints, such as prevention of cancer or surgery, is not established.

Open duodenotomy and polypectomy is associated with high recurrence rates and is not recommended.[51] Endoscopic resection is recommended for those with more severe

Table 3.2 Spigelman staging of severity of duodenal polyposis in FAP

	Points allocated		
	1	2	3
Number of polyps	1–4	5–20	>20
Polyp size (mm)	1–4	5–10	>10
Histological type	Tubular	Tubulovillous	Villous
Degree of dysplasia	Mild	Moderate	Severe

Total points	Spigelman stage	Recommended follow-up interval
0	0	5 years
1–4	I	5 years
5–6	II	3 years
7–8	III	1 year and consider endoscopic therapy
9–12	IV	Consider prophylactic duodenectomy

FAP, Familial adenomatous polyposis.

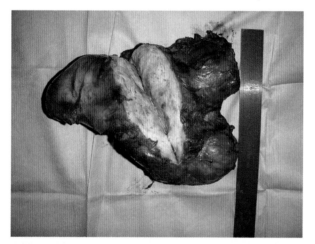

Figure 3.2 A desmoid tumour excised from the abdominal wall.

disease and may delay or prevent the need for definitive surgery; however, robust data on benefit are lacking.

While prophylactic pancreatico-duodenectomy or pylorus-preserving pancreatico-duodenectomy have been described with good outcomes, associated morbidity and mortality are substantial.[52] The poor prognosis once invasive disease is present and the high rate of progression to cancer of advanced polyposis (36% over 10 years in one series) mean that this aggressive approach can be justified in some cases with Spigelman stage IV disease. Cancer risk and hence the need for intervention is minimal in stage 0–II disease.

DESMOID TUMOURS

Desmoid tumours are fibromatous lesions consisting of clonal proliferations of myofibroblasts (Fig. 3.2). They occur in approximately 15% of individuals with FAP, with a mortality rate of about 10%.[53] Most exhibit cycles of growth and resolution and, while causing discomfort and being unsightly, may not cause significant problems. Most desmoids associated with FAP arise either intra-abdominally (usually within the small-bowel mesentery) or on the abdominal wall, although they can appear in the extremities and trunk. They are histologically benign, but within the abdomen can cause small-bowel and ureteric obstruction, intestinal ischaemia or perforation, all of which can be fatal.

The aetiology of desmoid tumours is multifactorial, with contributions from trauma (e.g., operative), oestrogens, specific *APC* gene mutations and modifier genes.

MANAGEMENT

The challenge in the management of these bizarre tumours is to identify the minority that are rapidly and relentlessly progressive, and to avoid harming patients with unnecessarily aggressive attempts to treat the rest. Ureteric obstruction is not infrequent, and as the consequences can be obviated by ureteric stenting it is wise to perform regular renal tract imaging every 6–12 months.

Computed tomography (CT) provides the best imaging with respect to size and relationship to surrounding structures. Ultrasound can be used to monitor the ureters.

✔ Treatment options include NSAIDs, anti-oestrogens, radiofrequency ablation, surgical excision and cytotoxic chemotherapy.[54] Small bowel or multi-visceral transplant is an option in severe mesenteric disease. Desmoid should be managed within a specialist centre.

Anecdotal successes with a variety of NSAIDs and/or anti-oestrogens abound, although good evidence of efficacy is lacking. Evaluation of these treatments is hampered by the natural history of desmoids, which have been documented to regress spontaneously and exhibit relentless growth in only a small minority of patients.

✔ Evidence[53] supports the use of surgery as first-line treatment for abdominal wall and extra-abdominal desmoids, although the recurrence rate is high.

There is no evidence to support the concern that recurrence might be increased by the use of prosthetic materials to repair any resulting defect. Historical evidence of significant morbidity and mortality has led to the recommendation that surgery should usually be avoided where possible for intra-abdominal desmoids. If surgery is required, because of progressive disease or desmoid-related complications, then referral to a specialist centre may lead to good outcomes with low morbidity and mortality, although recurrence remains a problem.[55]

MYH-ASSOCIATED POLYPOSIS

Study of patients with the phenotype of FAP but no identifiable *APC* mutation has led to the discovery of this form of adenomatous polyposis, which has considerable clinical overlap with FAP, but is genetically distinct.[56]

CLINICAL FEATURES

THE LARGE BOWEL

As in FAP, the most consistent feature of MAP is the development of colorectal adenomas and carcinomas. The number of polyps is very variable[57] with about half the patients in one series having a phenotype consistent with classical FAP (hundreds of polyps), and half having an attenuated phenotype with fewer than 100 polyps. Some cases of cancer have been reported in individuals with a definite genetic diagnosis of MAP, but very few polyps indeed, and the lifetime risk of CRC is almost 100% by the age of 60 years. CRC often develops at a slightly later age than FAP (an average of 47 years).

THE UPPER GASTROINTESTINAL TRACT

Duodenal adenomas and adenocarcinomas are seen in MAP but there is the suggestion of different disease pattern to FAP.[58] Duodenal polyposis occurs less frequently than in FAP (21% vs. 65–95%).[61] Data from a large international cohort has suggested that duodenal adenocarcinoma develops independently from advanced polyposis, suggesting that Spigelman staging, as used in FAP, fails to accurately predict patients at risk of cancer.[59] Data are lacking about gastric involvement in MAP.

OTHER MANIFESTATIONS

It has been suggested that there is an increased frequency of breast cancer in MAP, up to 18% in one series.[60] Osteomas and dental cysts have also been documented. To date, no MAP patient with desmoid has been reported.

GENETICS

This condition is caused by biallelic mutation of the MutY human homologue (*MYH*) gene on chromosome 1p. Thus, for the first time, autosomal recessive inheritance has been described in the context of inherited bowel cancer. The frequency of mutation carriage (heterozygosity) in the general population may be as high as 1 in 100–200, but individuals who are heterozygotes appear to be only at minimally increased risk of CRC.

Genetic testing is available and should be considered in individuals with adenomatous polyposis. The recessive inheritance means that there will often be no family history of CRC or polyps. This mode of inheritance also poses challenges in terms of genetic counselling and family testing strategies.

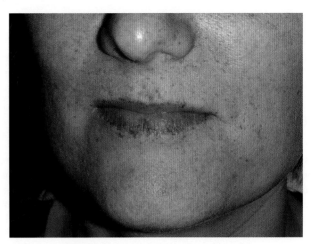

Figure 3.3   Peutz–Jeghers pigmentation.

MANAGEMENT

The management of an affected individual is essentially the same as for FAP, although as a higher proportion has an attenuated phenotype, and the age of onset may be a little later, it may be that more patients can be managed for longer with colonoscopy and polypectomy. Upper GI tract surveillance is started at age of 35 years.

There is insufficient evidence currently to support breast screening, but female patients should be informed of the potentially increased risk. Breast self-examination and participation in population-based breast cancer screening should be encouraged.

For a heterozygote carrier any increase in the lifetime risk of developing CRC is at worst modest (up to 1.5–2 times); surveillance is not recommended.

PEUTZ–JEGHERS SYNDROME

Peutz–Jeghers syndrome (PJS) is an autosomal dominant condition characterised by mucocutaneous pigmentation (Fig. 3.3) together with GI hamartomatous polyps. The gene responsible in most patients is *STK11* (*LKB1*) on chromosome 19p13.

A 78-year follow-up of the original family described by Peutz is instructive.[61] Survival of affected family members was found to be reduced as a result of bowel obstruction and the development of a range of cancers.

BOWEL OBSTRUCTION

The commonest polyp-related complication is small-bowel obstruction, often caused by intussusception. The risk is estimated to be 44% by age 10 years, and 50% by age 20 years. Repeated episodes result in increasingly difficult laparotomies and loss of bowel length.

✓ The incidence of subsequent small-bowel obstruction can be reduced by adequate intra-operative small-bowel enteroscopy, allowing identification and removal of all polyps at the time of initial laparotomy.[62]

CANCER RISK

Individuals with PJS are at significantly increased risk of a number of malignancies, however, the reported risks are likely to be significant overestimates because of ascertainment bias of the studies in rare conditions.[63]

SURVEILLANCE AND MANAGEMENT

A baseline colonoscopy and gastroscopy at age 8 years in asymptomatic individuals is recommended. If polyps are detected, surveillance continues 3 yearly. If baseline endoscopies are normal, repeat can be deferred to age 18 years. Small bowel surveillance should commence at age 8 years and continue at least 3 yearly in asymptomatic individuals. Symptoms should prompt more urgent investigations, irrespective of age.[64] It is unclear if endoscopic surveillance and polypectomy alters the risk of cancer development.[65] Surveillance identifies polyps that may become symptomatic; if large polyps (>15–20 mm) are seen in the small bowel or symptoms suggesting intermittent small bowel obstruction occur, or if there are small-bowel polyps with anaemia, a double-balloon enteroscopy or laparotomy with intraoperative enteroscopy and polypectomy is recommended to clear the small bowel of polyps and prevent frank obstruction.

As far as malignancy at other sites is concerned, where surveillance programmes have been shown to be useful in the general population, they should be used. Breast surveillance has been recommended because of the increased risk of breast cancer and PJS has been included in the conditions for which breast cancer surveillance is recommended by NICE; patients with PJS should be referred to their local high-risk breast screening centre.[66] There is currently no evidence to support ovarian or pancreatic surveillance in PJS.[66,67]

JUVENILE POLYPOSIS

Not to be confused with the finding of an isolated juvenile polyp (which has very low, if any, malignant potential), juvenile polyposis is an autosomal dominant condition where characteristic hamartomatous juvenile polyps occur, mostly in the colon but also in the upper GI tract. Some affected individuals harbour germline mutation in the *SMAD4* gene,[66] while others have germline mutation in the *BMPR1A* gene. Those with *SMAD4* mutation should be assessed for hereditary haemorrhagic telangiectasia, which up to 75% will have. They should be managed in a specialist centre due to the risk of asymptomatic arteriovenous malformations.

There is a risk of CRC approaching 40%; there is also an increased risk of gastric cancer, in those with an *SMAD4* mutation. Regular colonoscopy screening,[68] from age 12–15 years, with polypectomy for large polyps, is mandatory. Upper GI endoscopy is recommended from age 18 years for *SMAD4* mutation carriers and age 25 years for *BMPR1A* mutation carriers. Surveillance interval should be determined according to the phenotype. Occasionally, prophylactic colectomy or gastrectomy is required.

> **Box 3.5 2019 WHO clinical criteria for diagnosis of serrated polyposis syndrome**
>
> - Five or more serrated lesions/polyps proximal to the rectum
>   - all being at least 5 mm in size
>   - with two or more being at least 10 mm in size
> OR
> - More than 20 serrated lesions/polyps of any size distributed throughout the large bowel
>   - at least five being proximal to the rectum.

SERRATED POLYPOSIS SYNDROME

Serrated polyposis syndrome (SPS) is being diagnosed increasingly commonly and is probably a group of disorders. The 2019 WHO clinical criteria for diagnosis of serrated polyposis should be used (Box 3.5).[69] There is an association with smoking; a genetic component to the disease has been proposed but remains undefined. There is no clear pattern of inheritance in SPS, however, it is established that first-degree relatives of an individual with SPS have a three- to fivefold increased risk of CRC.[70]

Most patients can be managed endoscopically.[71] The British Society of Gastroenterology produced a position statement with guidelines covering diagnosis, endoscopic management and surgery,[72] updated in 2020.[5] There are few data about surgery in SPS. The choice of operation will be determined by the large bowel phenotype, but in the prophylactic setting, segmental resection or IRA are likely to be the operations of choice; there seems little rationale to consider RPC. Early data suggested a risk of metachronous cancer as high as 7% at 5 years. However, with rigorous surveillance and polypectomy, this risk appears much lower. In the setting of cancer, the extent of the resection will be in part determined by the density and distribution of the polyp burden and the site of the cancer, whilst also taking into account the age and comorbidity of the patient and the likely functional outcome from surgery.

OTHER INHERITED COLORECTAL CANCER SYNDROMES

There are a number of extremely rare syndromes where the phenotype and cancer risk are still being defined, but for which surveillance is recommended. The patients with these conditions are best referred to a specialist unit.

Cowden's syndrome, caused by mutations in the *PTEN* gene, consists of GI hamartomas and cancers, together with a high risk of cancer of the breast, thyroid, endometrium and cervix, benign fibrocystic breast disease, non-toxic goitre and varied benign mucocutaneous lesions, particularly trichilemmomas. European guidance recommends thyroid, breast and renal screening from ages 18, 30 and 40 years, respectively. One off colonoscopy at age 35–40 years will assess polyp burden and polyp type. Dysplastic polyp burden will guide future surveillance.[73]

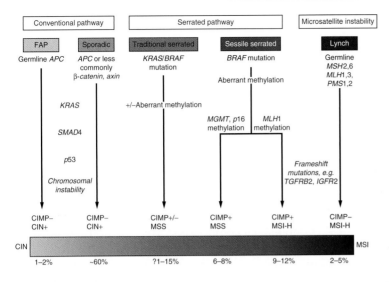

Figure 3.4 The pathways of development of colorectal cancer. *FAP*, Familial adenomatous polyposis. (Modified from East JE, Atkin WS, Bateman AC, et al. British Society of Gastroenterology position statement on serrated polyps in the colon and rectum. Gut. 2017;66:1181-96, with permission.)

NTHL1-associated polyposis (NAP) and polymerase proofreading associated polyposis (PPAP) and are recently described and very rare conditions. NAP is caused by pathogenic germline mutation in the base excision repair gene *NTHL-1* and is characterised by recessive inheritance, attenuated colonic adenomatous polyposis and CRC. PAPP is caused by a pathogenic germline mutation in the *POLE* or *POLD1* gene, has a variable phenotype but is associated with multiple adenomas, CRC and extra-colonic cancers. There are insufficient data to guide surveillance guidelines for these rare conditions.

MOLECULAR PATHWAYS OF COLORECTAL CANCER DEVELOPMENT

It has long been known that CRC develops through the adenoma–carcinoma sequence, with accompanying accumulation of genetic changes, in a process of evolution. It has become clear that there are several alternative pathways (Fig. 3.4), something that was first identified by studying the cancers arising in Lynch syndrome. While the study of cancers arising in the inherited syndromes has highlighted these different pathways, an appreciation and understanding of the differences between them is becoming increasingly important in managing all patients with CRC.

SUMMARY

The emerging complexity of the relationship between genetics and bowel cancer, coupled with rapid advances in knowledge, reinforce the need for the availability of experienced, informed and up-to-date opinion in the areas of diagnosis and management. Individual surgeons will rarely be able to meet all of these needs. Patients and their families are best served by the existence of good working relationships between managing clinicians, family cancer clinics and registries based in expert centres.

Key points

- Genetic factors make a significant contribution to colorectal cancer.
- High-risk families should be referred to specialised registries, genetics units or clinical groups.
- Lynch syndrome and FAP are the commonest autosomal dominant high-risk conditions.
- In the UK, NICE has recommended that all CRCs are tested for mismatch repair function using MMR immunohistochemistry or tumour DNA microsatellite instability assessment, to identify patients with Lynch syndrome.
- An understanding of these conditions is required to recognise and diagnose them.
- Individuals with these conditions are at risk of a range of extra-colonic tumours, so need specialised follow-up.

References available at http://ebooks.health.elsevier.com/

KEY REFERENCES

[13] Jarvinen HJ, Aarnio M, Mustonen H, et al. Controlled 15-year trial on screening for colorectal cancer in families with hereditary non-polyposis colorectal cancer. Gastroenterology 2000;118:829–34. PMID: 10784581.
  A prospective controlled trial showing that colonoscopic surveillance in Lynch syndrome led to a 63% reduction in colorectal cancer and a significant decrease in mortality.

[18] Burn J, Gerdes AM, Macrae F, et al. Long-term effect of aspirin on cancer risk in carriers of hereditary colorectal cancer: an analysis from the CAPP2 randomised controlled trial. Lancet 2011;378:2081–7. PMID: 22036019.
  A prospective, randomised trial whose primary endpoint was colorectal cancer development in patients with Lynch syndrome. It showed that taking 600 mg aspirin for 25 months significantly reduced risk of both colorectal and all Lynch syndrome-associated cancers after 55 months.

[49] Bulow S, Christensen IJ, Hojen H, et al. Duodenal surveillance improves the prognosis after duodenal cancer in familial adenomatous polyposis. Colorectal Dis 2012;14:947–52. PMID: 21973191.
  A series of 304 patients from a previous study were followed up. This is the first study to show a survival benefit from surveillance of the duodenum in FAP. Survival after a surveillance-detected cancer was significantly better than after a symptomatic cancer (8 years vs. 0.8 years; P <0.0001).

4 Surgery for colon cancer

Nicola Hodges | Danilo Miskovic

INTRODUCTION

The principles of surgery for colon cancer have been unchallenged for decades, and include a sufficient longitudinal resection margin, excision of the draining lymphatic territory and avoidance of unnecessary manipulation of the tumour before transection of the vascular pedicle ('no-touch technique'). Although these principles remain a mainstay of the surgical treatment for colon cancer, there is increasing controversy about the extent of resection, the definition of complete mesocolic excision (CME), and peri-operative treatment strategies, such as neoadjuvant chemotherapy and mechanical bowel preparation. Laparoscopic resection is nowadays regarded as the gold standard of care, but the value of novel concepts, such as robotic surgery and a complete minimally invasive approach, including intra-corporeal anastomosis and using natural orifices for access or specimen extraction is still debated. This chapter is focussed on current evidence and debates of the surgical principles of the treatment of colon cancer. Classification, tumour biology, genetics and oncological treatment options are discussed in previous chapters.

PERI-OPERATIVE RISK MITIGATION FOR ELECTIVE SURGERY

Colonic resection is classified within the National Institute for Health and Care Excellence (NICE) guidelines as major or complex surgery. Clear communication with the patient and their family regarding the diagnosis, risks and potential management options is required to facilitate shared decision making and formulation of an appropriate management plan for the individual. Pre-operative risk assessment is essential, not only to inform patients and surgeons regarding potential morbidity and mortality but also to address any reversible risk factors, which may be mitigated pre-operatively.

✔ There are a number of formalised risk assessment tools available including P-POSSUM, CR-POSSUM, SORT and NSQIP.[1] These may be used alongside multi-disciplinary team discussions with the surgeon, anaesthetic team and specialist physicians, as appropriate, to facilitate shared decision making.

PRE-OPERATIVE CONSIDERATIONS

Elderly patients should be screened for frailty using validated questionnaires.[2] Formalised exercise tolerance tests

(e.g., CEPEX) or stress echocardiography can be useful to further objectify increased risk. Medical optimisation of pre-existing cardiac or respiratory conditions should be considered promptly. Assessment of nutritional state, anaemia and lifestyle factors such as smoking must also be addressed. Patients with suspected malnutrition may benefit from high-calorie drinks pre-operatively. Intravenous iron or packed red blood cell transfusion, in severe cases, should be administered in cases of anaemia.[3,4] Smoking cessation must be encouraged, ideally at least 4 weeks before surgery, to avoid bronchial hypersecretion and normalise metabolic and immune function. Obese patients carry an increased risk of post-operative complications, but weight loss is often not feasible in the timeframe given in the cancer pathway. In selected cases of morbid obesity (BMI >40 kg/m^2), radical diet or the insertion of a gastric balloon can be considered. Each patient should be assigned a point of contact, such as a cancer nurse specialist, pre-operatively to answer any questions going forward and facilitate timely management.[1]

ENHANCED RECOVERY AFTER SURGERY

✔ Enhanced recovery after surgery (ERAS) protocols have been shown to reduce complications and length of stay in patients undergoing elective colonic resection.[5]

ERAS includes over 20 different elements of peri-operative care; minimally invasive surgery to reduce post-operative pain and the use of opioids, early mobilisation and early oral intake are some of the most relevant factors in a surgeon's practice. A detailed care protocol and informing patients about expected progression on a daily basis are equally important.

PRE-OPERATIVE MECHANICAL BOWEL PREPARATION AND ORAL ANTIBIOTICS

The use of pre-operative mechanical bowel preparation and non-absorbable oral antibiotics, in addition to intravenous antibiotics 30–60 minutes before knife-to-skin, has been shown to significantly reduce the incidence of surgical site infection (SSI) in patients undergoing surgery for colorectal cancer.[6–8] Large population-based, retrospective studies from the United States suggest that this regimen may be associated with lower anastomotic leak rates and ileus.[7] The results of a randomised controlled trial including 417 patients from Finland however, did not show a reduction of SSI rates in patients undergoing colon resection.[9]

Routine use of pre-operative mechanical bowel preparation and non-absorbable oral antibiotics before elective colorectal surgery is recommended by the World Health Organisation and American Society for Enhanced Recovery. An evidence review is currently being performed with the intention of updating the current NICE guidelines.

VENOUS THROMBOEMBOLISM PROPHYLAXIS

The incidence of post-operative venous thromboembolism (VTE) in patients undergoing colorectal surgery has been reported as 1.1–2.5%. This risk is higher for patients with colorectal cancer.

✓✓ Mechanical prophylaxis with graduated compression stockings and/or intermittent pneumatic compression and pharmacological prophylaxis with low-molecular-weight heparin is recommended. For cancer patients, it is recommended to extend the use of low-molecular-weight heparin 28 days post-operatively.[10,11]

SURGERY FOR COLON CANCER

BASIC PRINCIPLES

Surgery remains the mainstay of treatment for localised colon cancer. The operation performed is defined by the location of the primary and the tumour is resected en bloc with the lymphatic drainage by ligation of the arterial supply to that section of colon. To achieve optimal oncologic outcomes, any adjacent organ involvement must also be resected en bloc.

Unlike in rectal cancer, where the optimal surgical technique, total mesorectal excision (TME), is well established and standardised, very few national guidelines describe the optimal surgical technique recommended for colonic cancer resections.

The ESMO guidelines recommend a minimum of 5 cm of bowel to be resected either side of the tumour with at least 12 draining lymph nodes.[12] In practice, a greater longitudinal length of bowel resection is often mandated as a result of ligation of arterial supply.

SPECIMEN QUALITY CONTROL

Resection specimens can be assessed regarding the completeness and the quality of the resection margins.

✓ West et al. were the first to describe a grading system to assess the quality of colon cancer resection specimens based on the completeness of the mesocolic resection margin (mesocolic, intra-mesocolic and intramuscular) and demonstrated improved survival when surgery is performed in the ideal, mesocolic plane.[13]

It was also shown that the correct plane of dissection is more often achieved in left-sided colon cancer resections compared with right-sided colon cancer resections.[13] The length of the vascular pedicle is of limited use as it varies greatly between individual patients. A more recent grading system suggested by the German CME group also involves the completeness of the central extension of the mesocolic resection.[14] Its clinical validation is yet to be shown (Fig. 4.1).

EXTENT OF LYMPHADENECTOMY

The optimal extent of lymphadenectomy remains controversial. Colonic lymph node basins can be classified according to their proximity to the tumour-containing segment of bowel and supplying vasculature. Epicolic and paracolic lymph nodes (within 5 cm of the tumour containing bowel) may be termed *group 1* or *N1 lymph nodes* and are resected in a D1 resection. Intermediate lymph nodes (5–10 cm from the tumour bearing colon segment) are termed *group 2* or *N2 lymph nodes*. A D2 colonic resection refers to the resection of both N1 and N2 lymph nodes en bloc. Central lymph nodes at the root of the named vasculature are termed *N3 lymph nodes* and are resected with a D3 colonic resection.[15] Japanese guidelines recommend a D3 resection is performed for all patients with pre-operative radiological suspicion of node positive disease or for those tumours radiologically staged as T4 without obvious nodal involvement on computed tomography (CT).[16] Patients with tumours that do not meet these criteria are offered a D2 resection. No such guidance on extent of lymphadenectomy is provided in European guidelines. A potential pitfall for selective use

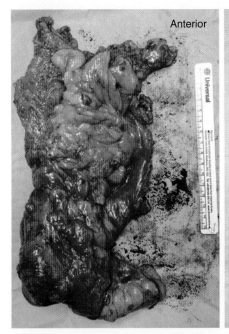
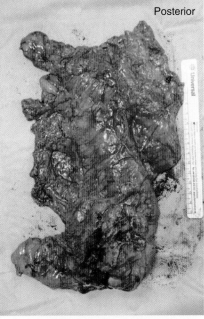

Figure 4.1 Example of right hemicolectomy specimen with intact mesocolic plane and central ligation of ileocolic and middle colic vessels. Note the intact mesocolic window.

D2 vs D3 lymphadectomy (each with CVL)

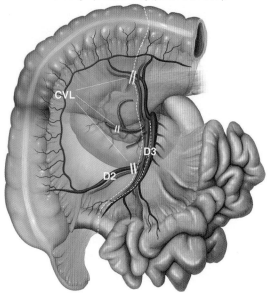

Figure 4.2   Excision levels for true D2 vs. D3 resections. *CVL*, central vascular ligation.

of D2/D3 resection based on pre-operative radiological staging is the inaccuracy of CT scans in determining accurately the depth of tumour invasion and the presence or absence of positive lymph nodes. In a meta-analysis by Nerad et al., the sensitivity and specificity of CT to distinguish between T1/T2 versus T3/T4 disease was 90% and 69% while the accuracy of prediction of lymph node involvement was only 78% and 68%, respectively (Fig. 4.2).[17]

COMPLETE MESOCOLIC EXCISION

First described by Hohenberger,[18] the term combines the principles of:

1. Sharp dissection in the mesocolic plane.
2. Adequate longitudinal bowel resection.
3. Central ligation of the supplying vessels.

Some consider central vascular ligation as optional or in combination with CME. Central vascular ligation can be thought of as being analogous to a D3 lymphadenectomy. This has become routine practice for left-sided colon cancers (central ligation of the inferior mesenteric artery and vein) but has not been adopted widely in the Western world for right-sided colon cancers because of the increased technical complexities associated with the procedure, potential morbidity associated with close dissection of the superior mesenteric artery and vein (SMA and SMV) and lack of conclusive data showing superiority over a high quality D2 resection.

Bertelsen et al. recently published their 5-year outcomes comparing CME over standard right hemicolectomy (non-CME) for right-sided colon cancer in a Danish based cohort study. They showed an absolute risk reduction in cumulative incidence of local and distant recurrence of 8.2% in the CME group after 5.2 years of follow-up. This risk reduction was present across all stages of tumours (stage I-III), albeit profound in stage III cancers (17.5%) and there was no difference in major complications or 30-day mortality.[19] There was a trend towards improved survival in the CME group although this did not reach statistical significance.

✓ This Danish study suggests routine CME may have a role in improving outcomes for patients with right-sided colon cancer. It remains unclear, however, which component of the CME approach is the significant contributor to improved outcomes.

West et al. have previously demonstrated that the correct plane of colonic resection is more often achieved when a CME or D3 lymphadenectomy is performed.[20] The question of whether or not a high quality D2 resection, in the correct mesocolic plane, could have the same outcomes as a CME with central vascular ligation/D3 resection remains unanswered. The RELARC trial is a Chinese randomised controlled trial comparing laparoscopic D2 versus D3 (CME) right hemicolectomy and aims to address this question.[21] Short-term outcomes of the RELARC trial were recently published. These demonstrated no overall difference in post-operative complications between the two groups. Clavien-Dindo III-IV complications were significantly less in the CME group compared with the D2 group (1% vs. 3%; P = 0.022) but intra-operative vascular injury was significantly more common in the CME group (3% vs. 1%; P = 0.045).[21] Interestingly, the quality of mesocolic excision was superior in the D2 group compared with the CME group.[21] A multicentre Russian trial (COLD trial) is addressing a similar question, and is reaching the end of its recruitment phase.[22] The long-term oncological outcomes of these trials are eagerly awaited.

There is concern CME may lead to greater long-term bowel dysfunction compared with a more limited resection because of the combination of the greater length of bowel resected and potential damage to the superior mesenteric nerve plexus with central vascular ligation. A Danish retrospective questionnaire-based study found no difference in bowel function or quality of life in those patients with right colon cancer managed with CME or conventional right hemicolectomy.[23] It is hoped future studies will address this prospectively.

PRACTICAL GUIDANCE ON THE EXTENT OF RESECTION

Right hemicolectomy is performed for tumours of the caecum, ascending colon and hepatic flexure; extended right hemicolectomy for tumours of the transverse colon (transverse colectomy may also be considered); left hemicolectomy for descending colon cancers and a sigmoid colectomy/high anterior resection for sigmoid colon cancers.

The surgical management of non-obstructed splenic flexure tumours is controversial due to the variable blood supply and lymphatic drainage of this segment of bowel. Surgical options include an extended right hemicolectomy, left hemicolectomy or segmental colectomy. A recent meta-analysis of retrospective studies showed no difference in overall complication rate or overall survival when comparing these procedures.[24] There is evidence however, that an extended right hemicolectomy when performed for a splenic flexure tumour results in longer operative time and an increased incidence of post-operative ileus.[25] The functional impact of such an extended resection must also be considered. The extent of bowel resection and vascular ligation for each procedure is shown in Fig. 4.3.

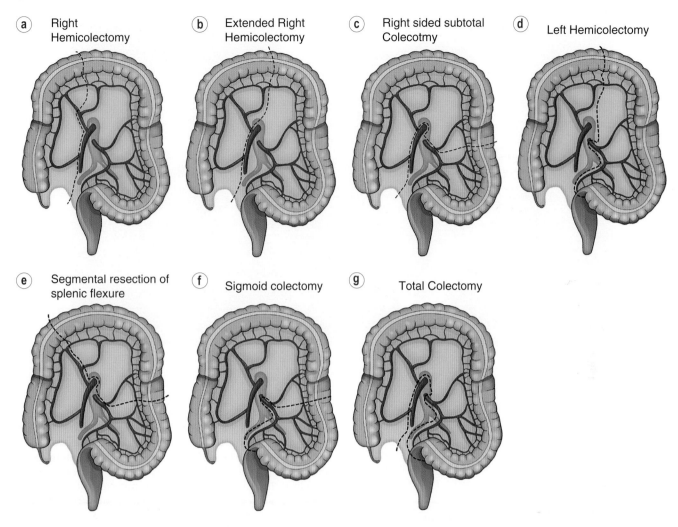

(a) Right Hemicolectomy

(b) Extended Right Hemicolectomy

(c) Right sided subtotal Colecotmy

(d) Left Hemicolectomy

(e) Segmental resection of splenic flexure

(f) Sigmoid colectomy

(g) Total Colectomy

Figure 4.3   Resection types for different tumour locations.

DIFFERENCES BETWEEN RIGHT AND LEFT SIDED COLON CANCER

The embryologic differences between the right (midgut) and left (hindgut) colon with the associated developing mesentery may underlie many of the differences observed between right- and left-sided colon tumours and outcomes.

DIFFERENCES IN TUMOUR BIOLOGY

Large population-based studies suggest that the survival for right-sided colon cancer is significantly worse than for left-sided tumours. A meta-analysis by Peterelli et al. showed a significantly reduced risk of death for those patients with a left-sided primary tumour compared with those with a right-sided primary (hazard ratio [HR], 0.82; 95% confidence interval [CI], 0.79–0.84; P <0.001).[26] This difference also remains, when adjusted for age, co-morbidities and tumour stage. The fact that surgery for the left side is more likely to be carried out along the CME principles explained earlier may play a role, but there are also biological differences associated with proximal colon adenocarcinomas, suggesting a poorer prognosis. Right-sided adenocarcinomas are more likely to be mucinous, poorly differentiated and possess microsatellite instability, *BRAF* mutations, methylated

phenotype and *RAS* mutations.[26–29] These findings suggest that a CME approach may be even more important on the right side.

ANATOMICAL VARIATIONS

Anatomical variations in the arterial supply and venous drainage of the colon are common and are of particular surgical significance when operating on the right colon. Having said that, there are also important variations on the left side, such as the occurrence of a centrally positioned meandering artery of Moskowitz, connecting the SMA and inferior mesenteric artery territory at the base of the left colonic mesentery. It is important for the surgeon to be aware of such variations to minimise intra-operative complications. This is best achieved by studying the patient's pre-operative staging CT scan. Three-dimensional (3D) reconstruction of the colonic vascular anatomy is already being used for such a purpose and it is hoped the more widespread use of this technology will aid surgeons in their operative planning (Fig. 4.4). One of the more complex variations on the right side is related to the common trunk of Henle and often source of anatomical misconception. This venous confluence may involve veins from the pancreas (anterior superior pancreaticoduodenal vein), the colon (superior right colonic vein and branches of the middle colic vein) and the stomach (right gastroepiploic

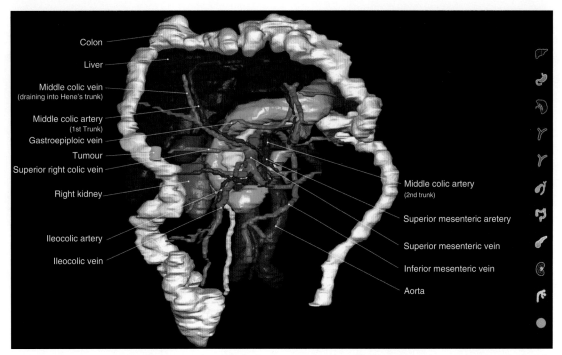

Figure 4.4   Example of three-dimensional reconstruction of superior mesenteric artery (SMA) and superior mesenteric vein (SMV) anatomy with surface rendering.

vein). All of these branches can drain into a common trunk (trunk of Henle), which leads into the SMV, but it is also possible that several can drain individually into the SMV or other associated veins (e.g., splenic vein, jejunal vein). A deeper understanding of patient-specific anatomy is crucial for the CME surgeon (Figs. 4.5 and 4.6).

COMPLICATIONS OF SURGERY FOR COLONIC CANCER

ANASTOMOTIC LEAK

Anastomotic leak is one of the most harmful complications after colonic surgery and has a significant impact on both short- and long-term morbidity, mortality and length of hospital stay. The true incidence of anastomotic leak in patients undergoing surgery for colon cancer has likely been underreported historically because of differences in definitions of anastomotic leaks, variable use of imaging post-operatively and the retrospective nature of most reported studies. Benign and malignant cases have often been grouped together in the same studies. Indeed the reported leak rates in a systematic review published in 2015 reported a leak rate of 1–4% for ileocolic anastomosis and 2–3% for colocolic anastomosis.[30] Two recent prospective cohort studies suggest these leak rates may in fact be higher. The European Society of Coloproctology (ESCP) right hemicolectomy snapshot study reported a leak rate of 7.4% in patients operated on for right colon cancer[31] while a sub-analysis of the ANACO study reported a leak rate of 8% for patients undergoing left hemicolectomy for left-sided colon cancer.[32] The ESCP snapshot study demonstrated a significantly greater mortality (10.6% vs. 1.6%; *P* <0.001) in those patients who suffered an anastomotic leak versus those without.[31]

DEFINITION AND CLASSIFICATION

An anastomotic leak is defined by Frasson et al. as 'the leak of luminal contents from a surgical join between two hollow viscera diagnosed (1) radiologically by CT (including a peri-anastomotic collection) or water soluble contrast enema; (2) clinically with evidence of extravasation of bowel contents or gas through a drain or wound; (3) by endoscopy; or (4) intra-operatively'.[33] The severity of an anastomotic leak can then be graded according to management as described by the International Study Group of Rectal Cancer as Grade A: no change in a patient's management; Grade B: requiring intervention but no relaparotomy and Grade C: requiring relaparotomy.[34]

DIAGNOSIS

A high index of suspicion and low threshold for investigation is required to diagnose and manage an anastomotic leak early to improve patient outcomes. Any deviation from an expected post-operative recovery should raise suspicions. Signs can include a subtle tachycardia, raised respiratory rate, failure to mobilise or open bowels as expected in addition to more classical signs of pyrexia, abdominal distension, pain and peritonism.[35]

✔ C-reactive protein (CRP) should be measured daily. Various cut-off values for CRP on differing days post-operatively (POD) have been reported in the literature with high negative predictive values but low positive predictive values.[36] Singh et al. reported a CRP cut-off of 172 mg/L on POD 3, 124 mg/L on POD 4 and 144 mg/L on POD had a negative predictive value of 97%.[36] Clinical concerns should prompt immediate CT scan of the chest, abdomen and pelvis with water-soluble contrast enema if appropriate.

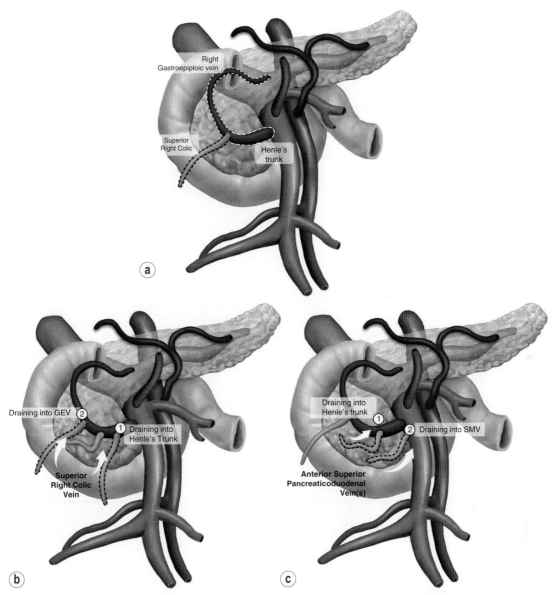

Figure 4.5 Venous drainage of the Henle trunk. All or several branches may drain into the confluence of the superior mesenteric vein (SMV). *GEV,* right gastroepiploic vein.

MANAGEMENT

Although some patients with a contained leak and minimal physiological disturbance can be managed with IV antibiotics, the vast majority of patients with an anastomotic leak will require urgent re-operation. Patients with significant physiological impairment, complete disruption of the anastomosis or peritoneal soiling will require take-down of the anastomosis and end stoma formation. If the patient has minimal physiological disturbance and the anastomosis appears intact with no soiling at the time of re-operation, it may be appropriate to perform a washout, preserve the anastomosis and defunction upstream with a stoma. Partial disruption can be managed with Endosponge® treatment and defunctioning stoma. A quick response and swift surgical intervention within hours are crucial to salvage the anastomosis and prevent significant pelvic sepsis. The latter often leads to long-term functional issues, even if the anastomosis can be preserved.

EMERGENCY MANAGEMENT

Almost one fifth of colorectal cancer patients in the UK will present as an emergency. Those presenting as an emergency, as opposed to electively, are more likely to have advanced disease (stage III/IV), and be under 50 years or over 85 years of age.[37] As a result only half of patients presenting as an emergency undergo surgery with curative intent. The 90-day post-operative mortality for colorectal cancer patients presenting as an emergency is significantly higher compared to those managed electively (10.5% vs. 1.8%).[37] The most common emergency presentation of colon cancer is obstruction.

OBSTRUCTION

Diagnosis of mechanical obstruction (in contrast to pseudo-obstruction) is confirmed with a CT scan on presentation

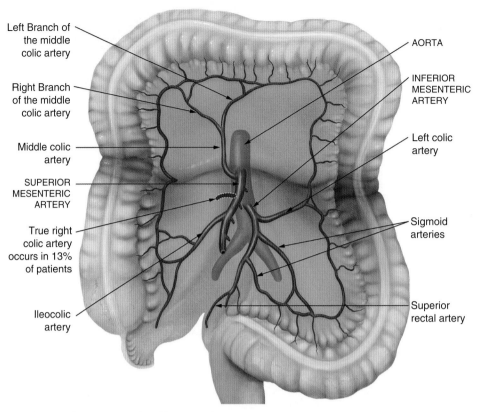

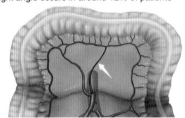

Artery to the transverse colon with artery to the right angle occurs in around 12% of patients

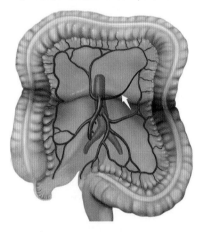

Accessory to the left colic artery originating from the SMA occurs in 7% of patients

Accessory artery to the transverse colon occurs in 2% of patients

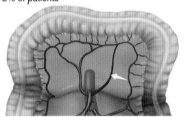

Figure 4.6 Examples of variations of superior mesenteric artery (SMA) and superior mesenteric vein (SMV) anatomy.

with flexible endoscopy/water-soluble contrast enema where necessary. Treatment options include emergency surgery or stenting with a self-expandable metal stent.

SURGERY

Timing of surgery depends on the patient's physiological condition and clinical signs. If signs of sepsis, peritonism or impending perforation are present surgery will need to be expedited. Almost all cases will require an open approach because of the significant bowel distension.

Decompression and on table lavage can be performed in either an antegrade (via the appendix or caecum) or retrograde (via incision 5–10 cm proximal to tumour) fashion.

Decisions regarding extent of resection and whether to perform a primary anastomosis need to consider the location of the tumour, viability of the proximal colon (particularly caecum with a competent ileocaecal valve), disparity in size of the proximal and distal bowel ends and physiological condition of the patient. Most cases presenting with obstruction in the emergency setting will require defunctioning when a primary anastomosis is performed. In the severely compromised patient, a proximal defunctioning stoma without resection may be most appropriate.

STENTING

✅ Stenting may be used as a bridge to elective surgery or as a definitive procedure in the palliative setting and is most commonly performed for left-sided tumours.

In 2020 a NICE evidence review found 84% of patients were able to be decompressed successfully in the palliative setting compared with 69% of patients being managed with curative intent with a perforation rate of 10%.[38] There was no clinically significant difference in 3-year progression free survival or anastomotic leak rates. Patients managed with a stent as a bridge to surgery had a significantly lower stoma rate than those managed with emergency surgery.[38]

EMERGING TECHNOLOGIES

ROBOTIC SURGERY

Robotic platforms provide the surgeon with stable enhanced 3D vision and increased versatility and precision of hand movements compared to traditional laparoscopic surgery. Despite these promising features, there is a lack of high-quality evidence supporting robotics for colon cancer. The only randomised controlled trial to date was from Korea and included only 71 patients undergoing right colectomy from 2009 to 2011.[39] Apart from higher costs for robotic surgery, no differences were found. In a follow-up study, the authors could not find any differences in long-term survival.[40] Not surprisingly, and despite the lack of current evidence, the adoption rate of robotics in colorectal surgery is increasing. Ergonomic advantages and superior results from case series seem to be some of the main drivers for this development. The Australian-led multicentre RoLaCaRT trial, comparing robotic and laparoscopic right hemicolectomy, involving centres from Australia, the UK and the United States is currently in the recruitment phase.

INTRA-CORPOREAL ANASTOMOSIS

Although intra-corporeal anastomosis is not a novel concept, it has gained wider adaption recently, possibly alongside the increased use of robotic surgery. The preferred technique by most surgeons is an isoperistaltic side-to-side anastomosis using a linear stapling device. The enterotomies need to be closed with sutures, which may explain the wider adoption alongside robotic surgery, since robotic platforms facilitate laparoscopic suturing for most surgeons. The advantage of intra-corporeal anastomosis lies mainly in the selection of the specimen extraction site and allows for a Pfannenstiel extraction for all resection types, but also a reduction in length of hospital stay and surgical site infection have been reported in a meta-analysis of published case series.[41] The incisional hernia rate for Pfannenstiel extractions is close to zero, whereas other extraction sites have reported hernia rates of 17%.[42]

SINGLE INCISION LAPAROSCOPIC SURGERY AND NATURAL ORIFICE TRANSLUMENAL ENDOSCOPIC SURGERY

Single incision laparoscopic surgery (SILS) and natural orifice translumenal endoscopic surgery (NOTES) are not widely adopted techniques for colon cancer surgery. Most published case series are small and only performed in selected patients. For NOTES, both a transvaginal and transrectal specimen extraction and transvaginal resection techniques have been described. Most case series are small and in selected patients. SILS and NOTES may become more prevalent in the future with the introduction of single port robotic systems.

INDOCYANINE GREEN FLUORESCENCE ANGIOGRAPHY

Indocyanine green fluorescence angiography (ICG-FA) enables real-time assessment of colonic blood supply and can be used to assess the vascular perfusion of an anastomosis in colorectal surgery. Several studies have demonstrated reduced anastomotic leak rates when ICG-FA is used.[43] The majority of these studies have evaluated its use in the setting of rectal cancer rather than colon cancer and further studies, ideally randomised controlled trials are required in colonic surgery to assess the efficacy of its use. There are several off-license applications of ICG that are currently used in an experimental setting. Laparoscopic or endoscopic injection of ICG into the tissue around the tumour can successfully highlight the lymph node chain. This might be useful for the localisation of the central lymph node compartments, but a true sentinel lymph node approach has so far failed to be of use in routine practice. Intra-ureteral ICG may also be used to facilitate ureteral visualisation during minimally invasive colorectal surgery and may be especially useful in retroperitoneally expanding advanced cancers.[44]

ENHANCED IMAGING

Three-D reconstructions of CT or magnetic resonance imaging scans can be a useful adjunct to identify patient-specific vascular variations and tumour localisation for planning before and guidance during an operation. Attempts to integrate such images into laparoscopic or robotic platforms and create a truly augmented reality environment have not been successful so far because of the soft and flexible tissues of the colonic mesentery.

FUTURE DEVELOPMENTS

Focus of research into improving the quality of colon cancer surgery and patient outcomes is long overdue. The refinement of pre-operative risk stratification techniques with improved radiological staging methods, tissue biomarkers, including liquid biopsies, should enable personalisation of treatment with neoadjuvant therapy and tailored surgery.

Key points

- Pre-operative risk assessment is essential to identify any reversible risk factors, which may be mitigated pre-operatively.
- Enhanced recovery after surgery (ERAS) programmes reduce complications and length of stay in patients undergoing surgery for colon cancer.
- The use of mechanical bowel preparation and oral antibiotics may reduce the incidence of surgical site infection in patients undergoing surgery for colon cancer.
- Surgery in the ideal, mesocolic plane is associated with improved survival.
- The optimal extent of lymphadenectomy in right colon cancer (D2 vs. D3/central vascular ligation) has yet to be determined.
- Vascular variations, particularly in relation to the right colon, are common and can be identified on pre-operative imaging.
- Surgeons should have a high index of suspicion and low threshold to investigate for the possibility of an anastomotic leak post-operatively.

 References available at http://ebooks.health.elsevier.com/

ACKNOWLEDGEMENT

The authors and editors would like to thank Jordan Fletcher for developing and providing the illustrations for this chapter.

KEY REFERENCES

[5] Spanjersberg WR, Reurings J, Van Laarhoven CHJM. Fast track surgery versus conventional recovery strategies for colorectal surgery. Cochrane Database Syst Rev 2011. https://doi.org/10.1002/14651858.CD007635

Cochrane review. Meta-analysis of trials comparing ERAS to conventional management of patients requiring colorectal resection. ERAS group had a significant reduction in all complications (RR 0.50; 95%CI 0.25-0.72) and significantly reduced length of stay (MD -2.94 days; 95% CI -3.69 to -2.19).

[10] Venous thromboembolism in over 16s: reducing the risk of hospital-acquired deep vein thrombosis or pulmonary embolism. NICE Guidel; 2018. https://www.nice.org.uk/guidance/ng89

NICE guideline recommendations for patients having abdominal surgery: (1) start mechanical VTE prophylaxis on admission with either antiembolism stockings or intermittent pneumatic compression (2) add pharmacological VTE prophylaxis for a minimum of 7 days in those whose risk of VTE outweighs that of bleeding (3) consider extending pharmacological VTE prophylaxis to 28 days post op for people who have had major cancer surgery in the abdomen.

[11] Vedovati MC, Becattini C, Rondelli F, et al. A randomized study on 1-week versus 4-week prophylaxis for venous thromboembolism after laparoscopic surgery for colorectal cancer. Ann Surg 2014;259:665–9.

RCT of 225 patients undergoing laparoscopic surgery for colon cancer. VTE occurred in 11 of 113 patients (9.7%) randomised to short (1 week) VTE prophylaxis and in none of the 112 patients randomised to extended (4 weeks) heparin prophylaxis (P = 0.001). The incidence of VTE at 3 months was 9.7% and 0.9% in patients randomised to short or to extended heparin prophylaxis, respectively (relative risk reduction: 91%, 95% CI, 30–99%; P = 0.005). The rate of bleeding was similar in the two groups.

Surgery for rectal cancer

5

Alexander Heriot

INTRODUCTION

Rectal cancer is defined as adenocarcinoma within 15 cm of the anal verge, and accounts for around 30% of colorectal cancers. There were 14 555 cases of rectal cancer in 2017 in the UK.[1] Surgical excision remains the primary treatment modality for rectal cancer, with selected application of neo-adjuvant therapy with radiotherapy, chemoradiotherapy or chemotherapy for advanced cases. Surgery is technically challenging as a result of operating within the bony confines of the pelvis and the necessity to undertake anastomoses in the depths of the pelvis, particularly with the increasing prevalence of obesity. The role of total mesorectal resection in reducing local recurrence is firmly established,[2,3] however, the optimal approach to radical resection, whether open, laparoscopic, robotic or transanal total mesorectal resection (ta-TME) remains controversial.

Surgery may result in significant short-term morbidity, including anastomotic leak, and the longer-term impact on quality of life is now increasingly recognised. This includes impairment of genitourinary and bowel function with low anterior resection syndrome.

OBJECTIVES OF SURGERY

There are three main aims of surgery:

- To maximise the potential for cure by removal of the local tumour with clear resection margins, including all the draining lymph nodes
- To avoid a permanent colostomy, if feasible in terms of oncological and functional outcomes
- To maintain functional outcomes and quality of life, including bowel and genitourinary function.

Every patient should be discussed in a multi-disciplinary meeting, with relevant staging investigations, to determine the optimal management plan, including the need for neo-adjuvant therapy. This should include the extent of resection required and the approach to be used. Radical resection of rectal cancer is major surgery and is associated with morbidity and mortality. Mortality is determined by patient factors, tumour factors, and surgeon factors, with an elderly patient over 80 years with significant co-morbidities having a mortality risk of 6–16%[4] as compared to a younger patient having a mortality of 1–8%.[5] There is increasing evidence that assessment and optimisation of patient's fitness

pre-operatively, including the use of prehabilitation,[6] improves post-operative outcome.

MULTI-DISCIPLINARY MEETING

Management of rectal cancer requires a multi-disciplinary approach and formal investigation and discussion in a multi-disciplinary meeting is essential. The members of the multi-disciplinary team should include colorectal surgeons, gastrointestinal radiologists, radiation oncologists, medical oncologists, pathologists and specialist nurses. The required investigations are listed in Box 5.1 and are important to determine the local extent and relationship of the primary tumour, determination of any local and locoregional lymphatic spread and the presence of distant disease.

CIRCUMFERENTIAL RESECTION MARGIN AND LOCAL RECURRENCE

The importance of the circumferential resection margin (CRM) of the rectum is well recognised and is intimately associated with the risk of local recurrence. Quirke et al. identified that tumour involvement of the resection margin of the resected rectum significantly increased the risk of development of local recurrence,[7] in a period when the risk of local recurrence following rectal resection was up to 32%.[8] At a similar time, Heald was demonstrating exceptional low local recurrence rates following rectal cancer resection and advocating the importance of sharp dissection of the rectum in the pelvis and the preservation of the fascia propria, the natural 'embryological' envelope, around the rectum.[9] Through this approach, the risk of a resection margin involved by the local tumour, and hence one of the factors leading to local recurrence, can be significantly reduced. This finding was confirmed through training programs in total mesorectal excision in a number of countries.[10]

The relationship of the primary tumour to the fascia propria is one of the key determinants of the management plan for specific rectal tumours. It is related to both the tumour stage and tumour position within the rectum. For example, a T2 tumour in the mid-rectum will be well away from the CRM as it has not penetrated through the muscularis propria of the rectum and is surrounded by the fatty mesorectum around the rectum. The same T2 tumour, if very low in the rectum in the muscle tube at the point beyond where the mesorectum is present, will be very close to

Box 5.1 Rectal cancer assessment

Digital rectal examination/rigid sigmoidoscopy/flexible sigmoidoscopy

- Local extent and fixity of rectal tumour
- Position in the rectum and relationship to the dentate line and sphincter complex
- Functional assessment of the sphincter

Colonoscopy

- Assessment of synchronous polyps and cancers

Imaging

- Pelvic magnetic resonance imaging: assessment of the extent of the primary tumour and associated local and locoregional lymphatic spread
- Chest/abdominal/pelvic CT: assessment of distant disease
- +/- PET-CT: assessment of locoregional and distant disease

CT, Computed tomography; *PET*, positron emission tomography.

the CRM. Whilst the CRM can be threatened by the local extent of the primary tumour, it can also be threatened by tumour deposits in involved mesorectal lymph nodes, or deposits of extra-mural venous invasion (EMVI) by tumour, which must all be assessed when determining the risk to the circumferential resection margin.

Multi-disciplinary management of rectal cancer is essential with staging magnetic resonance imaging (MRI) important to assess the requirement for neoadjuvant therapy for threatened circumferential resection margins or high-risk features such as EMVI.

The key tool for pre-operative assessment of the CRM is the pelvic MRI scan.

Fundamental work by Brown[11,12] and Beats-Tan[13] demonstrated the predictive value of the MRI in determining the relationship of the rectal tumour to the CRM; tumours within 1 mm of the fascia propria are considered to threaten the CRM. It does allow accurate T staging of the primary tumour, but the relationship of the tumour to the CRM is much more important when determining management. The MRI can also identify tumour involvement of mesorectal lymph nodes and the presence of extra-mural venous invasion in the mesorectum. More recently, the potential importance of pelvic sidewall lymph nodes has been highlighted and these can be identified and measured on pelvic MRI.

NEOADJUVANT THERAPY

Definitive description of the application and options for neoadjuvant therapy are described elsewhere in this book. In brief, rectal tumours considered to threaten the CRM or have high-risk features such as mesorectal or pelvic sidewall nodal involvement, or EMVI, may benefit from neoadjuvant therapy, whereas early stage disease can be treated with surgery alone. Selective application of neoadjuvant therapy is important as it does have negative longer-term functional impacts.

Early-stage disease, such T1 or T2 tumours, which do not threaten the CRM can be managed by primary surgical resection. This is also true for early T3 tumours, with less than 5 mm of mesorectal invasion and a clear CRM, as was demonstrated by the MERCURY study,[14] where excellent results were obtained in these tumours through surgery alone, without the use of neoadjuvant therapy. Rectal tumours threatening the CRM, or with nodal involvement, or EMVI,[15] will benefit from neoadjuvant therapy, including short-course radiotherapy, long-course chemoradiotherapy, or total neoadjuvant chemotherapy. Individualisation of care is essential.

RESTAGING

The concept of restaging after neoadjuvant therapy has been adopted more recently.[16] Whilst it is unusual for tumours to progress during neoadjuvant therapy, it can happen, and in some cases where there is uncertainty over the presence of distant disease such as small lung nodules, size change can give an indication of pathology through restaging. Local and locoregional disease, however, may show more distinct changes following neoadjuvant therapy and this may directly influence surgical intervention. Whilst the planned surgical procedure is usually determined on the initial staging, as it may be difficult to distinguish downstaging fibrosis following neoadjuvant therapy from persisting tumour, there are situations where downstaging can alter the surgical plan. Tumours threatening the CRM may show distinct downstaging and a clear CRM following neoadjuvant therapy. A good example is development of a clear anterior plane between the rectum and the prostate in the case of a bulky anterior tumour in a narrow pelvis where a clear anterior plane was not visible pre-neoadjuvant therapy, hence avoiding the need of a total pelvic exenteration. Downstaging may result in a complete clinical response and allow the consideration of a 'watch and wait' approach to management, with the potential to avoid surgical resection altogether.

The response of potentially involved pelvic sidewall lymph nodes is also important, with consideration of resection of persisting enlarged and potentially involved pelvic sidewall nodes following chemoradiotherapy, at the same time as the radical resection of the primary tumour.

PATIENT OPTIMISATION AND PREHABILITATION

Surgery for rectal cancer is major surgery and advances in anaesthesia and surgical technique have made surgical intervention safer and more accessible for patients with rectal malignancies. Patients are now older and have increasing co-morbidities, including obesity. Post-operative complications in patients undergoing major abdominal surgery are seen in up to 30% of cases,[17] and even without complications, a reduction in functional capacity during the first post-operative month is seen in one-third of patients. Furthermore, post-operative fatigue has been demonstrated to be associated with the pre-operative functional status, particularly affecting patients with poor pre-operative exercise capacity, the elderly, the nutritionally deplete and those with an associated malignancy. 'Prehabilitation' of the surgical patient is the pre-operative optimisation of functional capacity before an incoming stressor.[18] This typically occurs between the diagnosis and elective surgical intervention. Optimisation of patients with malignant disease poses an extra set of challenges because of the functional decline associated with neoadjuvant therapy. Patient-centred risk assessment can identify multiple factors that can be optimised in a tailored prehabilitation program (Box 5.2).

Cardiopulmonary exercise testing is the gold standard for evaluating functional capacity and plays an essential role in pre-operative risk stratification.[19] Interventions such as exercise therapy, optimisation of nutrition and immunonutrition, abstinence of smoking and alcohol, haematinic optimisation and psychological support have been investigated in the surgical population and have demonstrated benefits in isolated studies.[6] Prehabilitation has been demonstrated to improve physical fitness and reduce morbidity in patients with rectal cancers undergoing neoadjuvant therapy.[20]

Immediate preparation for surgery should include bowel preparation with oral antibiotics, which have demonstrated to reduce surgical site infection. Prophylactic intravenous antibiotics should be given at induction and thrombophylactic therapy with intra-operative intermittent calf compression and post-operative low-molecular-weight heparin should be used. An Enhanced Recovery after Surgery program (ERAS) should be used to reduce post-operative complications and shorten length of hospital stay (Box 5.3).

EXTENT OF EXCISION – TOTAL MESORECTAL EXCISION VERSUS MESORECTAL TRANSECTION, LEVEL OF VASCULAR LIGATION AND PELVIC LYMPHADENECTOMY

TOTAL MESORECTAL EXCISION VERSUS MESORECTAL TRANSECTION

The impact of TME in facilitating a resection margin that is clear of tumour, an R0 resection, through preservation of an intact fascia propria around the rectum, and the subsequent dramatic reduction in the risk of local recurrence has already been discussed, and sharp dissection in the TME plane to achieve this is an essential component of rectal cancer surgery. The extent of mesorectal resection is another important consideration. Tumour deposits have been demonstrated in the mesorectum distal to the primary tumour, up to 4-cm caudally in poorly differentiated tumours.[21] The mesorectum, however, does narrow and eventually disappears as it approaches the naked muscle tube that extends to the anal sphincter complex, and distal margins from low rectal tumours at this level of only 1 cm have not been associated with any increase in local recurrence.[22,23]

For tumours in the upper third of the rectum, it is reasonable to divide the mesorectum, tangentially to the rectal wall, and the rectum itself, 5 cm distal to the primary tumour, maintaining the lower part of the rectum, with subsequent benefits to bowel function, and potential reduction in anastomotic leak, with no negative oncological consequences.

For mid- and low-rectal cancers, TME is required to both obtain adequate distal clearance and also because of the technical difficulty in dividing the low rectum above the muscle tube (Fig. 5.1). For TME, the muscle tube is usually divided with a stapler following vascular ligation

and complete rectal mobilisation. Use of a stapler greatly facilitates division of the low rectum following TME, but some very low-lying tumours may require transanal division of the rectum or abdominoperineal resection as discussed later.

 TME is optimal for mid- or low-rectal cancer.

LEVEL OF VASCULAR LIGATION AND ABDOMINAL MOBILISATION

The predominant lymphatic drainage of the rectum follows its major arterial supply, the inferior mesenteric artery (IMA), arising from the aorta. It may be ligated directly on the aorta, however, this risks damage to the autonomic nerves running along the aorta and hence may be ligated a short distance off the aorta, preserving the sympathetic nerves whilst ensuring complete resection of the draining lymph nodes along the IMA. Ligation just below the origin of the left colic artery, a low ligation, has not demonstrated an inferior oncological outcome, however.[24] The sigmoid and left colon must be mobilised to allow bowel to be available to anastomose following the rectal resection. The sigmoid is considered less optimal for anastomosis because of the higher pressures generated within it, which may increase the risk of anastomotic leak, and the poor marginal artery flow, increasing the risk of ischaemia. Hence the sigmoid colon should be resected with the rectum and the descending colon used for the rectal anastomosis. To allow the left colon to reach down to the low pelvis, the inferior mesenteric vein needs to be divided below the base of the pancreas and the splenic flexure needs to be mobilised. The inferior mesenteric vein and origin of the left colic artery must also be divided adjacent to the ligation of the IMA to provide an adequate length of left colon to facilitate a tension-free anastomosis.[25]

As well as the risk to the autonomic nerves adjacent to the origin of the IMA, there are two other sites at risk of nerve injury during rectal resection. The hypogastric nerves on the pelvic brim posterior to the mesorectum may be inadvertently damaged, as may the nervi erigentes in the deep pelvis, which lie anterior to Denonvilliers' fascia, lateral to the prostate.

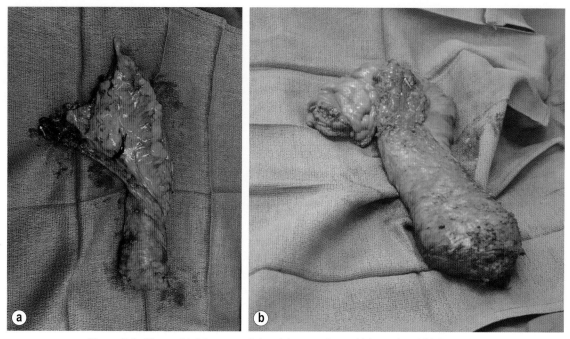

Figure 5.1   Views of total mesorectal excision specimen. (a) Lateral and (b) Posterior.

LATERAL PELVIC LYMPH NODES DISSECTION

The primary lymphatic drainage of the rectum is to the mesorectum and then along the IMA. There is also, however, a proportion of drainage to the lateral pelvic sidewall lymph nodes, which increases distally down the rectum.[26] This has been well recognised in Japan and has directed management policy for low-rectal cancer, with lateral pelvic lymph node dissection (LPLND), in conjunction with TME, considered standard of care for extra-peritoneal rectal cancers. The Japanese guidelines highlighted that in locally advanced low-rectal cancers, up to 30% of patients had involved lateral pelvic sidewall lymph nodes, sometimes in the absence of mesorectal nodal involvement.[27] The approach in the Western world has been to use neoadjuvant chemoradiotherapy before surgical resection with TME, with the assumption that neoadjuvant therapy will sterilise any nodal metastasis present outside the mesorectum, thus negating the requirement for LPLND.[28] There is now realisation that neither individual approach completely addresses the problem of lateral pelvic recurrence, with lateral recurrence gaining more prevalence as overall rectal cancer treatment improves.[29,30]

Oguru et al.[31] reported that persisting pelvic sidewall lymphadenopathy following chemoradiotherapy was associated with increased local recurrence, and that the risk of local recurrence could be reduced by selective pelvic side wall dissection following chemoradiotherapy. LPLND, however, does result in higher morbidity with increased blood loss and longer operating time, even in the hands of experienced surgeons, as demonstrated by a Japanese randomised controlled trial (RCT) of LPLND.[32] Pelvic sidewall dissection requires en bloc resection of the pelvic sidewall nodal tissue rather than 'cherry picking' of the enlarged nodes. Therefore when considering the potential benefit for some patients, at the expense of increased morbidity, the selection of patients for LPLND becomes a very important factor. Pre-therapy pelvic sidewall lymph node size of 7 mm was considered significant, and post-neoadjuvant therapy 4 mm

should be the criteria for persistent involvement,[32] with another study reporting 5 mm.[33]

Pelvic sidewall dissection has not yet become standard of care in the West but is highly likely to have increasing penetration in selective patients, with those with persisting pelvic sidewall nodes following neoadjuvant chemoradiotherapy undergoing pelvic side wall dissection at the time of resection of the primary tumour. Williamson et al.[34] and Peacock et al.[35] provide excellent reviews of the subject (Fig. 5.2).

✔ Lateral pelvic sidewall lymph nodes should be resected in selected cases.

SURGICAL APPROACH FOR RECTAL CANCER RESECTION

LAPAROSCOPIC

Whilst a laparoscopic approach to colon cancer has become standard of care since the mid 2000s, the optimal approach to rectal cancer remains controversial, which is a reflection of the challenge of undertaking rectal resection. Open resection remains the oncological gold standard to which other approaches are compared. Whilst rectal resection was included in the CLASSIC study,[36] which compared laparoscopic to open approach for both colon and rectal cancers, it was only in the 2010s that a number of large, well designed, multicentre studies comparing laparoscopic to open resection for rectal cancer began to report (Table 5.1).

✔✔ Both open and laparoscopic approaches can be considered to be appropriate for rectal cancer resection, though laparoscopic surgery may be better in a subset of patients when performed by surgeons with advanced laparoscopic skills. Patients that could be considered to be particularly challenging for a laparoscopic approach would be those with low, bulky tumours, particularly in obese, male patients.

COLOR II from Europe[37] and the COREAN study from Korea[38] both had endpoints of 3-year survival and demonstrated equivalent oncological outcomes between a laparoscopic and an open approach, with COLOR II actually reporting a significantly lower local recurrence rate for low-rectal tumours with a laparoscopic approach. Complication rates were similar between the two approaches but post-operative recovery was quicker, quality of life better, and length of stay shorter in the laparoscopic groups. ACOSOG

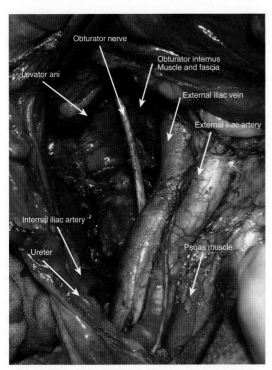

Figure 5.2 Right pelvic sidewall anatomy following pelvic sidewall lymph node clearance.

Z6051 from the United States[39] and ALaCart from Australasia[40] were both non-inferiority studies based on a combination of pathological outcomes including CRM involvement, completeness of TME, and distal margin involvement. Both the studies failed to demonstrate that a laparoscopic approach was oncologically non-inferior to an open approach (see Table 5.1). Longer-term follow-up at 2 years demonstrated no difference in local recurrence or disease-free survival, however, the studies were not powered to detect differences in disease-free survival or local recurrence.[41,42]

ROBOTIC

There has been increasing interest in the application of a robotic approach to rectal cancer resection. The provision of a stable platform, three-dimensional vision, and a greater range of movement does provide the potential to overcome some of the limitations of a laparoscopic approach, though currently at a greater financial cost; up till recently, the market has been dominated by a single monopoly industry provider. A number of small cohort studies have demonstrated potential advantages of a robotic approach over a laparoscopic approach. There has only been one RCT, the ROLAAR trial, which recruited 471 patients undergoing rectal cancer resection, randomised in a 1:1 fashion, with an endpoint of conversion rate.[43] The study did not demonstrate any difference in conversion rate between the two approaches, nor in pathological outcome, or morbidity. Subgroup analysis demonstrated a potential advantage in obese male patients, which are the most challenging cases, however, further data are lacking. Subjectively, there do seem to be advantages to a robotic approach, including range of movement and opportunities for training using a dual console platform, and it is very likely that there will be increasing penetration of robotics into rectal cancer resection in the future, particularly with the entry of new robotic providers into the market. Currently however, the data on

Table 5.1   Randomised controlled trials of laparoscopic vs. open resection for rectal cancer

Trial	Dates	No. of patients	Conversion rate	Operative time LR vs. OR	Post-operative complications	Positive CRM		Recurrence rate	DFS
						LR	OR		
COLOR II [37]	2004–2010	699 LR 345 OR	17%	240 vs. 188	LR=OR 40% vs. 37%	10%	10%	LC = OC	LC = OC
COREAN [38]	2006–2009	170 LR 170 OR	1.5%	244.9 vs. 197	LR=OR 21.2% vs. 23.5%	2.9%	4.1%	LC = OC	LC = OC
ACOSOG Z6051 [39]	2008–2013	240 LR 222 OR	8.8%	266.2 vs. 220.6	LR=OR 22.5% vs. 22.1%	12.1%	7.7%	LC = OC	LC = OC
ALaCart [40]	2010–2014	238 LR 237 OR	11.3%	210 vs. 190	LR=OR 18.5% vs. 26.4%	7%	3%	LC = OC	LC = OC

CRM, Circumferential resection margin; *DFS,* disease free survival; *LC,* laproscopic colectomy; *LR,* laproscopic resection; *OC,* open colectomy; *OR,* open resection.

clinical outcomes are limited, as is the availability of access to robotic platforms and costs are high.

TRANSANAL TOTAL MESORECTAL EXCISION

The persistent conversion rate in the major laparoscopic rectal studies and the difficulty of resection of low-rectal tumours in a narrow male pelvis has led to the introduction of an alternative approach to rectal cancer, taTME. Whilst the abdominal and upper rectal mobilisation is as for a standard laparoscopic rectal resection, the lower one to two thirds of the rectum is mobilised transanally. This requires the low rectum to be closed with a purse string and then a full thickness rectotomy to be performed distal to the purse string, allowing entry to the mesorectal plane from below. Carbon dioxide insufflation is then used to allow dissection of the mesorectal plane, and the transanal dissection meets the abdominal dissection. This approach does facilitate low-rectal dissection, particularly anteriorly on the prostate, and provides excellent identification of the distal resection margin.

Despite early enthusiasm related to the technique, and large registry studies showing pathological equivalence and superiority compared with the abdominal approach,[44] a number of procedure specific concerns have been raised. These include a unique complication profile including urethral injury and carbon dioxide embolisation,[45,46] a potentially higher anastomotic leak rate[47] (though the anastomoses are often very low and equivalent to a handsewn coloanal anastomosis), and there is a significant learning curve associated with transanal approach.[48] More recently, concerns have been raised over oncological safety. Initially, the Norwegian registry reported a high local recurrence rate and multifocal pattern of local recurrence.[49] This was hypothesised to be a consequence of purse-string failure leading to direct seeding or aerosolisation of tumour cells to the pelvis,[50,51] with a similar pattern reported by some small cohort studies in the Netherlands. Conversely, a multicentre consecutive case study of 767 patients showed a local recurrence rate of 3% at 2 years,[52] and the Australiasian experience of 308 cases of taTME has reported a local recurrence rate of 1.9% and an anastomotic leak rate of 5%.[53]

Rectal resection using taTME does facilitate low coloanal anastomoses and provides excellent views for low-rectal dissection, however, some oncological concerns remain. COLOR III, a multicentre randomised controlled study comparing laparoscopic and taTME approaches to rectal cancer resection is currently recruiting and may provide further evidence as to the role and equivalence of taTME in rectal cancer resection.[54]

✔ Surgeon, tumour and patient factors should all be considered when determining the optimal surgical approach to radical resection of rectal cancer. Open surgery and minimally invasive approaches have demonstrated equivalent oncological outcomes.

DISTAL CLEARANCE AND COLOANAL ANASTOMOSES

A major change over the last 30 years has been the increasing proportion of restorative resections undertaken for rectal cancer. A major driver was the introduction of circular staplers, but another has been a clearer understanding of the required distal resection margin. Whilst for higher rectal tumours, a 5-cm distal margin is recommended as a result of tumour deposits being found in the mesorectum distal to the primary tumour, for low-rectal tumours a distal clearance of 1 cm is considered adequate, and results in no increase in rate of recurrence. Assessment of the tumour position and ability to apply a transverse stapler across the distal rectum following mobilisation is best determined by careful digital rectal examination and sigmoidoscopy to identify the relationship of the lower edge of the tumour to the sphincter complex and dentate line. The variability in length of the anal canal may mean that a tumour sitting at 7 cm from the anal verge in a bulky male is actually anatomically lower than a tumour at 3 cm from the anal verge in a thin female patient. Assessment should also be undertaken intra-operatively if required to ensure adequate clearance from the lower edge of the primary tumour. In some cases, there is clear distal rectal muscle tube below the tumour, but it is impossible to technically apply a transverse stapler below the tumour because of the depth and narrowness of the pelvis. In these cases, it may be necessary to release the distal edge by incising at the dentate line, performing a mucosectomy and then dividing the internal sphincter as it becomes the inner layer of the muscularis propria of the rectum, to enter the pelvic cavity and detach the rectum from the sphincter complex. This may be an area where taTME is helpful in performing a rectotomy under vision as operating without a pneumorectum in a male patient with a long sphincter can be very challenging. A hand sewn coloanal anastomosis can be used to reconstruct. Tumours even lower, which involve the upper part of the internal anal sphincter can be excised in a similar manner but including excision of the involved internal anal sphincter. As the proportion of internal sphincter that needs to be excised increases to obtain a clear margin, the risk of local recurrence increases and the ultimate functional bowel outcome becomes poorer, hence there needs to be careful consideration balancing the ability to reconstruct using a very low anastomosis against performing an abdominal perineal resection, which may result in a lower risk of recurrence with better quality of life, but results in a permanent colostomy.[55]

RECONSTRUCTION (COLONIC POUCH, END-TO-SIDE OR END-TO-END ANASTOMOSIS)

The rectum acts as a reservoir and has intrinsic capacitance so it is unsurprising that resection will impact on bowel function and contribute to anterior resection syndrome. A straight anastomosis is simplest but provides the least capacitance of the reconstructive techniques, though sometimes it is the only option in a very narrow pelvis. Reconstruction to provide increased capacitance can use a colonic J pouch, an end-to-side anastomosis, or a coloplasty.[56] Construction of a 5–6 cm J pouch is probably the most commonly used.

✔✔ All reservoir options provide similar functional benefits as compared to a straight anastomosis, though the additional functional benefits usually become equivalent at around 1–2 years, when the neorectum in a straight anastomosis has distended, providing similar capacitance.[57]

DEFUNCTIONING STOMA

Anastomotic leak is a significant concern for any rectal anastomosis. The risk increases with lower anastomoses, with an incidence between 5% and 10%. A defunctioning stoma may reduce the risk of an anastomotic leak, as demonstrated by a Swedish RCT.[58] It may also increase the likelihood of preserving an anastomosis if a leak occurs.[59] A loop ileostomy is the most common option. A left-side colostomy is an alternative, but it may be difficult to bring the colon up to the abdominal wall following resection and anastomosis in the pelvis and there is a potential risk of damaging the marginal artery, which is the blood supply to the neorectum.

ABDOMINOPERINEAL EXCISION

Whilst there has been a proportionate increase in restorative procedures over time, in some cases, this is not possible, either because of the close position of the tumour to the sphincter complex (Fig. 5.3), or because of poor preexisting sphincter function, such as secondary to sphincter injury at childbirth. The lack of clear anatomical planes and historically poor pathological outcomes, with involved resection margins and intra-operative rectal perforation, have resulted in an increased focus on the technical and anatomical aspects of abdominal perineal excision. The tendency to 'cone' into the specimen just above the sphincter complex by not dividing levator ani widely, reduces the resection margins at this site, particularly for tumours sitting in the naked muscle tube directly above the sphincter complex.[60] Holm demonstrated improved pathological outcomes by undertaking wide resection of the pelvic floor with extra-levator

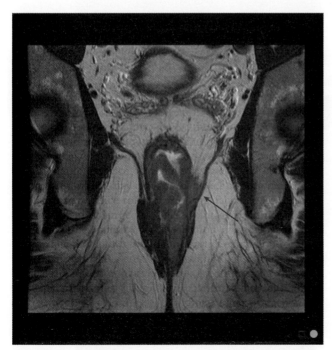

Figure 5.3 Coronal view magnetic resonance imaging demonstrating tumour extending onto levator ani *(red arrow)* necessitating an extra-levator abdominoperineal excision.

abdominoperineal excision (ELAPE) and also highlight the technical challenge of anterior dissection on the prostate and the potential for optimising the view of this plane by placing the patient in a prone position.[61] Whilst this is not mandatory, it may definitely facilitate the view in selected cases. ELAPE may increase perineal wound issues, raising the potential for use of either a myocutaneous flap or of prosthetic material for reconstruction. The focus on abdominoperineal excision has also led to 'tailoring' of the operation, rather than 'one size fits all' (Fig. 5.4). Dissection in the inter-sphincteric plane for tumours away from the sphincter complex in patients with pre-existing poor sphincter function, necessitating a permanent colostomy, should be differentiated from patient with tumours situated in the muscle tube and encroaching on levator ani, which require an ELAPE. Extended resection of the ischiorectal fossa is not usually required unless there is direct tumour extension or perforation into this area.

The English National Low Rectal Cancer Program has highlighted the challenge of low-rectal cancers, with a focus on appropriate staging, selective use of neoadjuvant therapy, particularly in cases with threatened resection margins, and appropriate choice of operation.[62]

✅ Abdominoperineal resection, when required, should be tailored with consideration of the tumour extent.

BEYOND TOTAL MESORECTAL EXCISION SURGERY

If tumours extend beyond the fascia propria, standard TME with dissection in the TME plane will result in an involved margin. To obtain a clear margin, by necessity 'beyond' TME surgery must be undertaken, with an extended resection outside of the mesorectal plane to obtain a clear margin; the concept and approach was defined by a working group in 2013.[63]

NON-RADICAL RESECTION OF RECTAL CANCER

Whilst radical resection of rectal cancer is the primary curative approach, there are other options available. Local excision of rectal cancer, using transanal resection, transanal minimally invasive surgery or transanal endoscopic microsurgery, may be applied to early stage rectal tumours. Colonoscopic techniques such as endoscopic submucosal dissection may be applied to the rectum, but a direct surgical approach using one of the transanal platforms described is preferable as the depth of dissection in the rectal wall may be determined directly, particularly if full thickness excision is required.

Many of the challenges have already been discussed with management of a malignant polyp. Whilst preserving the rectum, the limitations of local excision include technical difficulties of ensuring clear resection margins are achieved and the lack of excision of the draining lymphatic tissue. Accurate pre-operative imaging, including MRI and endorectal ultrasound and multi-disciplinary discussion are essential, with discussion of the balance between the benefits of rectal preservation, stoma avoidance and reduced operative morbidity, with increased risk of local recurrence and failure to identify involved lymph nodes. The risk of local recurrence increases as the T stage progresses from T1sm1, to T1sm2, to T1sm3, with a significant increase with T2 tumours to a local recurrence rate of up to 20%.[64,65] Local excision is an option to consider for Stage 1 rectal tumours, particularly low tumours otherwise necessitating an abdominoperineal excision in elderly co-morbid patients.

At the other end of the spectrum, a proportion of patients with locally advanced tumours undergoing neoadjuvant therapy will undergo a complete clinical response, raising the consideration of a 'watch and wait' approach.[66]

Some patients are not appropriate for consideration of radical resection, in view of severe co-morbidities or the presence of extensive metastatic disease, and a palliative approach is required. Radiotherapy or chemoradiotherapy will often provide good local control for 6 to 9 months, and a defunctioning stoma may manage or prevent obstruction or local symptoms such as high frequency of defaecation.

COMPLICATIONS OF RECTAL CANCER SURGERY

Radical resection of the rectum is major surgery, regardless of patient optimisation and surgical approach and is associated with morbidity. This includes general complications of surgery as well as more specific ones related to rectal surgery. Overall complication rates are reduced with minimally invasive approaches, with lower pulmonary complications and incisional hernia rates, but decisions over surgical approach should be carefully considered as described earlier.

Haemorrhage is a potential risk associated with the technical challenges of operating low in the pelvis, however, anastomotic leak is probably the most feared complication. The risk is between 5% and 10% and is increased by the use of neoadjuvant therapy. Standard considerations to reduce the risk of anastomotic leakage include those applied to any bowel anastomosis such as adequate blood supply, minimisation of tension with adequate mobilisation, and careful

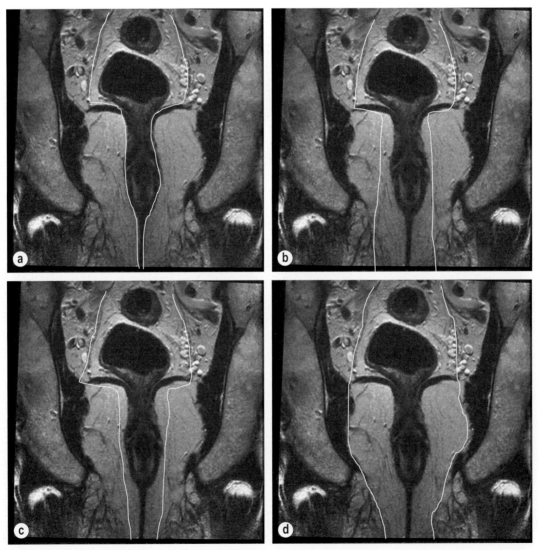

Figure 5.4   Options for abdominoperineal excision, demonstrated on a coronal view magnetic resonance imaging image. (a) Interspincteric. (b) 'Standard'. (c) Extra-levator. (d) Ischioanal.

tissue handling. A defunctioning ileostomy should also be considered, particularly for low anastomoses.

Management of a low rectal anastomotic leak may require a defunctioning stoma, if not already present, and adequate drainage of the abscess cavity. A negative pressure dressing may be inserted into the cavity, which may speed healing and preserve anastomotic integrity.[67] With major anastomotic breakdown, particularly in the absence of an existing defunctioning ileostomy, the whole anastomosis may need to be taken down, with a significant risk that it may never be re-anastomosed, emphasising the importance of consideration of a defunctioning ileostomy at the original resection when undertaking an anastomosis at the pelvic floor.

QUALITY OF LIFE

Improvement in oncological outcomes has led to an increased focus on survivorship of patients following treatment for rectal cancer, including bowel, sexual and urinary function, and quality of life.

BOWEL FUNCTION AND LOW ANTERIOR RESECTION SYNDROME

Bowel function is a complex multi-component entity, and it is unsurprising that resection of the rectum has a major impact on function. There is significant heterogeneity in outcome measures addressing this dysfunction and the collective has been termed *low anterior resection syndrome (LARS)*, describing 'disordered bowel dysfunction following rectal resection, leading to a detriment in quality of life'.[68] This heterogeneity has been addressed recently through an international consensus on the definition of anterior resection syndrome.[68] The consensus involved surgeons, healthcare professionals and patients, and

defined LARS as a combination of one or more symptoms, in a patient who has undergone an anterior resection or restorative rectal resection, which results in one or more consequences (Fig. 5.5). Function and impact may be measured through a LARS scoring system and there is a wide spectrum of degree of dysfunction and impact of quality of life.[69] Approaches to address LARS include use of reservoirs for rectal reconstruction, application of bulking agents and drugs to reduce intestinal motility, pelvic floor training, and for severe dysfunction, insertion of a sacral nerve stimulator, or formation of a defunctioning stoma.[70]

SEXUAL AND URINARY DYSFUNCTION

Pelvic autonomic nerves are responsible for normal sexual and urinary function and are at risk from pelvic dissection for rectal resection, with damage resulting in subsequent sexual and urinary dysfunction. The pre-sacral autonomic nerves form the inferior hypogastric nerves, which lie like a wishbone at the sacral promontory, containing predominantly sympathetic autonomic nerves, which are important for ejaculatory function in males. They may be damaged at this point and should be identified during the initiation of dissection of the mesorectal plane.

The nervi erigentes are formed predominantly from parasympathetic autonomic nerves arising from the S2, S3 and S4 nerve roots, and passing to the pelvic hypogastric autonomic plexus. The nervi erigentes lie between the seminal vesicles and the prostate and supply erectile function in males. They may be damaged by dissection in this area. Judicious haemostasis in the advent of bleeding is essential and decisions over the optimal dissection plane are important. Denonvilliers' fascia passes posterior to the vesicles and fuses with the back of the prostate. Dissection posterior to this fascia will reduce the risk of inadvertent damage to the nervi erigentes, however, with

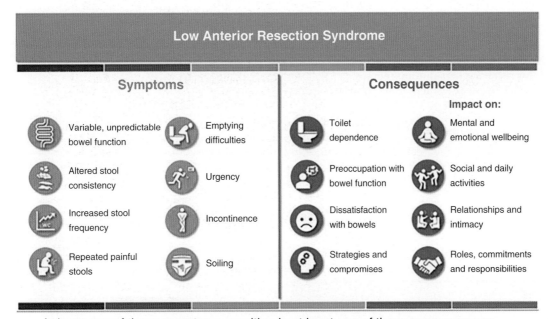

At least one of these symptoms resulting in at least one of these consequences

Figure 5.5 Symptoms and consequences of low anterior resection syndrome.[68]

a tumour sited in the anterior rectum, dissection anterior to Denonvilliers' fascia may be essential to maximise the resection margin from the tumour, with the oncological priorities overriding the functional risks. There are mixed data on whether the type of surgical approach impacts on the risk of nerve damage, with early data demonstrating an increased risk from laparoscopic approaches, not repeated in later studies. Pelvic sidewall dissection, however, is definitely associated with an increased risk of nerve dysfunction.

Urinary function is dependent on both sympathetic and parasympathetic nerve innovation and can be impacted by damage to the innervation at all the sites described. This may result in urinary retention, a particular risk on males with pre-existing prostatic issues. Neoadjuvant therapy may also increase the risk of both sexual and urinary dysfunction in both male and female patients.[71]

The advent of an increase in rectal cancer in younger patients also raises the impact of rectal cancer therapy on fertility. Whilst a detailed review of this is beyond the scope of this chapter, it should be noted that neoadjuvant therapy and surgery will both impact on fertility. The former may necessitate consideration of egg harvest or sperm banking pre-therapy.[72] The latter, in terms of any pelvic surgery, will directly reduce fertility in women, presumably because of pelvic adhesions, and may affect erectile and ejaculatory function in male patients as discussed earlier.

✔ Functional outcomes including anterior resection syndrome and urogenital dysfunction should be considered following anterior resection for rectal cancer.

FOLLOW-UP

Despite progressive improvement in oncological outcomes for rectal cancer, patients may still develop recurrence and are also at risk of developing further colorectal tumours. Intensive follow-up after curative treatment of rectal cancer can improve survival and increase the potential for resection of recurrent disease. The risk of recurrence is highest in the first 2 years after surgery but may occur later, particularly in patients receiving neoadjuvant therapy.[73,74] Follow-up should include clinical assessment, tumour markers, and cross-sectional imaging.

Regular colonoscopy is also important in follow-up. It is essential that the whole colon is assessed by colonoscopy before surgery, or in the case of an obstructing tumour, soon after surgery, even if CT colonoscopy has been performed. It would be considered usual to perform a complete colonoscopy at 1 year after surgery and then 3 years following this.

✔✔ Two meta-analyses[73,74] of all randomised trials of follow-up have shown improved survival with intensive follow-up.

THE FUTURE

There is likely to be increased personalisation of therapy for rectal cancer going forward. This may include selection of neoadjuvant therapy including short-course radiotherapy, long-course radiotherapy, and total neoadjuvant chemotherapy. Surgical resection will become increasingly tailored in both extent of resection and approach, with a proportion of patients undergoing 'watch and wait'.

Key points

- Multi-disciplinary management of rectal cancer is key, with staging MRI important to assess the requirement for neoadjuvant therapy for threatened circumferential resection margins or high-risk features such as EMVI.
- Total mesorectal excision is essential for rectal cancer resection.
- Surgeon, tumour and patient factors should all be considered when determining the optimal surgical approach to radical resection of rectal cancer. Open surgery and minimally invasive approaches have demonstrated equivalent oncological outcomes.
- Lateral pelvic sidewall lymph nodes should be resected in selected cases.
- Abdominoperineal excision, when required, should be tailored with consideration of the tumour extent.
- Functional outcomes including anterior resection syndrome and urogenital dysfunction should be considered following anterior resection for rectal cancer.

 References available at http://ebooks.health.elsevier.com/

KEY REFERENCES

[37] Bonjer HJ, Deijen CL, Abis GA, COLOR II Study Group, et al. A randomized trial of laparoscopic versus open surgery for rectal cancer. N Engl J Med 2015;372(14):1324–32. 2.
   RCT of 1044 patients with rectal cancer. Three-year locoregional recurrence was the same in laparoscopic and open groups.
[38] Jeong SY, Park JW, Nam BH, et al. Open versus laparoscopic surgery for mid-rectal or low-rectal cancer after neoadjuvant chemoradiotherapy (COREAN trial): survival outcomes of an open-label, non-inferiority, randomised controlled trial. Lancet Oncol 2014;15(7):767–74.
   RCT of 340 patients with mid- or low-rectal cancer having surgery after neoadjuvant chemoradiotherapv, showing non-inferiority of laparoscopic resection.
[39] Fleshman J, Branda M, Sargent DJ, et al. Effect of laparoscopic-assisted resection vs open resection of stage II or III rectal cancer on pathologic outcomes: the ACOSOG Z6051 randomized clinical trial. JAMA 2015;314(13):1346–55.
   RCT of 486 patients with rectal cancer randomised to open or laparoscopic surgery after neoadjuvant therapy; the results failed to meet the criterion of non-inferiority for pathological outcomes.
[40] Stevenson AR, Solomon MJ, Lumley JW, ALaCaRT Investigators, et al. Effect of laparoscopic-assisted resection vs open resection on pathological outcomes in rectal cancer: the ALaCaRT randomized clinical trial. JAMA 2015;314(13):1356–63.
   RCT of 475 rectal cancer patients did not demonstrate non-inferiority of laparoscopic resection using oncological endpoints.
[41] Fleshman J, Branda ME, Sargent DJ, et al. Disease-free survival and local recurrence for laparoscopic resection compared with open resection of stage II to III rectal cancer: follow-up results of the ACOSOG Z6051 randomized controlled trial. Ann Surg 2019;269(4):589–95.
   Follow Follow-up of the ACOSOG Z6051 showing no significant difference in disease-free survival and recurrence between open and laparoscopic groups.
[42] Stevenson ARL, Solomon MJ, Brown CSB, et al. Australasian Gastro-Intestinal Trials Group (AGITG) ALaCaRT investigators. Disease-free survival and local recurrence after laparoscopic-assisted resection or open resection for rectal cancer: the Australasian Laparoscopic Cancer of the Rectum randomized clinical trial. Ann Surg 2019;269(4):596–602.

Follow-up report of ALaCaRT study showing laparoscopic surgery for rectal cancer did not differ significantly from open surgery in effects on 2-year recurrence, disease-free survival and overall survival.

[57] Heriot AG, Tekkis PP, Constantinides V, et al. Meta-analysis of colonic reservoirs versus straight coloanal anastomosis after anterior resection. Br J Surg 2006;93(1):19–32.

Meta-analysis showing that all reservoir options provide similar functional benefits as compared to a straight anastomosis, though this additional functional benefits usually disappears at around 1–2 years.

[73] Jeffery M, Hickey BE, Hider PN. Follow-up strategies for patients treated for non-metastatic colorectal cancer. Cochrane Database Syst Rev 2007:CD002200. PMID: 17253476.

[74] Renehan AG, Egger M, Saunders MP, et al. Impact on survival of intensive follow up after curative resection for colorectal cancer: systematic review and meta-analysis of randomised trials. Br Med J 2002;324:813.

Meta-analysis showing significant benefit for intensive follow-up.

6 Chemotherapy and radiotherapy for colorectal cancer

Beshar Allos | Ian Geh

INTRODUCTION

Colorectal cancer is the fourth most common cancer in the UK, with around 42 000 cases diagnosed each year. About two-thirds arise in the colon and one-third in the rectum. Between 1971 and 2011, there has been a steady increase in overall survival (OS) from 25% to 59%.[1] Improved staging, peri-operative care, surgical technique and adjuvant therapies have all contributed to this improvement. Therefore multi-disciplinary management is of key importance to successfully integrate the various medical and surgical disciplines.

ADJUVANT CHEMOTHERAPY FOR COLON CANCER

Clinical trials performed in the 1980s consistently demonstrated improved disease-free survival (DFS) and OS with the use of post-operative 5-fluorouracil (5FU)-based chemotherapy in stage III colon cancer and by the late 1990s, 6-months of adjuvant 5FU was standard.[2] Oral fluoropyrimidines, namely uracil-tegafur and capecitabine, have been shown to be as effective as intravenous 5FU and are licensed for adjuvant use.[3,4] The most commonly used oral agent is capecitabine.

Oral capecitabine is at least equivalent to intravenous 5FU as adjuvant chemotherapy for colon cancer.[4]

Adding oxaliplatin to fluoropyrimidine chemotherapy in stage III colon cancer reduces recurrence risk further (Table 6.1). Two phase III trials (MOSAIC and NSABP C-07) examining the addition of oxaliplatin to 5FU[5,6] and a third (NO16968) looking at its addition to capecitabine[7] have consistently demonstrated this advantage. Long-term follow-up of the MOSAIC trial showed an 8.1% 10-year OS improvement in stage III (59.0% vs. 67.1%, hazard ratio [HR] 0.80, $P = 0.016$) but no difference in stage II patients (79.5% vs 78.4%, HR 1.00, $P = 0.98$).[8]

The addition of oxaliplatin to fluoropyrimidine chemotherapy improves DFS and OS in stage III colon cancer.[5–7]

Unlike oxaliplatin, the addition of irinotecan to fluoropyrimidine chemotherapy in stage III colon cancer has not been shown to improve outcomes in three phase III trials.[9,10] Although the routine use of targeted agents in addition to oxaliplatin-based chemotherapy in advanced colorectal cancer is well established, multiple phase III trials examining the addition of bevacizumab (vascular endothelial growth factor [VEGF] inhibitor) and cetuximab (epidermal growth factor [EGFR] inhibitor) in the adjuvant setting have not demonstrated further improvement in outcomes.[11,12]

There is no evidence to support the addition of targeted agents to adjuvant oxaliplatin-based chemotherapy.[11,12]

ACUTE AND LONG-TERM TOXICITY

Fluoropyrimidine chemotherapy is commonly associated with lethargy, mucositis, diarrhoea and hand-foot syndrome. Although the risk of neutropenic sepsis is generally low, a very small proportion of patients (<1%) are deficient in the enzyme dihydropyrimidine dehydrogenase (DPD) and consequently may develop severe and life-threatening toxicity, usually within the first 3 weeks of treatment. This deficiency can be detected by either identifying *DPYD* gene variants (genotype) that encode DPD activity or by phenotyping (e.g., measuring DPD activity in peripheral blood mononuclear cells or endogenous uracil levels). Fluoropyrimidines are contraindicated in patients with complete DPD deficiency, and should be used with caution in patients with partial deficiency. Routine testing before commencing fluoropyrimidines is currently recommended in guidelines.[13]

The addition of oxaliplatin increases risk of diarrhoea and neutropenia. Oxaliplatin also causes neurotoxicity, particularly cumulative peripheral sensory neuropathy (PSN), developing in the latter cycles of adjuvant chemotherapy but with some recovery over time. In the MOSAIC trial, grade 3 PSN (functional impairment) reduced from 12.5% during treatment to 0.7% by 18 months, however, a further 15% reported permanent grade 1-2 symptoms.[5]

Therefore the potential risks should be weighed against the potential survival benefits of adding oxaliplatin. In general, higher-risk patients with good performance status should be considered for an oxaliplatin-based combination, as their risk of death from cancer significantly outweighs their risk of death from unrelated causes.

OLDER PATIENTS

Whilst it is accepted that selected older patients with colon cancer benefit from adjuvant fluoropyrimidine chemotherapy,[14] a meta-analysis suggested no further benefit with the addition of oxaliplatin to 5FU.[15] However, data from the most recent XELOXA trial suggest that patients over 70 years gained as much as younger patients.[7] Due

Table 6.1 Disease-free and overall survival from trials testing the addition of oxaliplatin or irinotecan to fluoropyrimidine chemotherapy

	Oxaliplatin + 5FU	5FU		Irinotecan + 5FU
MOSAIC				
All patients n = 2246	73.3%	67.4%	–	HR 0.80 (0.68–0.93)
5 y DFS	78.5%	76.0%	–	HR 0.84 (0.71–1.00)
6 y OS				
Stage III n = 1347	66.4%	58.9%	–	HR 0.78 (0.65–0.93)
5 y DFS	72.9%	68.7%	–	HR 0.80 (0.65–0.97)
6 y OS				
Stage II n = 899	83.7%	79.9%	–	HR 0.84 (0.62–1.14)
5 y DFS	86.9%	86.8%	–	HR 1.00 (0.70–1.41)
5 y OS				
NSABP C07				
All patients	69.4%	64.2%	–	HR 0.82 (0.72–0.93)
n = 2,409	80.2%	78.4%	–	HR 0.88 (0.75–1.02)
5 y DFS				
5 y OS				
Stage III	64.4%	57.8%	–	Not stated
5 y DFS	76.5%	73.8%	–	Not stated
5 y OS				
Stage II	82.1%	80.1%	–	Not stated
5 y DFS	89.7%	89.6%	–	Not stated
5 y OS				
NO16968				
n = 1886	66.1%	59.8%	–	HR 0.80 (0.69–0.93)
5 y DFS	77.6%	74.2%		Not stated
5 y OS*				
PETACC-03				
PETACC-03	–	54.3%	56.7%	HR 0.90 (0.79–1.02)
Stage III	–	71.3%	73.6%	P = 0.094
n = 2094				
5 y DFS				
5 y OS				
CALGB 8903				
n = 1264	–	61%	59%	Not stated
5 y DFS	–	71%	68%	Not stated
5 y OS				

*After 57 months follow-up only. Further longer-term follow-up data awaited.
5FU, 5-Fluorouracyl; *DFS*, disease-free survival; *OS*, overall survival; *HR*, hazard ratio.

to the higher risk of grade 3-4 toxicity in older patients, careful individual assessment must be made of the competing risks of toxicity, death from cancer and death from unrelated causes to make the most appropriate recommendation.

STAGE II COLON CANCER

The main evidence to support the use of adjuvant chemotherapy in stage II (lymph node negative) disease comes from the UK QUASAR 1 trial, which randomised 3239 patients (91% with stage II) to 5FU or observation. Use of chemotherapy reduced risk of recurrence by 22% (HR 0.78, P = 0.008) and improved OS by 3.6%.[16]

A number of clinical and pathological features indicate increased risk of systemic recurrence in stage II cancer,

including TNM pT4, extra-mural vascular invasion, obstructed or perforated cancers, poor or mucinous differentiation, and fewer than 12 lymph nodes assessed in the specimen. A stage II cancer with multiple high-risk features will be associated with a similar or higher recurrence risk than a stage III cancer with none of these features. Although oxaliplatin is not licensed or usually recommended for routine use in stage II cancers, it can be considered in selected high-risk patients.

Approximately 15% of stage II colon cancers have defects in the deoxyribonucleic acid (DNA) mismatch repair system (MMR) leading to microsatellite instability (MSI), which is associated with a better prognosis than microsatellite-stable tumours.[17] A meta-analysis suggested that patients with MSI tumours do not derive benefit from adjuvant chemotherapy using 5FU alone.[18] The UK Royal College of Pathologists recommends routine assessment of MSI either genetically or by immunohistochemistry for the four MMR proteins in stage II patients who are being considered for adjuvant therapy.

✅✅ Single-agent fluoropyrimidine improves DFS and OS in stage II colon cancer with high-risk features.[16]

TIMING AND DURATION OF ADJUVANT CHEMOTHERAPY

Most clinical trials recommend a 6–8-week time point for the commencement of adjuvant chemotherapy. A meta-analysis of 15 410 patients in 10 trials concluded that delay of 4 weeks beyond this time point was associated with a significant decrease in OS.[19] Chemotherapy should therefore start soon after surgery, although the authors acknowledge that a benefit for chemotherapy may still exist if a significant delay is needed.

Previous trials demonstrated that 6 months of chemotherapy was as effective as 12 months. Six concurrent international trials including a total of 12 834 patients compared 3 versus 6 months of oxaliplatin-based adjuvant chemotherapy using either CAPOX (capecitabine and oxaliplatin) or FOLFOX (fluorouracil, leucovorin [LV] and oxaliplatin). Through the International Duration Evaluation of Adjuvant Therapy (IDEA) Collaboration, a combined analysis of the stage III patients in these trials was performed to see if 3 months could be considered to be non-inferior to 6 months, thus reducing the duration, toxicity and cost of treatment.[20,21] Non-inferiority of 3 versus 6 months was not confirmed for DFS nor OS in the overall cohort by a very small margin (absolute 0.4% difference in 5-year OS, 82.4% vs. 82.8%). Although the selection of CAPOX or FOLFOX was not randomised, a pre-planned subgroup analysis showed an unexpected but strong interaction between choice of regimen and duration of treatment. Three months of CAPOX was non-inferior to 6 months (HR 0.98; 95% confidence interval [CI], 0.88–1.08). Although this finding was only confined to lower-risk (T1-3 and N1) tumours, the absolute difference in high-risk (T4 or N2) tumours remained small. Three months of FOLFOX was inferior to 6 months (HR 1.16; 95% CI, 1.07–1.26) in both groups. As expected, significantly more patients receiving 6 months experienced grade 3 neurotoxicity than 3 months of treatment (15.9% vs. 2.5% for FOLFOX and 8.9% vs. 2.6% for CAPOX, $P <0.0001$).

Fewer patients (3273) with high-risk stage II disease were included in the IDEA Collaboration. The results were similar to the data on stage III disease, although non-inferiority could not be established because of the lack of statistical power.

These data provide a framework for discussion of risks and benefits of individualised adjuvant therapy approaches, taking into consideration the risk factors present and the regimen used.

✅✅ For lower-risk (T1-3 and N1) stage III colon cancers, 3 months CAPOX should be the adjuvant chemotherapy regimen of choice. However, the additional benefit of 6 months CAPOX for higher risk (T4 or N2) is small.[20,21]

NEOADJUVANT CHEMOTHERAPY IN COLON CANCER

The UK FOxTROT trial (1053 patients) compared 6 weeks of neoadjuvant chemotherapy (NAC), surgery and 18 weeks adjuvant chemotherapy with surgery and 24 weeks adjuvant chemotherapy in CT-staged T3-4 N0-2 M0 colon cancer. NAC resulted in marked histological downstaging (lower T and N stage) and pathological complete response (pCR) in 4%, with fewer incomplete resections (R1/R2 4% vs. 9%; $P = 0.002$). Response to NAC was significantly less in MMR-deficient than MMR-proficient tumours (7% vs. 23%; $P <0.001$). Peri-operative morbidity and mortality were not increased. Early outcomes showed a trend towards less recurrent/residual disease at 2 years (HR 0.7; $P = 0.11$).[22] Current National Institute for Health and Care Excellence (NICE) guidelines recommend considering NAC in patients with T4a/b colon cancers.[23]

ADJUVANT CHEMOTHERAPY IN RECTAL CANCER

Historically, local recurrence was the predominant site of failure following surgery for rectal cancer and resources were focused on improving locoregional control. With improvements in the management of rectal cancer over the past three decades, distant metastases are now the most common pattern of failure.

There is a current lack of consensus in international guidelines on the use of adjuvant chemotherapy in rectal cancer. The UK QUASAR trial randomised 7559 patients with uncertain indications for adjuvant chemotherapy, including 29% with rectal cancer, and reported a 3.6% improvement in OS (HR 0.82), with no difference between rectal or colon cancers.[16] A Cochrane review of 9785 rectal cancer patients treated in 21 randomised trials (including QUASAR) showed improvements in DFS (HR 0.75) and OS (HR 0.83) with adjuvant chemotherapy.[24] However, most of these trials pre-dated the routine use of pre-operative radiotherapy or total mesorectal excision (TME).

More recent trials, which included patients who received pre-operative radiotherapy (with or without chemotherapy) and TME, have failed to demonstrate benefit from adjuvant chemotherapy. Several systematic reviews and meta-analyses have since been published, with conflicting conclusions.[25–27] Investigators have also looked at whether there is a role for adjuvant chemotherapy in patients who have or have not achieved significant downstaging from pre-operative chemoradiotherapy (CRT) and failed to convincingly identify a sub-group who would benefit.[28,29]

Several factors may contribute to reduce the effectiveness of adjuvant chemotherapy in rectal cancer, in contrast to colon cancer. Greater morbidity from pelvic surgery, recent pelvic radiotherapy and presence of defunctioning stomas (and associated complications) often result in slower recovery, leading to fewer patients being treated or a delay in commencing chemotherapy with poorer tolerance and compliance to treatment.

PRINCIPLES OF SYSTEMIC ANTI-CANCER THERAPY IN ADVANCED OR METASTATIC DISEASE

In patients with non-curative disease, clinical trials have shown that by using a combination of cytotoxic chemotherapy and biological agents, median OS can be prolonged to around 30 months.[30] Prior to commencing treatment, it is routine clinical practice to test tumours for *RAS* and *BRAF* mutations, as well as of MSI. This provides useful prognostic and predictive information and helps to individualise the optimal combination and sequence of treatments to the patient's molecular profile.

As with adjuvant chemotherapy, fluoropyrimidines remain the backbone in this setting. The addition of oxaliplatin (FOLFOX, CAPOX) or irinotecan (FOLFIRI) increases response rates and progression-free survival (PFS), although at the expense of some increased toxicity.[31,32] These doublet regimens can be switched at disease progression. A triplet regimen, namely FOLFOXIRI is an option for selected patients in whom a high response rate is needed, such as for potentially resectable liver metastases.

The addition of biological agents such as EGFR inhibitors or VEGF inhibitors to systemic chemotherapy, can be beneficial. The combination of EGFR inhibitors such as cetuximab or panitumumab to chemotherapy improves response rates and PFS, but only in patients with no *KRAS* or *NRAS* mutations.[33] The presence of a *BRAF* mutation predicts for poorer DFS and OS, unless associated with mismatch repair deficiency. Patients with mismatch repair deficient tumours often respond well to immune checkpoint inhibitors such as nivolumab or pembrolizumab despite being used after progression of conventional treatments.[34] Clinical trials are ongoing assessing their use in the first-line setting.

In patients who remain responsive to treatment, the options are to continue until progression or cumulative toxicity, or to step down from doublet to single-agent maintenance therapy, or to offer planned breaks with recommencement of treatment on progression. There are data to support all three approaches and decisions should be made on an individual basis, in discussion with the patient.[35]

There are two oral agents licensed for use in the third/fourth line setting. Trifluridine-tipiracil (TAS-102) and regorafenib (multitargeted tyrosine kinase inhibitor) have been shown to provide a modest benefit in median OS when compared to placebo, although their response rate is less than 5%.[36,37]

RADIOTHERAPY

Radiotherapy is delivered using linear accelerators (Fig. 6.1) to accurately target cancers (gross tumour volume, GTV) (Fig. 6.2) and any sites of potential cancer spread (clinical target volume, CTV). Newer techniques such as intensity-modulated radiotherapy (IMRT) and volumetric arc therapy (VMAT) enable better dose distribution of complex-shaped volumes with greater sparing of surrounding normal organs, thereby reducing acute and late toxicity compared to conventional 3-dimensional computed tomography (CT) planning. IMRT/VMAT also allows treatment of several

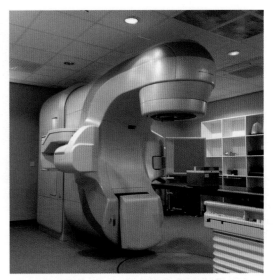

Figure 6.1 A modern linear accelerator.

dose volumes, such as simultaneous integrated boost to the GTV. Although it is now standard practice at most centres to deliver radiotherapy using IMRT/VMAT, the clinical benefit and optimal use of these techniques are yet to be fully defined in large scale prospective clinical studies.[38]

The role of radiotherapy in rectal cancer has evolved significantly over the past three decades. Radiotherapy can be given pre-operatively (neoadjuvant) or post-operatively, with or without synchronous chemotherapy. The current indications for radiotherapy are to reduce risk of local recurrence after surgery and to downstage locally advanced rectal cancers to facilitate curative surgery. The use of radiotherapy to enable sphincter-sparing surgery or to enable organ preservation (avoid surgery) is not yet fully established.

EVIDENCE FOR THE USE OF PRE- AND POST-OPERATIVE RADIOTHERAPY IN RECTAL CANCER

Systematic reviews have consistently concluded that both pre- and post-operative radiotherapy reduce the risk of local recurrence compared with surgery alone, although the impact on OS was not convincing.[39,40]

In North America, clinical trials initially focused on the use of post-operative radiotherapy and its integration with 5FU-based chemotherapy, resulting in a National Institute of Health consensus statement in 1990[41] recommending that patients with stage II and stage III rectal cancer should receive both systemic chemotherapy and concurrent CRT.

In contrast, a series of Scandinavian trials in the 1980s extensively evaluated short, accelerated radiotherapy schedules using 25Gy in five fractions given immediately pre-operatively.[42,43] The Swedish Rectal Cancer Trial (1168 patients) was the first to report an improvement in OS, without the use of systemic chemotherapy. This trial avoided the increase in early operative mortality seen in the previous trials by reducing the volume of the radiotherapy used.

Local recurrence rates have since significantly and consistently reduced with widespread adoption of TME as the optimal surgical technique.[44] Clinical trials to evaluate the role of pre-operative radiotherapy in addition to TME were required.

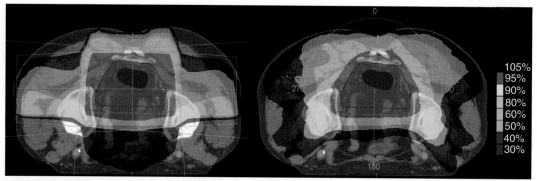

Figure 6.2 Modern radiotherapy planning using 3-dimensional computerised tomography (3DCT) (*left*) and volumetric arc therapy (VMAT) (*right*). The dose intended to be delivered to the 'Planning Target Volume' (PTV), containing the tumour, is 100% and the dose delivered to various regions of the pelvis is illustrated by colour-wash. VMAT delivers a more conformal high-dose volume and less dose anteriorly to the small bowel and anterior part of the bladder. 3DCT treats a slightly smaller volume of tissue to a low-dose 'bath' outside the high-dose region.

SHORT-COURSE PRE-OPERATIVE RADIOTHERAPY AND TOTAL MESORECTAL EXCISION

Two trials, the Dutch TME (1861 patients) and the MRC CR07 (1350 patients) trials addressed the role of short-course pre-operative radiotherapy (SCPRT, 25Gy in five fractions) followed by TME compared with TME and selective post-operative radiotherapy to patients with involvement of the circumferential resection margin (CRM). In the Dutch trial,[45] patients with involved CRM received post-operative radiotherapy alone and adjuvant systemic chemotherapy was not used in any of the patients. In the CR07 trial,[46] patients with involved CRM received concurrent 5FU CRT and the adjuvant systemic chemotherapy policy pre-determined by each centre was applied to both trial arms (Table 6.2). Although the short interval between commencement of radiotherapy and date of surgery did not allow time for any significant tumour downstaging to occur, both trials reported that the use of SCPRT reduced local recurrence to 4–5% compared to 11% in patients having surgery first, although there was no difference in OS. There was no difference in operative mortality or anastomotic leak between the treatment arms. The reduction in local recurrence occurred across all rectum subsites and the absolute difference between the treatment arms was more marked with increasing tumour and nodal stage. Both trials demonstrated that good-quality surgery in the mesorectal fascial plane was associated with the lowest recurrence risks.

✔✔ SCPRT halves the risk of local recurrence when combined with TME, but there is no impact on OS.[45,46]

PRE-OPERATIVE LONG-COURSE CHEMORADIOTHERAPY

Two trials tested the addition of concurrent chemotherapy (5FU/LV) to radiotherapy compared to long-course radiotherapy alone (45Gy in 25 fractions). The EORTC 22921 trial (1011 patients)[47] used a 2x2 factorial design to compare radiotherapy with or without concurrent 5FU/LV with a second randomisation of post-operative systemic 5FU/LV versus no chemotherapy. The FFCD 9203 trial (762 patients)[48] compared radiotherapy with or without concurrent 5FU/LV with all patients recommended to receive post-operative adjuvant 5FU/LV.

Both trials reported similar findings, showing that the addition of concurrent 5FU/LV reduced local recurrence to 8–10% from 15% with radiotherapy alone. Although the addition of concurrent chemotherapy increased acute toxicity, this was considered acceptable. No difference in DFS or OS was seen.

The German Rectal Cancer Group trial (823 patients)[49] compared pre-operative CRT versus post-operative CRT. Patients receiving pre-operative CRT had a lower rate of local recurrence (6% vs. 13%; $P = 0.006$) as well as reduced acute and late toxicity compared to post-operative CRT but no difference in DFS or OS (see Table 6.2).

These three trials led to a shift from the use of post-operative CRT to pre-operative CRT. Two subsequent trials demonstrated equivalence of using oral capecitabine instead of intravenous 5FU with pre-operative CRT.[50,51]

✔✔ The addition of 5FU/LV as a radiosensitiser to long-course radiotherapy halves the risk of local recurrence but has no impact on OS.[47,48]

✔✔ Pre-operative CRT is more effective and less toxic than post-operative CRT.[47–49]

SHORT-COURSE PRE-OPERATIVE CHEMORADIOTHERAPY VERSUS PRE-OPERATIVE LONG-COURSE CHEMORADIOTHERAPY

Two trials have directly compared SCPRT with pre-operative CRT. The Polish trial (312 patients)[52] was designed to see if pre-operative CRT could increase the rate of sphincter-preserving surgery, with comparison of local recurrence as a secondary endpoint. The Trans-Tasman Radiation Oncology Group trial (326 patients)[53] used local recurrence as the primary endpoint. Both trials showed no difference in local recurrence or OS. Therefore both approaches are considered suitable options when the aim is to reduce local recurrence risk, without the need for tumour downstaging. However, the main advantages of using SCPRT are a shorter overall treatment time and less acute toxicity.

✔✔ SCPRT is as effective as long-course CRT in reducing local recurrence in resectable rectal cancers with less acute toxicity.[52,53]

Table 6.2 Key trials comparing outcomes following short-course pre-operative radiotherapy and radiotherapy and chemoradiation

Trial	No. pts	Randomisation	N	1 endpoint	LR	OS	DFS
Short-course pre-operative radiotherapy trials							
Dutch Trial CKVO 95-04 (2011) SCPRT	1861	25 Gy in 5 fractions + surgery Surgery + highly selective RT	897 908	LR	10 years 5% 11%	10 years 48% 49%	Not stated
CR07 (2008) SCPRT	1350	25 Gy in 5 fractions + surgery Surgery + highly selective CRT	674 676	LR	3 years 5% 11%	3 years 80% 79%	3 years 78% 72%
Pre-op long-course RT ± chemotherapy trials							
EORTC 22921 (2006)	1011	45 Gy in 25 fractions vs. 5FU/FA + 45 Gy	505 506	OS	5 years 17% vs. 9%	5 years 65% vs. 66%	5 years 54% vs. 56%
FFCD 9203 (2006)	762	45 Gy in 25 fractions vs. FUFA + 45 Gy	367 375	OS	5 years 17% vs. 8%	5 years 68% vs. 67%	No data
Pre-op CRT vs. Post-op CRT trial							
CAA/ARO/AIO-94 (2004)	823	Pre-op 50.4 Gy + 5FU vs. Post-op 55.8 Gy + 5FU	421 402	OS	5 years 6% vs. 13%	5 years 76% vs. 74%	5 years 68% vs. 65%

5FU, 5-Fluorouracil; *CRT*, chemoradiotherapy; *DFS*, disease-free survival; *FA*, folinic acid; *LR*, local recurrence; *OS*, overall survival; *RT*, radiotherapy; *SCPRT*, short-course pre-operative radiotherapy.

SHORT-COURSE PRE-OPERATIVE CHEMORADIOTHERAPY WITH DELAYED SURGERY

Although the use of SCPRT followed by immediate surgery to reduce risk of local recurrence is well established, its effectiveness in downstaging locally advanced disease when the surgery is delayed by 6–12 weeks has not been appreciated until recently. Small series of patients[54,55] have reported acceptable toxicity and a complete pCR rate of 8–15% when this approach is used in elderly and poor performance status patients.

Stockholm III (840 patients) was a three-arm trial, consisting of SCPRT with immediate surgery, SCPRT with delayed surgery, and long-course radiotherapy with delayed surgery. An interim analysis of 120 patients receiving SCPRT with delayed surgery reported pCR in 12.5%.[56] A final analysis[57] reported that this same group experienced fewer post-operative complications when compared to SCPRT and immediate surgery (41% vs. 53%; $P = 0.001$), with no difference in local recurrence rates.

This strategy warrants wider evaluation as it offers an attractive compromise, when pre-operative CRT is not feasible (comorbidity, relative contraindications to 5FU). In addition, the use of SCPRT with delayed surgery has been incorporated into more recent randomised trials of 'total neoadjuvant therapy' (TNT) as discussed later in this chapter.

LATE TOXICITY AND SECOND MALIGNANCIES

Although pre-operative radiotherapy and CRT reduce the risk of local recurrence, there is no evidence of an improvement in survival when used with TME. This benefit must be weighed against the risks of late toxicity. Long-term side-effects of pelvic radiotherapy include bowel, sexual and urinary dysfunction and infertility.[58–60] An initial Swedish report using large volume radiotherapy suggested an increased risk of second malignancy,[59] however, more recent analysis has failed to confirm this.[61]

Quality-of-life data from MRC CR07 demonstrate a significant impairment in sexual function attributable to surgery and a further detriment because of radiotherapy.[60] Both the Dutch and CR07 trials show a similar pattern for faecal incontinence.[58,60] The Polish and TROG trials[52,53] have not shown a difference in clinician-assessed late toxicity when SCPRT was compared with pre-operative CRT.

SPHINCTER PRESERVING SURGERY

There remains insufficient evidence to support using pre-operative CRT to enable sphincter-preserving surgery. An anterior resection should be feasible in the majority of patients with mid- or upper rectal cancers without the need for tumour shrinkage. Very low tumours situated less than 4 cm from the anal verge usually require an abdominoperineal excision regardless of response to CRT. Therefore it is only in a very small group of patients whose distal tumour extent is 4–6 cm from the anal verge where pre-operative CRT may play a role in achieving a sphincter-preserving procedure.[62]

ORGAN PRESERVATION

There is global interest to develop non-surgical treatments for rectal cancer, to avoid major surgical resection. Firstly, elective surgical resection results in permanent stoma formation in up to 55% and is associated with a significant risk of immediate and long-term morbidities.[63] Secondly, patients who achieve complete clinical response (cCR) from pre-operative radiotherapy generally have a good prognosis and omission of surgery is an attractive concept. Thirdly, the proportion of early cancers detected through population-based bowel cancer screening programmes has increased and the optimal treatment for these cancers is yet to be defined.

The concept of organ preservation was pioneered by Habr-Gama. Patients who achieved cCR after pre-operative CRT for rectal cancer were intensively followed up by a 'watch and wait' (W&W) approach, with surgery reserved only for tumour regrowth. Approximately 25% had sustained local control without the need for major surgery.[64,65] A propensity-score matched analysis of 129 patients entered into the OnCoRe registry (four North West UK centres) who were managed by a W&W approach having achieved cCR from CRT, reported that most patients avoided major surgery.[66] Of the 44 (34%) with local tumour regrowth, 36 (82%) were surgically salvaged. When compared to a matched cohort of patients undergoing surgery, there was no difference in non-regrowth DFS or OS. Patients undergoing W&W were 26% less likely to have a permanent stoma.

Subsequent international registry data[67] and systematic reviews[68,69] suggested that the local tumour regrowth rate in cCR patients was 20–30%, most (85–90%) of which occurred within the first 2 years. Salvage surgery was possible in 90%. Patients undergoing W&W had an excellent prognosis (3-year OS over 90%). The majority of patients treated had locally advanced (≥cT3) cancers.

For early rectal cancers, local excision through the anus using transanal endoscopic microsurgery (TEMS) or other similar techniques, potentially allows for preservation of the rectum and its function, with a low risk of complications. However, stage for stage in all but the very earliest cancers, TEMS is associated with significantly higher local failure when compared to TME.[70] A logical strategy is to combine pelvic radiotherapy with local excision. Smart et al.[71] reported a cohort of 62 patients with cT1–2 N0 cancers, who were considered high surgical risk therefore were treated by SCRT followed by TEMS instead. Over 90% had R0 resection with four intra-luminal recurrences recorded at a median follow-up of 13 months. The Dutch CARTS trial (55 patients) used CRT followed by TEMS in cT1-3 N0 cancers and reported that organ preservation was achieved in half of the patients treated, although at the expense of significant toxicity including two deaths.[72] The UK TREC trial[73] was designed to investigate the feasibility of randomly assigning 55 eligible patients with T1-2 N0 rectal cancers to TME (surgery arm) or SCRT followed by TEMS 8–10 weeks later (organ preservation arm). In addition, a non-randomised

register allowed 61 patients who were considered high surgical risk for TME to be treated within the organ preservation protocol. Organ preservation was achieved in 70% of the randomised and 92% of the non-randomised patients, with pCR achieved by SCRT in 30% and 40%, respectively. TREC also demonstrated that patients randomised to organ preservation had better patient-reported bowel toxicity, quality of life and function scores compared to patients randomised to surgery.

Following completion of the CARTS and TREC trials, the STAR-TREC phase II/III trial[74] was developed in an international collaboration between the UK, Dutch and Danish investigators. This is a trial designed to establish the benefits of organ preservation and its associated risks, compared with standard TME. The initial phase II part of STAR-TREC was a three-arm feasibility trial, randomising patients with T1-3b N0 rectal cancer to standard TME or one of two organ preservation arms (SCRT or CRT, followed by either W&W, TEM or TME depending on the initial response). The ongoing phase III part is designed as a patient preference study. Patients who prefer an organ preservation approach are randomised to either SCRT or CRT. Patients who prefer surgery are offered TME.

Low-energy contact x-ray brachytherapy (CXB, the Papillon technique) involves insertion of a cylindrical x-ray tube through the anus and placing it in contact with the tumour.[75] It can be used to deliver high doses of radiotherapy to small superficial (T1) rectal cancers, or following external beam radiotherapy as a boost to T2-3a rectal cancers. NICE guidance (IPG532)[76] indicates that CXB is an option for patients with early rectal cancer (<3 cm) who are not considered suitable for surgery or decline surgery despite being suitable. The OPERA trial recently completed recruitment in 2020 and is assessing the benefit of CXB in addition to CRT.

ADDITION OF A SECOND CONCURRENT CHEMOTHERAPY AGENT DURING LONG-COURSE CHEMORADIOTHERAPY

The addition of oxaliplatin to fluoropyrimidine-based chemotherapy improves response to systemic therapy in the adjuvant and advanced setting in colorectal cancers. Five phase III trials have investigated the addition of oxaliplatin as a radiosensitiser to fluoropyrimidine-based CRT namely ACCORD-12,[77] CAO/ARO/AIO-04,[78] NSABP R-04,[79] STAR-01,[80] PETACC-6.[81] Radiation doses delivered ranged from 45–50.4Gy in most patients. Pathological CR with fluoropyrimidine CRT ranged from 11.6–19.1% and oxaliplatin/fluoropyrimidine from CRT 13.0–20.9%, with only one trial reporting a higher pCR rate (17.6% vs. 13.1%; $P = 0.033$) with the addition of oxaliplatin.[78] Although this trial also demonstrated improved DFS (from 71.2% to 75.9%; HR 0.79; $P = 0.03$), it is unclear if this advantage was caused by the adjuvant oxaliplatin patients in this arm received post-operatively. A meta-analysis of four trials concluded that adding oxaliplatin to standard 5FU-base CRT did not improve DFS or OS, although there appeared to be a reduction in distant metastases (HR 0.76; $P = 0.03$).[82]

The addition of irinotecan to fluoropyrimidine-based CRT has been investigated in one phase III trial (UK ARISTOTLE).[83] Early analysis showed that the addition of irinotecan was associated with increased toxicity and poorer compliance of radiotherapy, without improving pCR rates. Data on DFS are not yet mature.

✓✓ There is no convincing advantage of adding oxaliplatin or irinotecan to fluoropyrimidine-based CRT. Therefore single agent 5FU or capecitabine CRT remains the standard of care.[77–83]

NEOADJUVANT CHEMOTHERAPY AND TOTAL NEOADJUVANT THERAPY

The last three decades has seen significant advances in the multi-disciplinary management of rectal cancer, which has resulted in a dramatically reduced risk of locoregional failure and the prognosis of patients treated for rectal cancer is now better than for colon cancer.[84] However, these advances have hardly altered the risk of distant metastases, which now outnumber locoregional recurrence by a factor of 3 or 4 to 1.[25,46] The effectiveness of adjuvant systemic chemotherapy following surgery for rectal cancer (with or without SCPRT or CRT) appears limited, at best. Therefore the use of systemic NAC before local disease treatment is an attractive concept. Firstly, it allows for potentially more effective early treatment of micrometastases. Secondly, the compliance of NAC is likely to be better than with adjuvant chemotherapy, allowing a higher percentage of patients to receive treatment and to maintain a higher dose intensity. However, potential risks of NAC include disease progression in a proportion of patients, delayed time to definitive treatment (surgery) and increased surgical complications.

As clinical trials of NAC have been for locally advanced rectal cancers, most trials have also included pre-operative pelvic radiotherapy or CRT either before or after NAC, before the patient undergoing surgery. This is commonly referred to as 'total neoadjuvant therapy' or TNT.

Early phase II trials of NAC suggested acceptable toxicity and promising response rates, with low rates of disease progression whilst on NAC.[85,86] The German CAO/ARO/AIO-12 randomised phase II trial[87] reported that delivering NAC after CRT was less toxic and resulted in better compliance than delivering NAC before CRT. A number of phase III trials have recently completed recruitment. The Polish II trial (541 patients) compared SCRT followed by 6 weeks of FOLFOX then surgery, with standard CRT followed by surgery, in cT3-4 rectal cancers. Mature data showed no difference in R0 resection rate (primary endpoint) or DFS and OS.[88]

The Dutch-Scandinavian RAPIDO trial[89] (920 patients) compared SCRT followed by 18 weeks of FOLFOX or CAPOX then surgery with standard CRT followed by surgery, with or without adjuvant chemotherapy according to policy of participating centre, in magnetic resonance imaging (MRI)-defined high-risk locally advanced rectal cancer. The use of SCRT and 18 weeks of NAC met the primary endpoint of 3-year disease-related treatment failure (23.7% vs. 30.4%; HR 0.75; $P = 0.019$) and was associated with an improved pCR rate (28.4% vs. 14.3%; $P<0.001$).

The French PRODIGE 23 trial[90] (461 patients) compared 12 weeks of mFOLFIRINOX followed by CRT then surgery

and 12 weeks of mFOLFOX or CAPOX, with standard CRT followed by surgery and 24 weeks of adjuvant mFOLFOX or CAPOX, in cT3-4 rectal cancers. The use of NAC and CRT met the primary endpoint of 3-year DFS (75.7% vs. 68.5%; HR 0.69; $P = 0.034$) and was also associated with an improved pCR rate (27.5% vs. 11.7%; $P<0.001$).

Therefore there are emerging data supporting the use of TNT in locally advanced rectal cancers, particularly those with high-risk features for distant relapse, which include T4 disease, N2 disease, extra-mural venous invasion (EMVI), involvement of the mesorectal fascia (MRF) and the presence of pelvic side wall lymphadenopathy.

✓✓ The Dutch-Scandinavian RAPIDO trial shows that SCRT followed by 18 weeks of NAC significantly increases the pCR rate and improves 3-year disease-related treatment failure.[89]

PATIENT SELECTION

The absolute benefit of pre-operative radiotherapy in patients undergoing TME remains small (5–6% reduction in risk), meaning that the number needed to treat to avoid one recurrence is between 16–20.[45,46,49] The addition of radiotherapy to TME worsens functional outcomes. Therefore a more selective approach to avoid radiotherapy in patients who are least likely to benefit is needed. Pre-operative local tumour (T) staging by high-resolution

MRI has been demonstrated to accurately correlate with depth of extra-mural invasion on histology as well as predict that a CRM of >1 mm can be achieved (Figs. 6.3 and 6.4).[91,92] MRI can readily identify EMVI and tumour deposits, however, staging of mesorectal lymph nodes is less accurate.[93] MRI can also be used to identify patients at low risk of local recurrence despite not receiving pre-operative radiotherapy.[94]

Numerous national and professional society guidelines have been published for the management of rectal cancers. Whilst there are areas of overall agreement, there are also discrepancies between them, based on different interpretations of the same data. This has led to a wide variation in the use of pre- and post-operative radiotherapy in patients undergoing surgery for rectal cancer. Across 148 English NHS Trusts, the proportion managed with surgery alone varied from as little as 22–95%.[95]

The current principle in UK practice[96] is to stratify patients being considered for TME into low, moderate and high risk of local recurrence according to MRI staging; T stage and depth of extra-mural invasion, N stage (including presence of pelvic side-wall lymph nodes), presence of EMVI and tumour nodules and relationship of any disease with the MRF. Patients at low risk should proceed to surgery alone, unless eligible for organ preservation procedures or trials. Patients at moderate risk may be considered for SCPRT and immediate surgery or CRT and delayed surgery to reduce local recurrence risk. Patients at high risk should be offered downstaging treatment, which may consist of CRT and delayed surgery or TNT (based on the RAPIDO trial protocol) to improve likelihood of achieving a clear CRM as well as to reduce local recurrence risk. Patients who have significant co-morbidities may be offered SCRT and delayed surgery. Patients with cCR are potentially eligible for W&W.

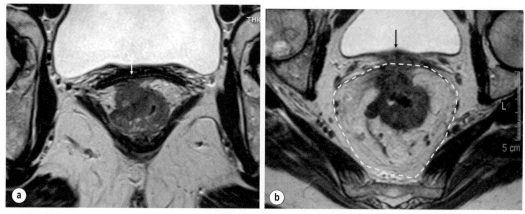

Figure 6.3   Magnetic resonance imaging (MRI) is now a standard pre-operative technique to identify rectal cancer that threatens, involves or breaches mesorectal fascia. Such patients can then be selected for more aggressive pre-operative treatment to try to downsize the tumour and facilitate complete resection. In **(a)** a low-rectal tumour threatens the mesorectal fascia anteriorly (*white arrow*) and also sits very close to the right levator ani at 8 o'clock. In **(b)** a mid-rectal cancer breaches the mesorectal fascia (*white dashed line*) to involve the bladder wall anteriorly (*black arrow*).

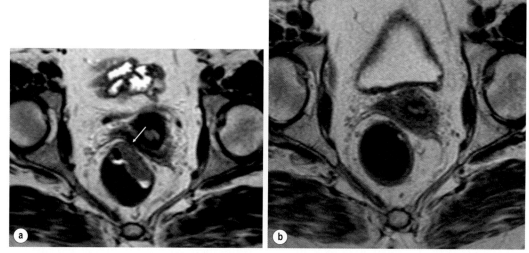

Figure 6.4   Response to neoadjuvant chemoradiotherapy. **(a)** A bulky mid-rectal tumour threatens the expected circumferential resection margin (CRM) anteriorly (*white arrow*). **(b)** Following an excellent response to neoadjuvant chemoradiotherapy (CRT), the CRM is no longer threatened.

In patients who undergo TME without receiving SCPRT or CRT may be considered for post-operative CRT if subsequently found to have an involved CRM. However, the data on use of post-operative CRT to reduce local recurrence risk were in trials, which predated TME, high-resolution MRI staging and assessment of CRM in rectal cancers.[39] The effectiveness of post-operative CRT in reducing local recurrence risk in this situation remains unproven and is likely to be small, at best.[97]

FUTURE DIRECTIONS

The past decade has seen the introduction of molecular profiling into routine clinical practice to prognosticate and to personalise systemic therapy in colorectal cancer. For example, we now use EGFR inhibitors for *RAS* wild-type tumours, immunotherapy for mismatch repair deficient tumours and encorafenib for *BRAF* mutated tumours.[33,34,98] As our understanding of the increasing number of molecular subtypes of colorectal cancer improves, we need pragmatic ways to manage our patients.

A proposed approach by the Consensus Molecular Subtypes (CMS) Consortium[99] is to classify cancers into four CMS groups, and a fifth unclassified group, based on mismatch repair status, chromosomal instability and other immunohistochemical analysis. However, it is likely that this will evolve as new markers will continue to emerge and become incorporated into routine clinical practice for many decades to come.

It is recognised that adjuvant chemotherapy benefits only a small proportion of stage II and III colon cancer patients treated but in the process many more patients will endure needless toxicity. Ways of identifying patients at the highest and lowest risk of recurrence are needed. The role of detecting circulating tumour cells (CTCs) is a promising way forward and can identify sub-groups of stage II and stage III patients at highest recurrence risk.[100,101] The use of CTCs during follow-up may detect recurrent disease at a significantly earlier stage to allow for more effective salvage therapy. Further randomised trials are ongoing.

Research into the gut microbiome and its role in the development and treatment of colorectal cancers remains in its infancy. There has been recent recognition of an association between certain gut microbiome alterations and colorectal cancer incidence, which may potentially lead to new therapeutic options to target this mechanism, such as faecal microbiota-transplantation, pre-/probiotics or phage therapy.[102]

Key points

1. Adjuvant single-agent fluoropyrimidine improves DFS and OS in stage II colon cancer but the benefit is marginal, thus it is only considered in those with high-risk features where that benefit is higher and as such the benefit-risk profile is improved. The addition of adjuvant oxaliplatin to fluoropyrimidine chemotherapy improves DFS and OS in stage III colon cancer.
2. SCPRT halves the risk of local recurrence in resectable rectal cancers when combined with TME, but there is no impact on OS. SCPRT is as effective as long course CRT in reducing local recurrence with less acute toxicity.
3. Long-course CRT is recommended over SCPRT in MRF involved or unresectable rectal cancers when tumour downstaging is required.
4. Emerging data support the use of TNT in locally advanced rectal cancers, particularly those with high-risk features for distant relapse; T4 disease, N2 disease, EMVI, involvement of the MRF and the presence of pelvic side wall lymphadenopathy.

 References available at http://ebooks.health.elsevier.com/

ACKNOWLEDGEMENT

This chapter in the sixth edition was written by Simon Gollins and David Sebag-Montefiore and we are grateful to them for those parts of the chapter, which we have kept in this edition.

KEY REFERENCES

[4] Twelves C, Wong A, Nowacki MP, et al. Capecitabine as adjuvant treatment for stage III colon cancer. N Engl J Med 2005;352(26):2696–704. PMID: 15987918.
The X-ACT study showed equivalence between bolus 5FU and folinic acid and oral fluoropyrimidine capecitabine after 6.9 years of follow-up.

[5] Andre T, Boni C, Mounedji-Boudiaf L, et al. Oxaliplatin, fluorouracil, and leucovorin as adjuvant treatment for colon cancer. N Engl J Med 2004;350:2343–51. PMID: 15175436.
Randomised controlled trial showing that addition of oxaliplatin to 5FU and leucovorin improved DFS at 3 years.

[6] Yothers G, O'Connell MJ, Allegra CJ, et al. Oxaliplatin as adjuvant therapy for colon: updated results of NSABP C-07 trial, including survival and subset analyses. J Clin Oncol 2011;29:3768–74. PMID: 21859995.
The NSABP C07 study demonstrated that the addition of oxaliplatin to infusional 5FU/LV resulted in a better 5-year DFS and OS. This benefit was at the expense of increased acute toxicity, including neurotoxicity.

[7] Schmoll HJ, Tabernaro J, Maroun J, et al. Capecitabine plus oxaliplatin compared with fluorouracil/folinic acid as adjuvant therapy for stage III colon cancer: final results of the NO16968 randomized controlled phase III trial. J Clin Oncol 2015;33(32):3733–40. PMID 26324362.
This study showed that capecitabine and oxaliplatin for stage III colon cancer resulted in better OS at median follow-up of 7 years compared to 5FU/folinic acid (73% and 67%, respectively).

[11] de Gramont A, Van Cutsem E, Schmoll HJ, et al. Bevacizumab plus oxaliplatin-based chemotherapy as adjuvant treatment for colon cancer (AVANT): a phase 3 randomised controlled trial. Lancet Oncol 2012;13:1225–33. PMID: 23168362.
OS data suggest a potential detrimental effect with bevacizumab in addition to oxaliplatin-based adjuvant therapy for resected stage III colon cancer.

[12] Huang J, Nair SG, Mahoney MR, et al. Comparison of FOLFIRI with or without cetuximab in patients with resected stage III colon cancer; NCCTG (Alliance) Intergroup trial N0147. Clin Colorectal Cancer 2014;13:100–9. PMID: 24512953.
The addition of cetuximab to FOLFIRI resected stage III colon cancer, was associated with a nonsignificant trend toward improved DFS and OS.

[16] Gray R, Barnwell J, McConkey C, et al. Adjuvant chemotherapy versus observation in patients with colorectal cancer: a randomised study. Lancet 2007;370:2020–9. PMID: 18083404.
Randomised trial of 3239 patients (91% with stage II) to 5FU or observation. Use of chemotherapy reduced risk of recurrence by 22% (HR 0.78, P = 0.008) and improved OS by 3.6%.

[20] Grothey A, Sobrero A, Shields A, et al. Duration of adjuvant chemotherapy for stage III colon cancer. N Engl J Med 2018;378(13):1177–88. PMID 29590544.
In patients with stage III colon cancer, 3 months of CAPOX adjuvant therapy was as effective as 6 months.

[21] Andre T, Meyerhardt J, Iveson T, et al. Effect of duration of adjuvant chemotherapy for patients with stage III colon cancer (IDEA collaboration): final results from a prospective, pooled analysis of six randomized, phase 3 trials. Lancet Oncol 2020;21(12):1620–9. PMID 33271092.
Non Non-inferiority of 3 months versus 6 months of adjuvant chemotherapy for patients with stage III colon cancer was not confirmed in terms of OS, but results support the use of 3 months of adjuvant CAPOX for most patients with stage III colon cancer. This conclusion is strengthened by the substantial reduction of toxicities, inconveniencies, and cost associated with a shorter treatment duration.

[45] van Gijn W, Marijnen CA, Nagtegaal ID, et al. Preoperative radiotherapy combined with total mesorectal excision for resectable rectal cancer: 12-year follow-up of the multicentre, randomised controlled TME trial. Lancet Oncol 2011;12:575–82. PMID: 21596621.
The Dutch TME trial demonstrated that the addition of short-course pre-operative radiotherapy halved the risk of local recurrence but with no evidence of an effect on OS.

[46] Sebag-Montefiore D, Stephens RJ, Steele R, et al. Preoperative radiotherapy versus selective postoperative chemoradiotherapy in patients with rectal cancer (MRC CR07 and NCIC-CTG C016): a multicentre, randomised trial. Lancet 2009;373:811–20. PMID: 19269519.
The MRC CR07 trial demonstrated that the addition of short-course pre-operative radiotherapy halved the risk of local recurrence but with no evidence of an effect on OS.

[47] Bosset JF, Collette L, Calais G, et al. Chemotherapy with preoperative radiotherapy in rectal cancer. N Engl J Med 2006;355:1114–23. PMID: 16971718.
The EROTC 22921 trial showed that the addition of 5FU/LV to long-course radiotherapy halved the risk of local recurrence but without any difference in OS.

[48] Gérard JP, Conroy T, Bonnetain F, et al. Preoperative radiotherapy with or without concurrent fluorouracil and leucovorin in T3–4 rectal cancers: results of FFCD 9203. J Clin Oncol 2006;24:4620–5. PMID: 17008704.
The FFCD 9203 trial showed that the addition of 5FU/leucovorin to long-course radiotherapy halved the risk of local recurrence, but without any difference in OS.

[49] Sauer R, Becker H, Hohenberger W, et al. Preoperative versus postoperative chemoradiotherapy for rectal cancer. N Engl J Med 2004;351:1731–40. PMID: 15496622.
Pre-operative chemoradiotherapy, as compared with post-operative chemoradiotherapy, improved local control and was associated with reduced toxicity but did not improve OS.

[52] Bujko K, Nowacki MP, Nasierowska-Guttmejer A, et al. Long-term results of a randomized trial comparing preoperative short-course radiotherapy with preoperative conventionally fractionated chemoradiation for rectal cancer. Br J Surg 2006;93:1215–23. PMID: 16983741.
Neoadjuvant chemoradiation did not increase survival, local control or late toxicity compared with short-course radiotherapy alone.

[53] Ngan SY, Burmeister B, Fisher RJ, et al. Randomized trial of short-course radiotherapy versus long-course chemoradiation comparing rates of local recurrence in patients with T3 rectal cancer: trans-Tasman Radiation Oncology Group trial 01.04. J Clin Oncol 2012;30:3827–33. PMID: 23008301.

No differences in rates of distant recurrence, relapse-free survival, OS or late toxicity were detected between the short-course radiotherapy and adjuvant chemotherapy group and long-course chemoradiotherapy group.

[89] Bahadoer R, Dijkstra E, Van Etten B, et al. Short-course radiotherapy followed by chemotherapy before total mesorectal excision (TME) versus preoperative chemoradiotherapy, TME and optional adjuvant chemotherapy in locally advanced rectal cancer (RAPIDO): a randomised, open-label, phase 3 trial. Lancet Oncol 2021;22:29–42.

A lower rate of disease-related treatment failure (23.7% vs. 30.4%) and higher rate of pathological complete response (27.7% vs. 13.8%) was achieved with pre-operative short-course radiotherapy, followed by chemotherapy and TME than by conventional chemoradiotherapy in high-risk locally advanced rectal cancer patients.

[96] Gollins S, Moran B, Adams R, et al. Association of Coloproctology of Great Britain & Ireland (ACPGBI): guidelines for the management of cancer of the colon, rectum and anus (2017) – multidisciplinary management. Colorectal Dis 2017;19(S1):37–66. PMID 28632307.

Current national evidence-based guidelines.

Advanced and recurrent colorectal cancer

7

Omer Aziz

INTRODUCTION

The treatment of advanced and recurrent colorectal cancer represents a significant challenge to oncologists and surgeons, requiring a multimodality treatment approach. As a result, the National Institute for Health and Care Excellence (NICE; 2020) colorectal cancer guideline recommends these patients are best managed in specialist centres by an advanced colorectal cancer multi-disciplinary team (MDT).[1]

For the purposes of this chapter, *advanced primary colon and rectal cancer* is defined as any or all of the following:

- Tumours that locally invade into adjacent organs or structures (T4a and T4b lesions according to the American Joint Committee on Cancer [AJCC] TNM classification 8th edition). In the case of rectal cancer, these are tumours that have grown beyond the facial plane removed in a total mesorectal excision (beyond-TME).
- Tumours that have spread to lymph nodes outside their regional lymphatic drainage area (AJCC TNM classification 8th edition, stage 4 disease).
- Tumours that present with systemic (e.g., liver or lung) or peritoneal (e.g., ovaries or omentum) metastases (AJCC TNM classification 8th edition, stage 4 disease).

Recurrent colorectal cancer is defined as any or all of the following:

- Local recurrence at site of previous surgery.
- Peritoneal recurrence (colon or rectal peritoneal metastases – CRPM).
- Systemic recurrence (non-locoregional nodal or solid organ metastases).

INCIDENCE

Despite improved access to screening, colorectal cancer still presents as advanced primary or recurrent disease. Population-based studies suggest surgery with curative intent for all-stage disease has a 5-year local recurrence cumulative incidence of 13% (23% for rectal cancer), and systemic metastasis cumulative incidence of 26%.[2,3] The timing and sites of distant metastases are important to consider:

- **Liver metastases**: Synchronous liver metastases are found in 15% of presenting colorectal cancers. Metachronous liver metastases within 5 years of diagnosis occur in 13% of cases.[4]

- **Lung metastases**: Synchronous lung metastases are found in 11% of presenting colorectal cancers. Metachronous lung metastases within 5 years of diagnosis occur in 6% of cases.[5]
- **CRPM** are found in 10.3% of primary right-sided cancers and 6.2% of left-sided cancers.[6] They are found in up to 27% of primary rectal cancers.[7]
- **Bone metastases**: The 5-year incidence is 10%.[8]
- **Brain metastases**: The 5-year incidence is 2%.[9]

Survival from surgery for advanced and recurrent colorectal cancer can be presented as *relative survival* (RS). This is the ratio of observed survival rate to the expected survival rate in a comparable population of patients without colorectal cancer. Longitudinal studies looking at Western populations over the last 40 years have suggested that the volume of surgery taking place for locally recurrent colorectal cancer with curative intent has risen from 16% of cases to 58%, with a 5-year RS of 36%. In the same population over the same time period, the volume of surgery with curative intent for metastatic colorectal cancer has risen from 7% to 24% of cases, with a 5-year RS of 24%.[10] The median overall survival (OS) for patients being treated for metastatic colorectal cancer reported in phase III oncology trials and large observational series is 30 months.[11]

DIAGNOSIS AND STAGING OF ADVANCED AND RECURRENT COLORECTAL CANCER

HISTOLOGICAL CONFIRMATION AND BIOMARKERS

✓ Histological confirmation through biopsy is important before treatment. Deoxyribonucleic acid (DNA)-based biomarker testing such as *RAS* and *BRAF* mutation analysis not only guides epidermal derived growth factor (EGFR)-based antibody therapy (cetuximab and panitumumab), but also has prognostic significance:[11]

Extended *RAS* analysis to include *KRAS* exons 2, 3 and 4, and *NRAS* exons 2, 3 and 4 is recommended. Tumours harbouring any of these *RAS* mutations respond poorly to EGFR antibody therapy. *BRAF* should accompany *RAS* analysis, as this is a significant negative prognostic indicator with regard to OS and may also predict EGFR antibody therapy response.

DNA mismatch repair (MMR) status (by microsatellite instability or MMR- immunohistochemistry) can assist genetic counselling, identification of Lynch syndrome, and have prognostic importance. NICE now recommends this testing in all newly diagnosed colorectal cancers.[12]

In patients with advanced disease and those with local recurrence, colonoscopy may be used to obtain these samples. Other options include radiologically guided biopsy or in selected cases of CRPM, laparoscopic biopsy.

✅ The serial enlargement of a lesion accompanied by either positive positron emission tomography–computed tomography (PET–CT) or rising carcinoembryonic antigen level may be accepted for tumour diagnosis.[13]

In cases where biopsy of the recurrence is not possible, biomarker testing of either the original primary tumour or liver and lung metastasis is adequate with high concordance rates.

RADIOLOGY

COMPUTED TOMOGRAPHY

CT scanning of the thorax, abdomen and pelvis with oral and intravenous contrast is the gold standard for disease staging. Oral contrast opacifies small bowel and identifies sites of extra-luminal disease (Fig. 7.1). CT also plays an important role in image-guided biopsy.[13]

MAGNETIC RESONANCE IMAGING

Magnetic resonance imaging (MRI) is a discriminatory test to stage tumours in the pelvis. In locally advanced/recurrent rectal cancer and CRPM involving the pelvis, MRI helps identify the planes of dissection and structures that require removal to achieve complete tumour clearance. Pelvic examination under anaesthesia is used alongside MRI to determine whether a clearance of over 1 mm (R0 resection for primary colorectal cancers) can be achieved. MRI liver is more sensitive for lesions over 10 mm in diameter than CT. Its diagnostic accuracy for liver lesions may be improved through contrast enhancers (gadoxetate).[13] MRI small bowel with diffusion-weighted imaging is increasingly used to determine operability of CRPM.[14]

POSITRON EMISSION TOMOGRAPHY

PET–CT is an investigation for the detection of extrahepatic metastases and local recurrence, and has been shown to change management in 8–30% of cases. Its role is limited to selected cases, with no consensus on its routine use.[13]

ULTRASONOGRAPHY

Ultrasonography (US) may include endorectal ultrasonography for targeted biopsy and assessment of sphincter involvement, and contrast-enhanced US for characterisation of liver lesions, surgical planning and biopsy.

THE ADVANCED COLORECTAL CANCER MULTI-DISCIPLINARY TEAM

Advanced colorectal cancer MDTs should include appropriately experienced colorectal surgeons, clinical and medical oncologists, radiologists, pathologists and clinical nurse specialists. In centres undertaking pelvic clearance (exenteration) surgery for locally advanced and recurrent rectal cancer, the MDT should be supported by urologists, gynaecological oncologists and plastic (reconstructive) surgeons. Units undertaking sacrectomy and pelvic bony excisions

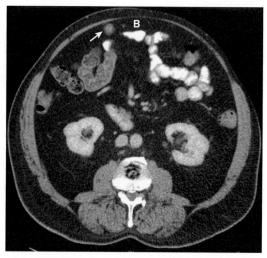

Figure 7.1 Computed tomography (CT) scan with oral and intravenous contrast demonstrating colorectal peritoneal metastases (CRPM) in the omentum (*arrow*) of a patient who previously had a right hemicolectomy for a T4N1M0 adenocarcinoma of the hepatic flexure. The distinction between this and the adjacent loop of small bowel (*B*), which has been opacified with oral contrast, can easily be made.

may be supported by spinal or orthopaedic surgeons. For CRPM, liver and lung metastases there should also be a defined pathway to discuss patients with peritoneal tumour, hepatobiliary and thoracic specialist MDTs.

The advanced colorectal cancer MDT plans appropriate diagnostic workup and establishes goals of treatment. A personalised approach accounting for previous treatment is required. If the disease is not potentially resectable with clear margins of at least 1 mm then neoadjuvant treatment such as chemo- and/or radiotherapy should be considered for downstaging. Fig. 7.2 shows a patient with a local recurrence of a previously resected splenic flexure tumour treated with neoadjuvant chemotherapy followed by en bloc left upper quadrant resection. In this case over 1 mm margin was obtained and the patient was recurrence free at 4 years. If greater than 1-mm resection clearance cannot be obtained, then the goal of treatment is to strike a balance between quality of life and duration of disease control. For chemotherapy, this involves taking into account toxicity, and for surgery, the procedural morbidity. Symptom control is important, and centres should have access to specialist palliative care teams. Information on interventions and patient outcome should be collected prospectively with a view to obtaining long-term follow-up data.

Patients with oligometastatic disease (more than one distant metastatic site) should be considered for systemic chemotherapy versus synchronous or staged resection of the sites. In the case of staged resections, the order in which these are undertaken is important. Despite the absence of high-quality data, patients with resectable oligometastatic disease are increasingly being considered for staged surgery. Finally, there is a role for local ablative techniques in treating lung and liver metastases. These include thermal devices (radiofrequency, cryo-, or microwave ablation), non-thermal devices (brachytherapy and external beam high-precision radiotherapy), embolisation (radioembolisation with selective internal radiation therapy or transarterial chemoembolisation) and locally delivered chemotherapy.

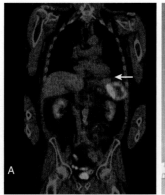
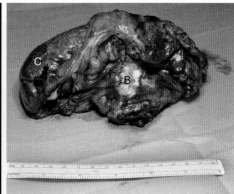

Figure 7.2   Local recurrence following previous resection of a splenic flexure tumour seen on a positron emission tomography/computed tomography (PET CT) (*A – arrow*) treated with neoadjuvant chemotherapy followed by en bloc resection of left upper quadrant tissues including tumour (*B*) and spleen (*C*) to achieve clearance.

LOCALLY ADVANCED PRIMARY AND RECURRENT RECTAL CANCER

'Locally advanced primary rectal cancers' are defined in this chapter as primary rectal cancers beyond the TME plane, a term coined by the 'Beyond TME Collaborative'.[13] These lesions range from being just beyond the circumferential resection margin of a TME (T4a) to infiltrating adjacent organs (T4b). 'Recurrent rectal cancer' in this chapter is defined as local recurrence following previous mesorectal excision. Whilst both groups potentially require multivisceral surgery beyond the traditional mesorectal excision (TME) planes to achieve a clear resection margin, it should be noted that only 50% of recurrent rectal cancer cases are selected for surgery, either because a 1-mm margin cannot be obtained, the patient is unfit for multivisceral resectional surgery, or the morbidity is unacceptable to the patient.[15] Patients should be appropriately counselled, setting realistic expectations. Data on outcomes from specialist centres suggest that in selected cases, R0 rates of around 86% can be achieved for locally advanced primary rectal cancer, with 5-year OS rates of 62%.[16] For recurrent rectal cancer, these figures are lower, with greater than 1-mm clearance rates of over 60% and 55% 3-year disease-free survival. R1 and R2 resections are associated with a poor prognosis.[17]

RADIOTHERAPY

✔✔ Patients should be considered for neoadjuvant chemoradiotherapy before surgery.[18]

An established regime is 45Gy in 25 fractions with concurrent fluoropyrimadine-based chemotherapy. The optimal timing of subsequent re-staging and surgery after completion is debatable. Whilst some have suggested re-staging at 6–8 weeks,[13] it is recognised that tumour regression can occur up to 12 weeks.

✔ A number of established groups (including the author's institution) re-stage at 10 weeks, with surgery undertaken at 12–14 weeks.[15]

Localised radiotherapy may have a role in the treatment of recurrent rectal cancer, although outcome data are scarce. Options include:

- Intra-operative radiotherapy at the time of surgery as either intra-operative electron beam radiotherapy or high-dose-rate brachytherapy at surgical sites where the resection margin is threatened.[15]
- Stereotactic body irradiation therapy (CyberKnife system) delivering multiple beams to well-defined targets in few fractions. Indications include irresectable pelvic sidewall and pre-sacral recurrences.[19]

PERINEAL EXCISION

For low rectal cancers, the concept of 'extra-levator abdominoperineal excision' (ELAPE) with a cylindrical specimen has gained acceptance. However, it is important to note that in the context of locally advanced primary low-rectal cancers, there may be a need for an extended excision of the ischio-anal fat akin to 'salvage' surgery for recurrent anal cancers after chemoradiotherapy. Fig. 7.3 illustrates the difference in these two procedures.

PELVIC MULTIVISCERAL EXENTERATION

Organs that may require removal with the rectum in locally advanced primary and recurrent rectal cancers include anterior structures (bladder, prostate, seminal vesicles, urethra, uterus, vagina), posterior structures (pre-sacral fascia and sacrum) and lateral structures (ovaries and associated structures, ureters and pelvic sidewall vessels, nerves and musculoskeletal tissue).

PATTERNS OF RECTAL CANCER RECURRENCE

Classification systems describing the patterns of recurrence in rectal cancer have been proposed, but standardisation of this nomenclature has not been achieved. A simplified version[15] has been described as:

- Central recurrence (Fig. 7.4) most commonly arising at a previous rectal anastomotic site or in the residual mesorectum. These can go on to involve the anterior urogenital structures and can also extend posteriorly to

Extralevator (ELAPE)

Ischio-anal resection

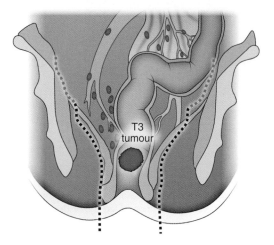
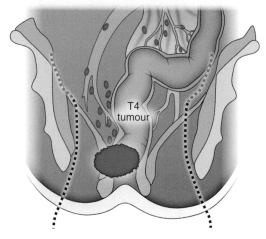

Figure 7.3 Approaches to perineal excision. **(a)** Standard extra-levator abdominoperineal excision approach. **(b)** A wider ischio-anal approach for low, locally advanced T4 rectal cancers.

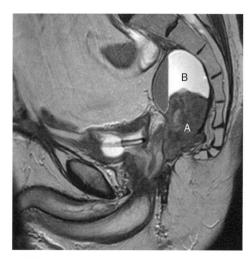
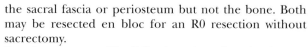

Figure 7.4 Magnetic resonance imaging (MRI) demonstrating central recurrence in a rectal stump following previous Hartmann's procedure (*A*) with associated cystic cavity (*B*).

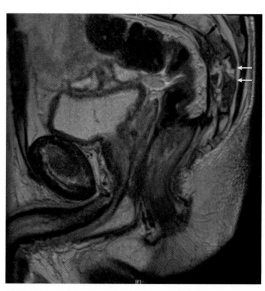

Figure 7.5 Magnetic resonance imaging (MRI) demonstrating sacral recurrence (*arrows*) extending up to the level of S3.

the sacral fascia or periosteum but not the bone. Both may be resected en bloc for an R0 resection without sacrectomy.

- Sacral recurrence (Fig. 7.5) where bony invasion is present and a >1-mm margin is only possible with a sacral resection through a two-stage combined abdominosacral approach.
- Lateral recurrence (Fig. 7.6) involves the lateral pelvic sidewall, encasing internal iliac vessels and branches, pelvic autonomic nerves and ureter and can extend through the greater sciatic foramen with or without invasion of the sciatic nerve. Of all the types of recurrence, this is the most difficult in which to achieve a >1-mm clearance, and is therefore associated with the poorest prognosis. Techniques to achieve clear lateral margins involving en bloc resection of the iliac vessels and other sidewall structures[20] and extended lateral pelvic sidewall excision[21] have been described with promising early results.

TYPES OF PELVIC CLEARANCE

Pelvic clearance (exenteration) surgery needs to be tailored to include:

- Total pelvic clearance (TPC) involves removal of the rectum, sigmoid colon, bladder, draining lymph nodes, pelvic peritoneum and lower ureters. In males, the prostate and seminal vesicles are also excised (Fig. 7.7). In females, the uterus, ovaries, fallopian tubes and required part of the vagina can be removed. The patient has an end colostomy and an ileal conduit as the most common urinary reconstruction technique.
- Anterior pelvic clearance involves removal of the distal ureters, bladder, prostate and seminal vesicles in a male, and in females also the uterus, ovaries, fallopian tubes and vagina as required. It is not a commonly performed operation for rectal cancer and reserved mainly

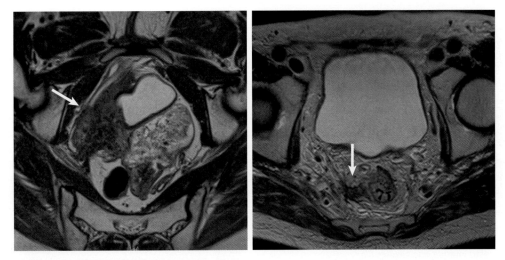

Figure 7.6   Lateral recurrences of the left pelvic side-wall involving left internal iliac vessels and ureter (left scan, *arrow*) or abutting left internal iliac artery branches (right scan, *arrow*).

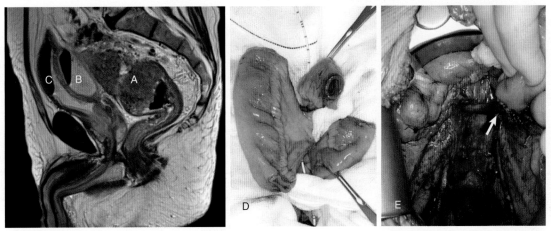

Figure 7.7   Magnetic resonance imaging (MRI) demonstrating locally advanced rectal cancer (*A*) with anterior perforation and associated abscess cavity (*B*) adjacent to bladder (*C*). The patient required total pelvic clearance. Urinary reconstruction was achieved with terminal ileum (*D*) brought out as a conduit with ureteric anastomoses (*E – arrow*).

for tumours of the upper rectum and rectosigmoid that invade into anterior structures. This operation is more commonly used for the treatment of advanced urological and gynaecological tumours. The distal rectum is spared and may be re-anastomosed. An ileal conduit is required for urinary reconstruction.

- Posterior pelvic clearance is a procedure performed in women, involving the removal of the rectum and uterus, required part of the vagina, ovaries and fallopian tubes. This may be with or without removal of the anus (perineal excision). The bladder is spared.

In undertaking lateral dissection of the pelvic sidewall, there are three planes of dissection used to get tumour clearance (Fig. 7.8):

- Mesorectal fascial plane – a continuation of the standard TME plane.
- Ureteric plane – deep to the lateral peritoneum where the ureter lies.

- Bony plane – lateral to internal iliac vessels along the obturator internus and piriformis muscles in the lateral pelvic compartments.

SACRECTOMY

✔ Resection of the sacrum at S1/S2 results in significantly poorer lower limb function compared to S3 or below[22] (Fig. 7.9) with equivalent reported survival rates in specialised units.[23]

S1 and S2 involvement is challenging because of the need for pelvic reconstruction and stabilisation as well as the resulting sensory and motor neurological deficit (the procedure involves ligation of the cauda equina and freeing the sacrum with sacrifice of sacral nerve roots below the level of resection). An international multicentre retrospective analysis of patients undergoing exenterative abdominosacrectomy has shown similar 5-year OS of above 40% for high versus low sacrectomy with negative margin rates of

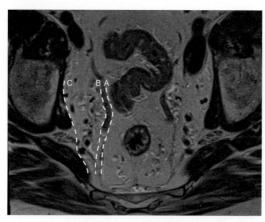

Figure 7.8 Magnetic resonance imaging (MRI) demonstrating planes of the right pelvic side-wall: mesorectal plane (A), ureteric plane (B) and bony plane lateral to internal iliac vessels (C).

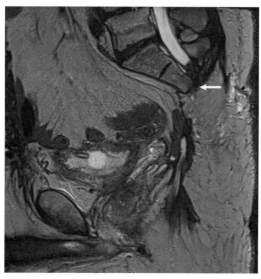

Figure 7.9 Magnetic resonance imaging (MRI) showing a sacrectomy below the level of S2 (arrow).

over 60%.[23] Patients undergoing high sacrectomy have a significantly worse lower limb motor function and poorer physical and mental health component quality of life scores.[22] Techniques such as unilateral sacral compartment excision also offer the prospect of high sacral resection without the need for pelvic stabilisation, but more data on these are awaited.[24]

PERINEAL RECONSTRUCTION

This may be required because of the size of the defect and impaired wound healing after previous chemoradiotherapy. Omentoplasty to the pelvis should be attempted where possible. Biological mesh reconstruction of the pelvic floor has been described for ELAPE; however, it is usually not appropriate in exenterative surgery because of the size of the defect and the fact that it also requires a flap of skin for closure. Pedicled flaps are most commonly used and include:

- Rectus abdominis myocutaneous flaps (unilateral with reconstruction of the abdominal harvest site often using mesh).
- Gracilis myocutaneous flaps (bilateral as they offer the least coverage).
- Gluteal myocutaneous rotational or advancement flaps (usually both sides) (Fig 7.10).
- Inferior gluteal artery perforator flap (usually both sides).

Where pedicled flaps are not an option, free flaps can be considered. The decision should be made with a plastic surgeon, and tailored to patient factors (comorbidity, tissue quality and perfusion) as well as previous surgery (abdominal and perineal incisions).[15] Vaginal reconstruction can be achieved and intercourse is feasible after this.[25]

COLORECTAL PERITONEAL METASTASES

CRPM (Fig. 7.11) can present synchronously (10.3% of primary right colon cancers, 6.2% of left colon cancers, and 27% of rectal cancers)[5,6] and metachronously (20% of colorectal cancers).[26]

✔✔ Systemic chemotherapy and palliative support used to be the mainstay of treatment for CRPM. Compelling data on outcomes from cytoreductive surgery with hyperthermic intra-peritoneal chemotherapy (CRS/HIPEC) from specialist centres using mitomycin or oxaliplatin HIPEC has emerged in the last decade showing a median survival of 46 months with CRS/HIPEC compared to 16.3 months with systemic chemotherapy.[27] A recent randomised control trial (Prodige 7) has compared CRS alone to CRS/HIPEC with a specific oxaliplatin regime. It has demonstrated an equivalent median OS (41.7 months) with CRS/HIPEC versus CRS alone (41.2 months) suggesting that a greater share of the effect of this outcome is from CRS.[28] More high-quality research is awaited on the optimal HIPEC regime.

CYTOREDUCTIVE SURGERY WITH HYPERTHERMIC INTRA-PERITONEAL CHEMOTHERAPY

This is an established treatment for peritoneal tumours (appendix neoplasms and pseudomyxoma peritonei [PMP]). PMP is a rare syndrome that arises from a low-grade appendiceal mucinous neoplasm that perforates, with leakage of mucin and cells into the peritoneal cavity, resulting in abdominal distension and organ compression.[29] The principle is to remove all visible tumour followed by administration of HIPEC using a cytotoxic drug with depth of penetration of approximately 3 mm. Hyperthermia itself also has a direct cytotoxic effect, probably through formation of heat-shock proteins.[30]

CRS can include peritonectomy, omentectomy, umbilectomy, excision of falciform ligament and ligamentum teres, cholecystectomy and any other required visceral resections. These may include segmental small- and/or large-bowel resection, splenectomy, total abdominal hysterectomy, bilateral salpingo-oophoerectomy and gastrectomy. HIPEC at 42 degrees is administered for 60–90 minutes with either

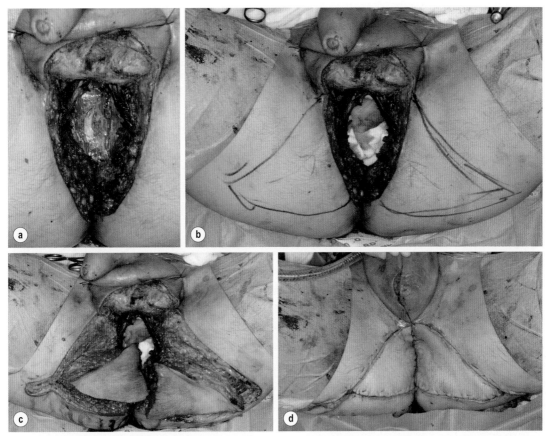

Figure 7.10 Ischi-oanal resection in a male with resection of the penile base **(a)**. The defect was closed with bilateral gluteal fold flaps **(b–d)**.

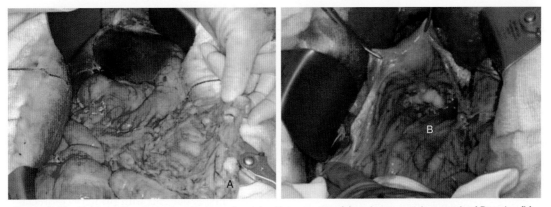

Figure 7.11 Colorectal peritoneal metastases involving the omentum **(a)** and recto-uterine pouch of Douglas **(b)**.

mitomycin C or oxaloplatin and intravenous 5FU. (See Video 1 for an outline of the CRS procedure.)

SCORING SYSTEMS

There are currently two main systems used to stratify outcomes from CRS/HIPEC, namely the Peritoneal Cancer Index (PCI), and the Completeness of Cytoreduction (CC) score, both developed by Sugarbaker.[31]

PCI is an intra-operative score accounting for both size and distribution of lesions (Fig. 7.12). Thirteen regions are each given a score of 0–3 based on lesion size, with final score ranging from 0 to 39. A higher PCI is associated with poorer short- and long-term outcomes.[30]

CC score is calculated at the end of the operation. CC = 0 indicates no residual disease, CC = 1 indicates nodules less than 2.5 mm in size remained, CC = 2 indicates nodules between 2.5 mm and 2.5 cm, and CC = 3 indicates that nodules over 2.5 cm remained.

PATIENT SELECTION

In England, CRS/HIPEC is a procedure that remains restricted to specialised units. Specialist peritoneal tumour MDTs in these centres take into account the patient's full treatment history, tumour type and biology, previous chemotherapy, prior surgery and future options. Patients are carefully selected and counselled for surgery. Laparoscopy

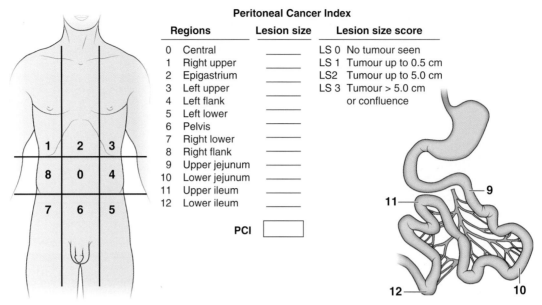

Figure 7.12   Peritoneal Cancer Index (PCI).

plays a role in some cases (see Video 2 for a diagnostic laparoscopy for CRPM). Annually audited results demonstrate a major morbidity rate of less than 20% and mortality of less than 1%.

COLORECTAL LIVER METASTASES

Certain 'technical criteria' have to be fulfilled in order for liver metastases to be considered resectable, as outlined in Table 7.1. In a proportion of patients, resection is made possible through portal vein embolisation, two-stage hepatectomy or hepatectomy combined with ablation. The finding that despite being technically resectable, approximately half of patients develop widespread systemic disease within 3 years, has led to 'oncological criteria' that should also be considered when selecting patients (see Table 7.1).[10]

✔✔ If a patient fulfils these criteria to undergo surgical resection, there is the option of either upfront surgery or peri-operative (pre- and post-operative) chemotherapy. The best available data from the EPOC study are not conclusive on whether peri-operative chemotherapy improves outcome. The study reported a 5-year OS rate of 51% (95% CI, 45–58) in the peri-operative chemotherapy group versus 48% (95% CI, 40–55) in the surgery-only group.[32] It would therefore not be unreasonable to consider upfront surgery for easily technically resectable liver metastases with favourable oncological criteria, but choose peri-operative chemotherapy for patients with favourable technical criteria, but unfavourable oncological criteria as outlined in Table 7.1. Data from the EPOC group also suggest that peri-operative chemotherapy should comprise 3 months chemotherapy before surgery and 3 months' chemotherapy post-surgery with FOLFOX or alternatively capecitabine with oxaliplatin – CAPOX.

Two further groups of patients with colorectal liver metastases should be considered.

Table 7.1   Technical and oncological criteria considered in surgery for colorectal liver metastases

Technical criteria	Oncological criteria
1. R0 resection possible	1. Five or fewer lesions
2. Maintenance of 30% of future liver remnant (FLR) or a remnant liver-to-body-weight ratio >0.5 (e.g., > 350 g of liver per 70 kg patient)	2. Presence (or suspicion) of extrahepatic disease
3. R0 resection possible only with complex procedures (portal vein embolisation, two-stage hepatectomy or hepatectomy combined with ablation).	3. The resectability of extrahepatic disease
	4. Evidence of tumour progression

The first is patients with primary colorectal tumours and synchronous liver metastases. In these patients, consideration should be given to synchronous versus staged resections, although the former is generally reserved for small isolated lesions. Ultimately, the combined morbidity of both procedures needs to be considered. In the case of staged resections, surgery for the primary tumour and liver metastases does not necessarily need to be interrupted with systemic chemotherapy.[33] These decisions need to be taken in consultation with a hepatobiliary MDT.

The second is patients with unresectable colorectal liver metastases in whom systemic chemotherapy renders the disease resectable. This has led to the introduction of the concept of 'conversion chemotherapy' into clinical practice. It is an area where data on long-term outcome from surgery after conversion versus continuation of chemotherapy are required.

Key points

- Advanced and recurrent colorectal cancers should be managed in specialist centres with the required multidisciplinary teams.
- Histological confirmation, biomarker (extended RAS, BRAF) and DNA MMR testing should be undertaken at the outset where possible.
- CT thorax, abdomen and pelvis with oral and intravenous contrast and MRI for pelvic tumours is the minimal recommendation for staging advanced and recurrent colorectal cancers.
- Radiotherapy should be considered for patients with locally advanced and recurrent rectal cancer before surgery.
- Locally advanced and recurrent rectal cancers require surgery beyond the TME plane through exenterative surgery that must be tailored to the patient.
- Sacrectomy should be undertaken in units with the required expertise and access to spinal orthopaedic or neurosurgeons.
- Perineal reconstruction should be planned with a plastic surgeon and the type of flap used tailored to the patient.
- CRS/HIPEC is an established treatment for CRPM and is undertaken in specialist centres in the UK with the required decision-making and operative experience. Whilst high-quality randomised evidence now exists demonstrating the effect of CRS, the optimal HIPEC regime is yet to be determined.
- All units treating advanced and recurrent colorectal cancer should collect, audit and present their long-term outcome data.
- Treatment of liver metastases should be planned with a specialist hepatobiliary MDT and based on both technical and oncological criteria.

🌐 References available at http://ebooks.health.elsevier.com/

▶ RECOMMENDED VIDEOS

- Cytoreductive surgery procedure – https://youtu.be/_WT8grwjzoQ
- Diagnostic laparoscopy for CRPM – https://youtu.be/aEHgQubDKNw

KEY REFERENCES

[18] McCarthy K, Pearson K, Fulton R, et al. Pre-operative chemoradiation for non-metastatic locally advanced rectal cancer. Cochrane Database Syst Rev 2012;12:CD008368. PMID: 23235660.

A meta-analysis of six randomized controlled trials comparing the efficacy of pre-operative chemoradiation to radiotherapy alone before surgery in the treatment of T3–4, node-positive (locally advanced) rectal cancer. While there was no difference in OS, chemoradiotherapy was significantly associated with less local recurrence.

[28] Quénet F, Elias D, Roca L, UNICANCER-GI Group and BIG Renape Group, et al. Cytoreductive surgery plus hyperthermic intraperitoneal chemotherapy versus cytoreductive surgery alone for colorectal peritoneal metastases (PRODIGE 7): a multicentre, randomised, open-label, phase 3 trial. Lancet Oncol 2021;22(2):256–66. PMID: 33476595.

A randomised, open-label, phase 3 trial of 17 cancer centres in France. Patients in whom complete macroscopic resection or surgical resection with less than 1 mm residual tumour tissue was completed were randomly assigned (1:1) to CRS with or without oxaliplatin-based HIPEC. After median follow-up of 63.8 months, median OS was 41.7 months in the CRS/HIPEC group and 41.2 months in the CRS group. Grade 3 or worse adverse events at 30 days were similar in frequency between groups however, at 60 days, grade 3 or worse adverse events were more common in the CRS/HIPEC group.

[32] Nordlinger B, Sorbye H, Glimelius B, et al. Perioperative FOLFOX4 chemotherapy and surgery versus surgery alone for resectable liver metastases from colorectal cancer (EORTC 40983): long-term results of a randomized controlled, phase 3 trial. Lancet Oncol 2013;14:1208–15. PMID: 24120480.

A randomised controlled trial that found no difference in OS with the addition of peri-operative chemotherapy with FOLFOX4 compared with surgery alone for patients with resectable liver metastases from colorectal cancer.

8

Anal neoplasia

Tamzin Cuming

INTRODUCTION

Anal cancer is predominantly (90%) squamous cell in origin, and 90% of anal squamous cell carcinoma (ASCC) is caused by the human papillomavirus (HPV).[1]

This chapter will outline what the surgeon needs to know about HPV infection, anal low- and high-grade intra-epithelial lesions (LSIL and HSIL) – otherwise known as anal intra-epithelial neoplasia (AIN) – as well as ASCC. Non-HPV origin and non-squamous rare anal cancers will be covered in a section towards the end of the chapter.

ANATOMY

The distal anal canal is lined by stratified squamous epithelium, the natural host tissue for HPVs. Stratified squamous epithelium is hair-bearing and keratinising in the perianus, becomes non-hair–bearing at the anoderm of the anal verge, and is non-hair–bearing and non-keratinising in the lower anal canal. The dentate line is the macroscopic marker of the junction of the embryological ectoderm and the embryonic hindgut at about one third along the length of the anal canal. However, the squamous epithelium of the lower anal canal forms a squamocolumnar junction (SCJ) with the upper anal canal more cranially than the dentate line. This zone of transition between two epithelial types is particularly susceptible to HPV-related disease in the anus, as it is in the cervix.[2]

The perianus is defined as 5 cm from the anal verge or margin (the edge of the anal opening visible with the buttocks gently parted) and, since 2018, the 8th edition of the American Joint Committee on Cancer (AJCC)[3] has defined perianal cancers as anal as opposed to skin cancers. Most ASCC arise from the squamous epithelium of the anal margin or anal canal, although a few arise from anal glands or ducts and the extremely rare rectal SCC is thought to arise from squamous metaplasia in the rectum.

The upper anal canal above the SCJ is lined with columnar epithelium, identical to rectal mucosa. The majority of cancers of the upper anal canal are therefore adenomatous in origin and are treated as extensions of low rectal cancer, although a rare anal-origin adenomatous cancer does occur.

HUMAN PAPILLOMAVIRUS

Papillomaviruses are a group of ubiquitous non-enveloped double stranded deoxyribonucleic acid (DNA) viruses of which a subset of around 150 are pathogenic to humans.

Those of interest here are mainly in the α-papillomavirus group with a predilection for the anogenital skin and mucosa.[4] As well as causing benign hyperproliferative lesions and flat pre-malignant change, HPVs are implicated in around 25% of oropharyngeal cancers, cause the majority of penile, vaginal and vulval cancers and cause 90% of cervical and anal invasive squamous cell carcinomas.[1]

HPV of the lower anogenital tract is sexually transmitted. This fact can lead to much distress among patients and needs to be managed carefully by the colorectal surgeon. Eighty-five to 91% of adults have met the HPV virus,[5] unless they were vaccinated against it prior to sexual debut and overall prevalence in US adults is 42%.[6] HPV is passed on orally, by genital touching, by finger or toys as well as penetrative sex; condom use reduces but does not eliminate the risk.[7] The prevalence of anal HPV is highest in men who have sex with men (MSM) living with human immunodeficiency virus (HIV) (90%) and HIV negative (60%),[8] however, anal HPV can also be found in men who have sex with women (MSW) (12%).[9] In women, anal HPV carriage is more common (42%) than cervical (27%)[10] and HPV prevalence in the anus is higher if the woman is living with HIV (68–87%).[11]

RISK FACTORS FOR HUMAN PAPILLOMAVIRUS DISEASE

Multiple partners, smoking and anoreceptive intercourse all increase the likelihood of anal HPV carriage[9,11] but are not necessary for it. In women, anal HPV is most often caused by self-inoculation (wiping after opening bowels) with a sixfold higher anal HPV carriage after front-to-back compared to back-to-front wiping.[12]

Anal pre-cancerous and malignant disease is higher in women with a previous history of genital HPV-related disease, particularly the vulva (Fig. 8.1).[13] Women with disease at multiple anogenital zones are termed to have multizonal intra-epithelial neoplasia, which poses a substantial risk of lower anogenital tract HPV-related SCC.[14]

Given that HPV causes the vast majority of anogenital warts, pre-cancer and squamous cell cancer, it stands to reason that patients susceptible to infection are at greater risk in particular those with innate and acquired immune defects. For persons living with HIV (PLWH), years living with undetectable viral load (VL) versus detectable VL reduces the risk of ASCC by 44% and for every rise of 100 cells/μL CD4 nadir, the anal cancer risk drops by 40%.[15,16]

Other at-risk groups include solid organ transplant recipients especially more than 10 years after transplant,[13] and patients on long-term pharmacological immune suppression for systemic lupus erythematosus, rheumatoid arthritis,

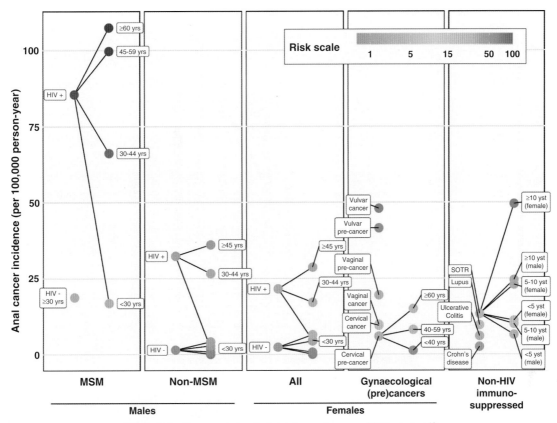

Figure 8.1   Groups at elevated risk for anal cancer. (Clifford et al.[13])

Crohn's and ulcerative colitis.[17] Immune suppression seems to bring the disease forward with an accelerated path to SCC in patients' 40s and 50s.[18] Nonetheless, age in the absence of immune suppression is a sufficient risk factor: the incidence of anal SCC is higher in women than men in the general population with a median age of over 80 years (Fig. 8.2).[19]

VACCINATION

There are increasing numbers vaccinated against HPV with substantial worldwide impact.[20] The UK and other high-income countries began vaccinating girls against the oncogenic HPV types, 16 and 18, in 2008. Additional protection against genital warts, HPV 6, 11, followed with the quadrivalent vaccine. Protection is almost 100% against vaccine types in the HPV-naïve. Already this has led to a reduction in cervical disease[21] and anogenital warts in not only women, but also men.[22] Boys have been vaccinated since 2019 in the UK and 2011 in the United States, and a nonavalent vaccine is available covering types 6, 11, 16, 18, 31, 33, 45, 52, 58.

Vaccine-related reduction in ASCC will happen later than cervical cancer because of the lengthy lead time from infection to disease in the anus (20–40 years). HPV vaccination of the already-exposed person has been trialled in HIV negative MSM aged between 18 and 26 years in a placebo-controlled randomised controlled trial (RCT).[23] Reduction of AIN by vaccine in the intention-to-treat arm was 50% and 77% in the per-protocol treatment group. However, no impact was seen when repeated in older MSM.[24] A modest impact of the vaccine in HPV-DNA negative women up to the age of 45 years has been found.[25] In the UK, HPV vaccination is available on

the National Health Service for MSM up to the age of 45 years as this group has no herd protection from the vaccination of girls.

✔✔ HPV vaccination against high-risk types 16 and 18 is reducing anogenital wart and cervical pre-cancer and cancer incidence.[21,22]

✔✔ HPV vaccination of HIV negative 18–26-year-old gay men results in at least a 50% reduction in anal HSIL.[23]

WARTS (CONDYLOMA ACUMINATA)

HPV types 6 and 11 are the main cause of anogenital warts, the vast majority of which have no malignant potential. Given the prevalence of anal HPV in unvaccinated adults, the majority must not form warts on first contact with HPV. Nonetheless, anogenital warts are common, with an incidence of 160–289/100 000 person years.[26] They tend to occur in the young and usually present to sexual health departments in the UK.

Immune clearance of HPV after infection can be incomplete, with integration of the viral genome into basal cells, which, given no viral reproduction and immune evasion, allows persistent virus to be present for many years, only to display pathological effects later in life.[4] Lesions can also develop soon after infection, producing small, often multiple, discrete outcrops of raised circular lesions, brown or skin colour with

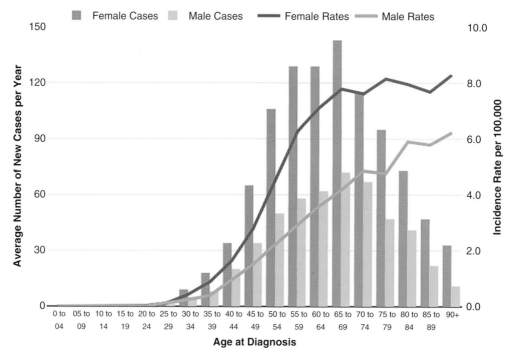

Figure 8.2   Cancer Research UK incidence anal cancer.

a corrugated surface, recognisable as warts, or condyloma acuminata (Fig. 8.3). Initially soft or nodular, both perianal and anal canal warts can grow large and confluent leading to irritation, bleeding and mucus production.

Warts are low risk and benign, although high-risk oncogenic HPV types can be involved in the immunocompromised.[27] The evidence for wart management is lower quality[28] in PLWH but the same range of treatments can be used as in the HIV negative. Warts in themselves are considered a risk factor for anal cancer in PLWH.[29]

MANAGEMENT

Diagnosis is by physical examination, with histological confirmation not necessary unless there is concern of a risk of cancer caused by age, risk factors or unusually intense symptoms. Pain is unusual, although very dense warts can fissure between them, and clinical examination should not discover deep attachment to the submucosa/subcutaneous layers. Simple unenhanced proctoscopy is recommended, particularly for MSM, for anal canal warts (Fig. 8.4). Vulvovaginal or penile examination may be indicated, and women should be sent for a cervical smear if not in the cervical screening programme.

A sexual health screen for other sexually transmitted infections (STIs) and counselling are suggested, with topical therapy and cryotherapy first-line treatments. For warts of the perianus, patient-applied creams are approved for external use and require 3–4 months of application: 5% imiquimod, a topical immune stimulant (toll-like receptor 7) is 35–75% effective,[26,30] and sinecatechins (green tea-derived immunomodulators, multiple pathways) have been shown to be 50–60% effective, albeit PLWH were excluded from trials.[31] Provider-administered therapy includes cryotherapy (success 44–87%),[26] and topical ablation with trichloroacetic acid, success 60–90%.[32] Recurrence rates are substantial for all

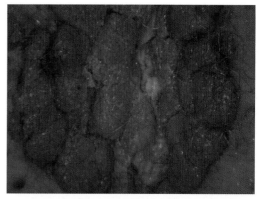

Figure 8.3   Extensive perianal warts.

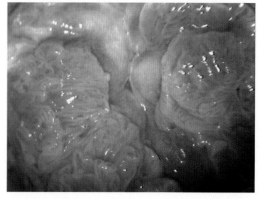

Figure 8.4   Anal canal warts covering squamous epithelium.

treatments (25–60% at a year) and most cause local irritation and burning.

Low-volume anal canal warts do not necessarily require treatment, albeit the patient will be more infectious with active lesions. Options include the aforementioned non-surgical therapies used for the perianus, however, these are not licensed for intra-anal use and are less successful in the anal canal. Cryotherapy is not used inside the anal canal.

Surgeons tend to be referred cases of warts that are recalcitrant to treatment. Surgical excision, electrocautery/hyfrecation and laser have a success rate of 95–100% with recurrence rate of 20%.[26,33] This can be achieved under local anaesthetic (1% or 2% lidocaine with adrenaline, or a posterior pudendal nerve block with 40 mL of 0.25% levobupivacaine), although a general anaesthetic will be required for large volume disease. Electrocautery and laser are less likely to penetrate the deep dermis and cause scarring. FFP3 masks should be used due to the risk of aerosolised particles with laser and electrocautery.[34] Site of excised lesions should be documented, and specimens sent for histology in the immune suppressed or patients over 40 years as warts can contain focal areas of high grade.[27]

Surgical excision should be considered carefully: do not leave any less of the mucosa than you would at a haemorrhoidectomy as life-changing anal stenosis can result, particularly if the patient is also defunctioned. If the multiple lesions have a narrow base, then the base or pedicle can be transected, leaving normal skin/mucosa between wounds, allowing full excision. If the lesions are confluent, there is no harm in staging the procedure over two, three or even four visits to minimise the risk of stenosis.

✔✔ First-line treatment of perianal warts is topical treatments of imiquimod or sinecatechins.[30,31]

✔ Surgical excision or ablation is successful but beware stenosis and stage large procedures.

BUSCHKE–LOWENSTEIN TUMOUR: GIANT ANAL CONDYLOMA

Buschke and Lowenstein described giant condyloma acuminata (GCA) in 1925. It is a highly recurrent locally invasive tumour of low malignant potential associated with low-risk HPV types 6 and 11. GCA is large in diameter (6–12 cm) and also in depth (up to 4 cm), appearing as densely packed firm warts, broad-based with a finely irregular surface (Fig. 8.5). Patients are predominantly male, often smokers. There is some overlap with verrucous SCC.[35] Magnetic resonance imaging (MRI) shows the tumour superficially infiltrating usually with no invasion of underlying muscle and T2 hyperintensitivity.[36]

There is no good evidence for treatment, but 5% imiquimod,[37] photodynamic therapy,[38] acitretin,[39] cidofovir,[40] chemotherapy combined with surgical excision,[41] and chemoradiation (CRT)[42] have all been tried. Patients often fail local ablation or excision, undergo skin grafts and end up with a defunctioning stoma, stenosis and eventual abdominoperineal excision.

ANAL INTRA-EPITHELIAL NEOPLASIA

AIN is an HPV-related, usually flat, dysplastic change in the squamous mucosa and skin of the anal canal and perianus. The Lower Anogenital tract Squamous Terminology

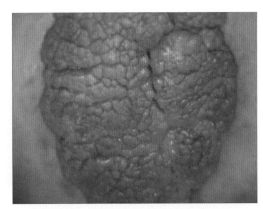

Figure 8.5 Buschke-Lowenstein tumour.

consensus statement in 2012[43] unified the terminology for HPV-related pre-cancerous dysplasia of the lower anogenital tract, reflecting the biological distinction between LSIL, the result of proliferative infection with HPV and not considered pre-cancerous, and HSIL, from oncological transformation of the cell, characterised by the expression of HPV genes E6 and E7.

So, AIN is anal LSIL or HSIL; -IN1 is the histological grade for dysplasia in the lower third of the epithelium. Histology, particularly -IN2 (dysplasia of the lower 2/3) is known to have low Cohen's Kappa values for histopathologists,[44] indicating significant diagnostic variation. The introduction of biomarker p16 with immunohistochemistry has enabled the distinction between LSIL, which is -IN1 and cases of -IN2 where p16 staining is negative, and HSIL, which is -IN2 with block positive p16 staining plus -IN3, full thickness epithelial dysplasia, confidently diagnosed without p16 staining and previously termed *carcinoma-in-situ.*

p16 is a tumour suppressor protein, which facilitates the binding of transcription factor E2F to the retinoblastoma protein (pRB) leading to cell cycle arrest.[45] The E7 protein of an oncogenic HPV binds preferentially to pRB, while the HPV E6 protein deactivates p53 preventing apoptosis. The cell, taken over by oncogenic HPV, is now driven by uninhibited E2F and goes into deregulated proliferation with p16 over-expression.

SYMPTOMS, SIGNS, EXAMINATION

Anal squamous intra-epithelial lesions (SIL) are usually asymptomatic while anal SCC is usually symptomatic. There are cases where extensive anal/perianal HSIL causes itching, soreness and pain, however, these should be carefully assessed and biopsied particularly at spots of ulceration or where the patient has pain to exclude focal SCC (Fig. 8.6). Macroscopically, anal SIL can appear as warts, or flat pink or red lesions, or grey or darker pigmentation in brown or black skin. The pigmented areas tend to be irregular in outline. Closer inspection shows dots visible (abnormal vasculature) and some more advanced lesions are thickened. Vascular patterns of SIL are similar to those seen in the cervix at colposcopy. Some are impossible to detect with the naked eye.

For both perianal and anal canal SIL, the technique of high-resolution anoscopy (HRA) is considered the gold standard worldwide to visualise the SCJ and identify SIL for targeted biopsies.[46] In a technique analogous to colposcopy, 5%

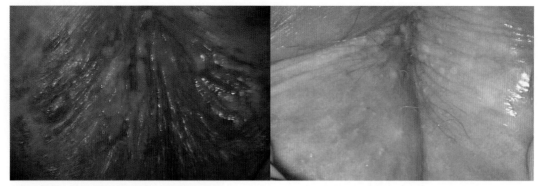

Figure 8.6 Extensive perianal high-grade intra-epithelial lesions (HSIL) field change with focal invasion and appearance after ablation and excision 8 months later.

aqueous acetic acid is used through an ordinary proctoscope with high-resolution real-time high-quality magnification by colposcope up to 30 times. Regions of active HPV mucosal infection turn cloudy white (acetowhite), and SILs are visible with abnormal vessel patterns showing as irregular lines (mosaic change), straight lines (striations) and dots (punctation) (Fig. 8.7). Standards have been set for carrying out the procedure.[47] Anal cytology can be carried out for detection of dysplasia from the anal canal before HRA (Floq swab in liquid-based cytology medium) as can swabs for high-risk HPV, but neither test yet has the sensitivity required for a screening programme for high-risk groups.[48]

Anal canal SIL can be detected and biopsied at endoscopy with a retroflexed view and relaxation of the anorectal junction plus narrow band imaging, with the diagnosis a surprise to most endoscopists.[49]

PREVALENCE

Anal HSIL is highly prevalent in high-risk groups. PLWH, especially MSM, have been the most studied with a prevalence of anal HSIL of 29–33%;[8,50] in women living with HIV prevalence is 27%, and 17% in those with no history of anal intercourse.[11] The odds ratio for renal transplant recipients having anal HSIL, controlled for factors of age, lifetime sexual partners, anal intercourse and smoking was 11.2 for men and 8.3 for women,[51] with an overall prevalence of 27/247 (11%). Of note, 4% of the female and 0.8% of the male non-transplanted controls had anal HSIL with no known risk factors.

PROGRESSION

Progression of anal HSIL to anal cancer is not inevitable and the diagnosis has to be put in context for patients. The risk of SCC varies from 1 in 456 per year for MSM living with HIV and 1:4000 per year for those without HIV[8] to 9.5% at 5 years.[52] There is also regression of anal HSIL, approximately 25% at 6 months.[53] A study from the specialist unit in San Francisco demonstrates photo documentation of anal HSIL lesions left untreated, returning as invasive lesions at the same location in 27 patients.[54]

DNA methylation of host and HPV genes in the anus – as for the cervix – seems to predict the progression of HSIL to cancer, and may enable the identification of at-risk lesions for treatment in the future, strengthening the case both for treatment and for screening.[55,56] In HIV-positive MSM,

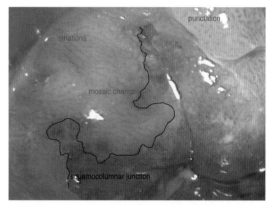

Figure 8.7 High-resolution anoscopy (HRA) image showing high-grade squamous intra-epithelial lesion (HSIL) and squamocolumnar junction (SCJ).

progression from LSIL or no SIL to HSIL was 55/1199 patients over 1–5 years.[57] At present, the evidence is that AIN3 is more likely to progress than AIN2 p16+ve and less likely to regress[53] and the relative risk of cancer for HSIL treated with ablation versus no treatment has been shown to be 0.3.[52]

TREATMENT

Although there has traditionally been an acceptance of non-treatment of anal HSIL due to a lack of evidence both of progression to anal SCC and also that treatment prevents that progression, this is likely to change in the near future. Previous studies have been poor in quality but shown a reduction in progression to cancer in long-term published series.[58,59] An RCT of HIV-positive MSM compared ablation to topical treatments, but numbers were low; both LSIL and HSIL were treated, and outcome included recurrence even in untreated areas. Electrocautery ablation was superior to 5% imiquimod and 5-flurouracil for anal canal treatment but recurrence (termed as such whether at the same site or a different site to that treated) was 67% at 2 years.[60] Excision of anal HSILs larger than 1 cm^2 in size is potentially highly morbid[61] and should be avoided but is a feasible technique for smaller lesions. Imiquimod was trialled in a small UK RCT showing 12/28 resolution or downgrading of HSIL to LSIL compared with one of the 25 placebo patients, a significant effect. A distinction between anal canal and perianal disease was not made but resolution was maintained at 33 months.[62]

Ablative techniques used for anal HSIL include laser,[59,63] electrocautery/hyfrecation,[64] radiofrequency ablation,[65] photodynamic therapy[66] and infrared coagulation (IRC), where an RCT of IRC versus active monitoring showed anal HSIL elimination in 71% at 12 months after one to three treatments compared with 27% in the placebo arm, with no further follow-up.[67]

Recent news prior to this chapter going to press, however, is likely to change this situation significantly. Although there is no peer-reviewed publication at the time of writing, the huge ANal Cancer/Hsil Outcome Research study, (ANCHOR) in the United States, randomising PLWH to HRA-guided treatment or watch (with HRA) and wait, was stopped early after the recruitment of 4446 of the planned 5058 patients due to the effectiveness of treatment in the prevention of anal cancer.[68] This is the first study to have shown that treating anal HSIL prevents anal SCC. Observation alone – at least in high-risk groups such as PLWH – will now become less acceptable.

Indicators affecting the clinical decision to treat include: perceived risk of progression; previous history of invasive SCC in any zone; risk factors including smoking and immune suppression; length of time with anal HSIL; volume/surface area of disease; advanced lesions, for example, thickened, symptomatic, ulcerated.

Flat anal LSIL and LSIL in warts does not have to be treated and patients are only followed up if considered to be in a high-risk group.

OBSERVATION

Surveillance of those at high risk for ASCC can be carried out with regular HRA where available, and where not, anal cytology and digital anorectal examination (DARE) are options.[69] Some take regular 12–24 'mapping biopsies' of the anus for untreated anal HSIL, but this is a morbid procedure that does not prevent cancer. Preferable is regular assessment of patients with anal HSIL paying close attention to symptoms and to a very careful DARE[70] with excision of concerning lesions. In the absence of HSIL treatment, the benefit of following up anal HSIL is to find invasive cancer,[71] most of which is detectable on DARE,[72] at an early stage when treatment is most effective. In the light of the recent ANCHOR study findings,[68] mere observation of anal HSIL without treatment may become less acceptable, and more clinicians will need to train in HRA and HSIL treatment.

✔ Anal and genital human papillomavirus-associated lesions may be identified clinically either by naked eye inspection or with high-resolution anoscopy with the application of acetic acid to the epithelium and targeted biopsy.[46]

✔ Anal high grade squamous intraepithelial lesions (HSIL) have a conversion rate to anal cancer of around 10% at 5 years.[52]

✔ Ablation such as laser, electrocautery and infra-red coagulation can be used in the treatment of anal HSIL[60] and a recent large RCT in the United States has now shown that treatment of anal HSIL prevents anal SCC.[68] Management of AIN will need to change to more interventional in the light of this study's finding.

ANAL CANCER

All anal cancer should be referred to a dedicated anal cancer multi-disciplinary team (MDT), of which the UK has a regional network, combining the expertise of surgeons, radiation oncologists, pathologists and radiologists.[71]

ANAL SQUAMOUS CELL CARCINOMA

ASCC is rare, 1.8/100 000 or 2000 cases/year in the UK;[19] incidence is rising in Western populations, with a 76% increase since the 1990s, notably in women.[19,73] The incidence of anal cancer overtook that of cervical cancer in the United States in white women over 65 years in 2016, although the cervical cancer incidence remained high in Black and Hispanic populations.[74]

There is wide geographical variation in the incidence of anal cancers around the world. Areas with a high incidence of anal cancer usually also have a high incidence of cervical, vulval and penile tumours, as well as other indicators of HPV presence such as anogenital warts. Increasingly, geographical variation will reflect adequacy of HPV vaccination coverage.

Aetiological factors follow those of HPV-related disease in 90%. Of HPV-positive cancers, 96% are caused by the types included in the nonavalent HPV vaccine (16,18, 33, 45, 56, 58, 6, 11) with HPV 16 being the most oncogenic (86%).[75] PLWH and other immunosuppressed groups are at higher risk of ASCC (see earlier),[8] although the rise of ASCC in older women in the last 30 years may be caused by societal changes in sexual behaviour.[74] ASCC incidence is 60% (women) and 89% (men) higher in the most socially-deprived quintile in the UK than in the least.[19]

It is accepted that ASCC develops most commonly within a field of anal HSIL,[54] and anal HSIL is found in ASCC specimens, and it is expected that the ANCHOR study will add further strong evidence that anal HSIL is a pre-requisite for anal HPV-related SCC when published. Superficially invasive SCC, particularly a SISCCA (defined as a fully-excised with 1-mm margin, maximum 7-mm diameter, maximum 3-mm depth of invasion SCC)[43] is increasingly described (Fig. 8.8).

✔ The incidence of anal cancer is increasing in both males and females with a greater increase in females.[73]

✔ The immunosuppressed, particularly HIV-positive MSM are at higher risk of anal cancer than the general population[8] but ASCC remains more common in women than men.[74]

HISTOLOGICAL TYPES

ASCC is an epidermoid tumour. Older terms such as *basaloid* or *cloacogenic carcinomas* refer to HPV-driven aggressive subsets of anal canal SCC near the ducts, (not to be confused with basal cell carcinomas of the perianal skin),[76] however, such terms were removed from the 4th World Health Organisation classification of anal cancers.[77] Perianal SCCs tend to be well-differentiated and keratinising, whereas those arising in the canal are more commonly poorly differentiated and generally have a worse prognosis. There are a small number of ASCC that while squamous, are non-HPV related (10–12%).[78] As

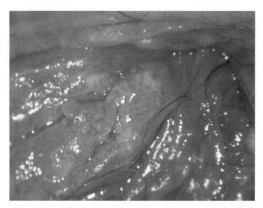

Figure 8.8 Superficially invasive squamous cell carcinoma (SISCCA) of the perianus on a background of perianal high-grade intra-epithelial lesions (HSIL); successfully treated with excision only.

in the oropharynx, these seem to have a worse response to treatment and poorer prognosis. If these are also negative for p16 over-expression, the prognosis is even worse,[79] with HPV DNA positivity and p16 expression now being considered to predict for locoregional control.[80]

Verrucous carcinoma (VC) is a separate, slow-growing form of SCC, macroscopically similar to Buschke-Lowenstein tumour but often smaller, either HPV-negative or having non-6 and 11 HPV types, is negative for p16 on immuno-histochemistry, and histologically characterised by a push-ing border. VC has a low propensity for distant spread but is extremely destructive locally if neglected.[35,81] It is often difficult to diagnose as it lacks the usual cytological features of malignancy.

PROGNOSIS AND SPREAD

The current 8th edition of AJCC staging is the most wide-ly used[3] and follows the TNM classification, which maps to prognosis[82].

Lymph node spread depends on location. Upper anal canal tumours tend to spread to mesorectal/internal iliac lymph nodes, and lower/perianal tumours to inguinal/exter-nal iliac lymph nodes. Prognosis is worse if the external iliac nodes are involved, especially in combination with other sites of lymph node spread.[82] Fifteen to 30% of patients will pres-ent with inguinal lymph node involvement.[83]

ACT 1[84] and RTOG-98-11[85] trials showed that male sex and positive lymph nodes predict for worse overall survival, but since then stage migration has reduced the prognostic im-pact of positive lymph nodes.[83] Overall lymph node negative survival is 72–80% in contrast to 49–65% with positive lymph nodes.

Haematogenous spread tends to occur late and is usually associated with advanced local disease or poorly differentiat-ed or non-HPV histology with lymphovascular invasion. The principal sites of metastases are the liver, lung, para-aortic nodes and bones. However, metastases have been described in the kidneys, adrenals and brain.

CLINICAL PRESENTATION

Unfortunately, the majority of symptomatically presenting ASCC are large tumours, often misdiagnosed in primary care, and even by surgeons, as haemorrhoids. In a cohort of 8640 PLWH, 38% of the 60 ASCC diagnosed were larger than 5 cm

(T3),[86] while 52/171 (31%) US cancers were ≥T2 stage.[52] In ACT 1, of 585 patients only 13% anal canal and 10% perianal SCC presented with T1 disease (≤2 cm).

The predominant symptoms of anal cancer are pain, bleed-ing or the presence of a mass. Pruritus and discharge occur in early disease, but pain can be present in even small invasive lesions. Beware the older patient presenting with anal fissure: an examination under anaesthetic (EUA) is preferable to topical fissure treatment with a delayed repeat clinic visit. Ad-vanced tumours, often presenting in the very elderly, may in-volve the sphincter mechanism, causing faecal incontinence. Invasion of the posterior vaginal wall can occur and present as a fistula.

Cancer of the perianus can present as a malignant ulcer, with a raised, everted, indurated edge but also as an unusual firm or erythematous tag (Fig. 8.9). Lesions within the canal may not be visible but almost all will be palpable, with the smallest feeling like a grain of rice and larger, a button. Exten-sive lesions spread from the canal to the anal verge, with ul-ceration and induration (Fig. 8.10), and DARE is often pain-ful. Large anal canal tumours involve the lower rectum and can be diagnosed at colonoscopy, otherwise EUA is standard. Small lesions can be biopsied under local in the clinic (under HRA guidance if available) or excised at EUA with a knife – not diathermy, or margins cannot be assessed – aiming for 3-mm clinical margin.

All ASCC patients are routinely tested for HIV and female patients should have consideration of other lower anogen-ital tract zone assessment and be up to date with cervical screening.

✔ Routine clinical examination of inguinal lymph nodes is expected, however, palpable lymph nodes may represent in-flammation not malignant spread.

STAGING INVESTIGATIONS

All patients should be staged with MRI of the pelvis and computed tomography (CT) of the chest, abdomen and pelvis for locoregional and metastatic staging respective-ly.[71] 18 F-FDG positron emission tomography (PET)/CT is commonly used for staging, with sensitivity of 93% for lymph node metastasis and 76% specificity;[87] although not mandated in guidelines, many feel PET/CT adds to plan-ning of radiotherapy.[88]

Enlarged inguinal lymph nodes can be characterised by clinical and radiological features as to whether they may be reactive or metastatic. In cases where PET/CT shows avid uptake, they are assumed to be positive. The inguinal region is routinely treated with prophylactic radiation so only before radical lymph node dissection after recurrence in the groins is an ultrasound-guided fine-needle aspira-tion mandated, although this can also be requested in sit-uations of diagnostic uncertainty. Serum tumour markers are unhelpful.

TREATMENT

The standard of care for invasive ASCC is CRT. This was first used in 1974 by Nigro and replaced the first-line treatment of ASCC with abdominoperineal excision of the rectum and anus (APER) with improved mortality and a chance of avoid-ing a permanent colostomy.[89]

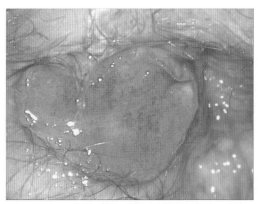

Figure 8.9 Stage 2A perianal cancer; patient was successfully treated with chemoradiation.

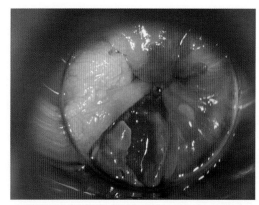

Figure 8.10 Stage 3A anal canal cancer in a human immunodeficiency virus (HIV)–positive patient; patient successfully treated with chemoradiation.

Some small T1 ASCC, particularly fully excised (1 mm) lesions of the perianus, are managed without CRT,[71,90] but CRT is otherwise the gold standard management for invasive disease.

✓✓ The current standard of care for ASCC is chemoradiotherapy with 50.4Gy radiotherapy in 28 daily fractions with mitomycin C and 5 fluorouracil (5FU) in all cases except where there are contraindications to radiotherapy.[91–93]

Chemoradiation or combined modality therapy

Radiation-alone compared with chemoradiation. Two trials in the 1990s randomised to CRT or RT alone, and showed improved local control and safety with CRT: EORTC[94] and ACT 1.[92] In EORTC, those in the mitomycin/5FU arm had an 18% higher locoregional control and 32% improved colostomy-free survival compared to RT alone. ACT 1 randomised 585 patients and confirmed that the standard therapy should be 50.4Gy of radiation with mitomycin-C and 5FU with a relative risk of 0.54 for locoregional control in the CRT arm, although no change in overall survival at 3 years. A follow-up study at 13 years showed that the benefit of CRT was maintained over RT alone, with local recurrence reduced by 25% (relative risk 0.46), and a significant improval in anal cancer deaths of 12% (hazard ratio [HR] 0.67) with a non-significant trend in overall survival (HR 0.86). This was despite a short-term increase in mortality in the chemotherapy arm.[95]

For small, good prognosis perianal tumours, a reduced dose of radiotherapy can be given with selective omission of chemotherapy and the inguinal prophylactic radiation dose.[71,96]

Chemotherapy

Capecitebine is a suitable alternative to 5FU, but mitomycin is required for the benefits of CRT.

The ACT II study randomised 940 patients to cisplatin/5FU or mitomycin/5FU and found equal 3 year progression-free survival 73–74%, with three deaths from CRT in the two arms and 90% complete response with no break in radiotherapy regime.[93] The RTOG 98-11 found a survival benefit for mitomycin over cisplatin.[97] Because of the high quality with which ACT II was conducted and its acceptable results, it has been the blueprint for CRT for

ASCC ever since. The 50.4Gy are given in 28 fractions with no break. Mitomycin is given on day 1 with 5FU infusions given days 1–4 and 29–32.

Cetuximab, an epidermal growth factor receptor inhibitor has been trialled in ASCC but has proven to have additional toxicity without a survival advantage.[98]

For those with reduced performance status, reduced dosage and reduction or change in chemotherapy agent can be used but with a reduction in effectiveness.[71]

Inguinal metastases

Irradiation of the groins may overtreat some patients, but at present, prophylactic radiotherapy to clinically uninvolved inguinal nodes is currently advised for all T2–4 tumours of the anal canal and margin due to the 30% risk of inguinal recurrence without it.[71] Sentinel node biopsy is used in vulval SCC but ASCC results are inconsistent.[99,100]

Complications

Complications of CRT for anal carcinoma include diarrhoea, mucositis, myelosuppression, skin erythema and desquamation. Late complications include anal stenosis and fistula formation.

Defunctioning before treatment is carried out for large symptomatic tumours and is suggested for anterior tumours in women as there is a high incidence of rectovaginal fistula formation in this group during radiotherapy treatment; only 50% of these stomas will ever be closed.[101]

Infertility is likely after CRT for ASCC and appropriate counselling should be given to relevant patients: sperm, oocyte, egg or ovarian tissue banking should be offered. Counselling should be offered regarding changes in sexual function particularly for women, and steps taken to address treatment-induced early menopause. Vaginal dilators should be given routinely for women undergoing CRT, with nurse-led advice on their prophylactic use.

Human immunodeficiency virus

PLWH with anal SCC are best treated with CRT, albeit with slightly worse outcomes (overall survival, OR 1.76), and increased toxicity.[102,103] There is some evidence that prognosis maps to prolonged lymphopenia in PLWH[104] but also in those without HIV.[105]

Improvements in radiotherapy

The one size-fits-all radiation dose in the ACT II protocol has recently been questioned, as possibly overtreating the early small lesions and under-treating large or T4 lesions. A series of UK trials grouped under the PersonaLising Anal cancer radioTherapy dOse (PLATO) are underway, named ACT 3, 4 and 5. Further improvements since ACT II have been made with intensity-modulated radiation therapy, which has allowed more accurate targeting of the tumour and a reduction of the dose to surrounding structures[106] and is now the usual mode of radiation delivery.

Excision alone of small perianal squamous cell carcinoma

Local resection is not recommended for ASCC of the anal canal because of the risk of incontinence and poorer prognosis. However, for a perianal or anal canal fully excised T1 or SISCCA in a haemorrhoid specimen, adjuvant CRT can be avoided if staging is negative. Close follow-up should be by radiological and clinical means, ideally with HRA, in view of the 74% rate of HSIL after excision only compared with 13% after CRT.[90] Metastasis and local recurrence are described after T1 cancer excision.[107,108] Positive <1-mm margins should result in adjuvant CRT.

✔ Small perianal T1 (<2 cm) completely excised (1-mm margin) lesions may be treated by local excision alone, obviating the need for CRT.[71]

Failure of primary chemoradiation

Ten percent of those undergoing CRT for invasive ASCC will have persistent disease by clinical examination on MRI and PET/CT restaging. If no progression is detected, it is advised to delay the diagnosis of persistence, as complete response is possible up to 26 weeks after CRT.[109] Histological proof of residual or recurrent disease is essential before radical surgery is recommended.

Early local recurrence can be managed with local excision, ideally in an HRA and HSIL treatment setting,[90] but the standard of care is salvage APER. Patient selection for salvage APER should be discussed at an anal cancer MDT and APER only used for curative-intent surgery. If margins are threatened, exenteration should be considered in appropriate patients.

APER is similar to that used for low-rectal cancer, but with wide excision of the perianal skin in combination with a meticulous total mesorectal excision of the rectum to achieve wide en bloc radical resection with negative surgical margins. Multi-disciplinary reconstruction is then used, with myocutaneous flaps recommended to avoid long-term perineal wound complications.[110,111]

Modern CRT has reduced salvage APER to only 8%, with improvement in R0 resection rates because of better patient selection and potentially 65-80% long term survival.[112]

Therapeutic groin dissection can be carried out at the same time for proven inguinal recurrence with a 50% long-term survival.[111]

✔ Persistent ASCC after CRT is diagnosed at 6 months,[109] and in the fit patient with no metastases is treated with salvage APER, with >60% survival for R0 resections.[112]

Palliative management

Management of recurrent disease in patients unsuitable for salvage surgery may involve a defunctioning stoma. Further local radiotherapy is usually avoided but has been described[113] and can be used for non-pelvic isolated lesions. The mainstay is palliative chemotherapy (carboplatin and paclitaxel). Second-line therapy is now immunotherapy with anti PD-1 antibodies nivolumab (24% response rate)[114] and pembrolizumab (response 17% with 42% stable).[115] Anal tumours are rarely mismatch repair deficient, and instead show high PD-L1 expression.

FOLLOW-UP

Clinical follow-up is recommended every 3–6 months for the first 2 years with median recurrence occurring at 11 months (range 3–92).[116] HRA is used if available to supplement DARE and unenhanced proctoscopy.

Radiological follow–up is variable: NCCN 2018 guidelines recommend annual CT and MRI for 3 years for T3/T4 or node positive disease only;[117] current UK guidelines suggest MRI for 1 year in high-risk cases, and CT for 1–2 years[71] with clinical assessment, although ACT 3 is 3-monthly clinical assessment and MRI at 1 and 3 years.[118,119]

SURVIVORSHIP

Whilst the prospect of clinical cure has been the focus of outcome reporting for patients treated by chemoradiotherapy, it is now evident that patients suffer a significant number of long-term consequences of CRT. In a follow-up study of 84 patients who underwent CRT for ASCC patients reported faecal (40%) and urinary (43%) incontinence and only 24% were satisfied with their sexual function.[120] Incontinence is often urge related and, if there is some sphincter integrity, can improve with functional management and over the first 2 years after CRT. The anatomic location of the peak radiation dose appears to influence post-CRT symptoms on the LARS scale.[121] A Delphi process undertaken with patients has produced a core outcome set for future studies in this field.[122] Fatigue and insomnia can continue for many years post-CRT and influence a reduction in quality of life for survivors.[123]

✔ Studies of outcomes after CRT for anal cancer should now follow the CORMAC dataset formed by Delphi process with patient involvement.[122]

RARER TUMOURS

Ten to 15% of anal cancers are not SCCs, 7% are adenocarcinomas arising from the glandular mucosa of the anal canal above the SCJ, or from the anal glands and ducts at the dentate line. A very rare and particularly aggressive tumour is anal melanoma. Neuroendocrine tumours of the anus make up less than 1% of anal cancers. Lymphomas and sarcomas of the anus are also described. Paget's disease and adenocarcinomas of the skin adnexae can affect the perianal skin. Basal cell carcinomas are extremely rare in the perianus. Management is by primary histological type.

ADENOCARCINOMA

True adenocarcinoma of the anal canal arises from the anal glands around the dentate line, which pass radially outwards into the sphincter muscles. This tumour appears to have a poorer prognosis than either low rectal adenocarcinoma or ASCC, with a median survival of 33 months (in contrast to 118 months for ASCC).[124] Due to its location, it often drains to the inguinal lymph nodes, spreads submucosally and should be treated aggressively with a combination of chemotherapy and radical surgery.[125] The impact of radiotherapy is uncertain.

PAGET'S DISEASE

Extra-mammary Paget's disease can present in the perianal region and be mistaken for dermatitis or anal HSIL. Biopsy provides the diagnosis, and the patient is then staged using radiology for metastasis and a search for a distant (e.g., breast, colon) or local (e.g., apocrine glands) primary site. Treatment is variable, from topical creams to excision and reconstruction, and prognosis appears to be worse with advanced age and whether the primary lesion is local or distant.[126]

MALIGNANT MELANOMA

Melanoma makes up 1% of anal malignant tumours, with incidence 0.34 per million in the United States; the anus is the site of 50% of gastrointestinal melanomas.[127] More common in women, the median age is 73 years and over 30% present with distant metastases.[128] The lesion may mimic a thrombosed external haemorrhoid because of its colour, although amelanotic tumours also occur. Historically, the prognosis was dismal, with median survival of around 18 months and 20% 5-year survival with combined surgical excision and radiotherapy.[129] Immunotherapy with tyrosine kinase inhibitors can improve survival and disease control in metastatic mucosal melanoma, however *KIT* oncogene mutations are less common in mucosal melanoma.[130]

FUTURE DIRECTIONS

Further details on the ANCHOR study in the United States after it was stopped early because of the effectiveness of treatment in the prevention of anal cancer are expected with publication over the next few years of papers from the study.[131]

Meanwhile in the UK, the PLATO series of trials is continuing in the tradition of the ACT 1 and 2 studies with ACT 3-5, aiming to personalise the radiation dose according to stage. ACT 3 is non-randomised, for small T1 N0 ASCC: if fully excised with a mm clear margin, for watchful waiting (without HRA), and CRT for less than 1 mm/positive margins; ACT 4, now closed to recruitment, was for invasive smaller ASCC – a lower dose of RT to reduce morbidity in good prognosis lesions; and ACT 5 is for dose escalation in the larger lesions.[118,119]

Screening for anal cancer precursors is advocated in for high-risk groups but no national guidelines exist;[132] Screening

for the Prevention of Anal Cancer (SEPAC) study is underway in the UK and blood-based biomarkers may detect HPV-related cancers in the near future.[133]

> ### Key points
>
> - The incidence of anal cancer is increasing although it remains rare except in certain high-risk groups.
> - HPV is the major aetiological factor in anal squamous cell carcinomas. Women with previous gynaecological HSIL or cancer particularly of the vulva are at risk of anal HSIL (AIN) and ASCC, as are MSM living with HIV and transplant recipients. Most ASCC arise on a background of HSIL.
> - Treatment of anal HSIL has recently been shown to prevent anal cancer in HIV positive individuals.
> - Chemoradiation is the treatment of first choice for most ASCC except for the most superficially invasive perianal lesions (≤T1N0).
> - Surgical excision with a 1-mm margin may be used for small perianal lesions with good prognosis but close follow-up is necessary due to background HSIL.
> - Melanoma, neuroendocrine tumour and adenocarcinoma of the anus are very rare and have a dismal prognosis.

 References available at http://ebooks.health.elsevier.com/

ACKNOWLEDGEMENT

With thanks to the authors of the sixth edition, Pasquale Giordano, David J. Humes and John H. Scholefield.

KEY REFERENCES

[21] Palmer T, Wallace L, Pollock KG, et al. Prevalence of cervical disease at age 20 after immunisation with bivalent HPV vaccine at age 12-13 in Scotland: retrospective population study. BMJ 2019;365:l1161. https://doi.org/10.1136/bmj.l1161. PMID: 30944092; PMCID: PMC6446188.
  Retrospective population study of 138 692 women showing 89% reduction in CIN3 or worse after introduction of bivalent HPV vaccine in Scotland.

[22] Ali H, Guy RJ, Wand H, et al. Decline in in-patient treatments of genital warts among young Australians following the national HPV vaccination program. BMC Infect Dis 2013;13:140. https://doi.org/10.1186/1471-2334-13-140. PMID: 23506489; PMCID: PMC3606327.
  Study of all in-patient care episodes in Australia showed a decrease of 85.3% in treatment numbers for vulval/vaginal warts associated with introduction of HPV vaccine.

[23] Palefsky JM, Giuliano AR, Goldstone S, et al. HPV vaccine against anal HPV infection and anal intraepithelial neoplasia. N Engl J Med 2011;365:1576–85.
  RCT of HPV vaccine in MSM showing 50% efficacy in intention to treat population and 77.5% in per-protocol population in preventing AIN/anal cancer.

[30] Grillo-Ardila CF, Angel-Muller E, Salazar-Diaz LC, Gaitan HG, Ruiz-Parra AI, Lethaby A. Imiquimod for anogenital warts in non-immunocompromised adults. Cochrane Database Syst Rev; 2014: CD010389.

[31] Stockfleth E, Beti H, Orasan R, et al. Topical Polyphenon E in the treatment of external genital and perianal warts: a randomized controlled trial. Br J Dermatol 2008;158(6):1329–38. https://doi.org/10.1111/j.1365-2133.2008.08520.x. Epub 2008 Mar 20. PMID: 18363746.
  RCT of polyphenon E showing about 50% response with active therapy compared with 37% with placebo, with low recurrence rate and good safety profile.

[91] Glynne-Jones R, Nilsson PJ, Aschele C, et al. Anal cancer: ESMO-ESSO-ESTRO Clinical Practice Guidelines for diagnosis, treatment and follow-up. Ann Oncol 2014;25(Suppl. 3):iii10–20. https://doi.org/10.1093/annonc/mdu159. Epub 2014 Jul 6. PMID: 25001200.
International evidence-based guidelines.

[92] UK Co-ordinating Committee on Cancer Research. Epidermoid anal cancer: results from the UKCCCR randomised trial of radiotherapy alone versus radiotherapy, 5-fluorouracil, and mitomycin. UKCCCR Anal Cancer Trial Working Party. Lancet 1996;348(9034):1049–54. PMID: 8874455.
RCT of radiotherapy versus chemoradiotherapy (CMT) showing a 46% reduction in the risk of local failure in the patients receiving CMT (relative risk 0.54, 95% CI, 0.42–0.69, p <0.0001). The risk of death from anal cancer was also reduced in the CMT arm (0.71, 0.53–0.95, P = 0.02).

[93] James RD, Glynne-Jones R, Meadows HM, et al. Mitomycin or cisplatin chemoradiation with or without maintenance chemotherapy for treatment of squamous-cell carcinoma of the anus (ACT II): a randomised, phase 3, open-label, 2 × 2 factorial trial. Lancet Oncol 2013;14(6):516–24. https://doi.org/10.1016/S1470-2045(13)70086-X. Epub 2013 Apr 9. PMID: 23578724.
RCT showed no advantage for cisplatin over mitomycin in chemoradiotherapy, and no improvement in outcome with maintenance chemotherapy.

Diverticular disease

9

Des Winter

HISTORICAL PERSPECTIVES

Colonic diverticulosis is a common anatomical disorder characterised by acquired, sac-like mucosal protrusions (diverticula) through the muscle wall.[1] They are false diverticula because they do not involve all colonic layers. The term '*diverticulum*' ('divertikel' in German) was originally used to describe what was an anatomical curiosity in the early 1800s and was not in widespread use until the recognition of 'perisigmoiditis' and related colovesical fistulae by the latter half of the 19th century.[2] It was Lord Berkeley Moynihan (1865–1936 Leeds) who propagated the term '*diverticulitis*' at the turn of the 20th century[3] while more latterly, diverticulosis was proposed as an umbrella term for asymptomatic individuals as well as symptomatic patients.[4] For decades much of what was written was based on erroneous assumption; a lack of evidence created a knowledge vacuum that was filled with the dogma of the era. We were left with variable terminology and a multiplicity of management protocols.

TERMINOLOGY

According to the European Society of Coloproctology (ESCP) guidelines,[5] the following terminology is used to define the various clinical scenarios with which colonic diverticula may be associated (Box 9.1).

ANATOMICAL AND PHYSIOLOGICAL PERSPECTIVES

Colonic diverticulosis and related disorders are traditionally thought to be a western world, industrialised country, mature age-group phenomenon with clearly defined origins in meat-rich, fibre-poor diets. Some of the earliest descriptions date only to the early 20th century[6] and the scientific basis for our current understanding is still limited. Parks described his findings on diverticulosis based on 300 cadaveric dissections in 1968.[1] He noted that diverticula tended to form rows in the lateral inter-taenial (rather than antimesenteric) areas that they were mainly in the sigmoid but could be anywhere in the colon, and that frequently, a blood vessel pierced the wall at the neck of the diverticulum. Much of what was determined about the incidence of diverticulosis was from this and other mid-20th century post-mortem studies.[7–9] Population-based studies confirm diverticula are rare before 30 years, more common after 40 years, found in one third after 60 years and over 50% of those older than 70 years of age. The age-related phenomenon gives clues to the aetiology and points to general ageing processes including declining collagen strength or repair.

INCIDENCE AND GEOGRAPHICAL DIFFERENCES

RACE AND GEOGRAPHY

Geographic disparities in the incidence of diverticulosis imply that it is predominantly in industrialised societies associated with an ageing population and western diet. Moreover, the incidence has increased in North America by up to 50% in the past two decades, and more so in younger people.[10-12] In contrast, diverticulosis is uncommon in Asia and Africa compared to Europe and the USA with a reported prevalence as low as 0.5–1.7% in China and Korea.[13,14] Industrialisation or immigration to western countries results in a higher prevalence.[15,16] This has been best described in Japanese immigrants to Hawaii where necropsy studies demonstrate a dramatic increase in diverticulosis compared to age-matched mainland Japanese controls (52% vs. 0.5–1%).[16] Similar increases are apparent among the urban, industrialised, black population in South Africa compared with their rural counterparts.[17]

However, the increasing incidence is not solely due to adoption of a western lifestyle and genetic factors may play a role. There are distinct differences in prevalence within ethnic groups living in the same region. For example, studies of ethnic groups living in Israel demonstrate differences in Ashkenazi Jews (16.2%), Sephardic Jews (3.8%) and Arabs (0.7%).[18,19] Aside from variances in prevalence between different ethnicities, anatomical variations also exist with a reported frequency of right-sided diverticulosis of 20% in patients <40 years increasing to 40% in patients >60 years old in Asian populations.[20,21] Furthermore, while the incidence of diverticular disease increases as these countries become more westernised, the anatomical location (right colon) remains the same.[22,23]

AGE AND GENDER

Recent studies point towards age- and gender-related differences in patients presenting with diverticulitis. Males are more likely to develop diverticulitis at a younger age whereas there is a female predominance in older patients.[24,25] In western populations, approximately one fifth of patients with diverticulitis are under the age of 50 years (reported incidence 18–34%).[26–28] There was a trend towards a more

Box 9.1 Terminologies used to define the various clinical scenarios with which colonic diverticula may be associated

Diverticulosis – the presence of colonic diverticula.
Diverticular disease – clinically significant and symptomatic diverticulosis and may be caused by:
- Diverticulitis or
- Other less well-described manifestations (e.g., visceral hypersensitivity without evidence of inflammation).

Symptomatic uncomplicated diverticular disease (SUDD) – persistent abdominal symptoms attributed to diverticula without diverticulitis or bleeding.
Diverticulitis – acute or chronic symptoms in the presence of inflamed diverticula.
- Uncomplicated – Computed tomography (CT) shows only colonic wall thickening with fat stranding.
- Complicated – CT shows abscess, peritonitis, obstruction, fistula or haemorrhage.

Diverticular bleeding – haemorrhage from diverticula (right- or left-sided)
Segmental colitis associated with diverticulosis (SCAD) – inflammation resembling inflammatory bowel disease isolated to areas marked by diverticulosis.

aggressive surgical approach in younger patients based on the hypothesis that the disease was more virulent in this subgroup.[29,30] Younger age may be a risk factor for recurrent disease rather than an indication for early intervention in the acute setting, as these patients are just as likely to settle with conservative management.[31,32]

DIET

Painter and Burkitt[2] described diverticular disease as a deficiency of dietary fibre proposing that consumption of a refined western diet led to longer colonic transit times, decreased stool volume and increased intra-luminal pressures.[32] Although a role for dietary fibre in the pathogenesis of diverticular disease is plausible, there is little evidence to support this hypothesis. Conclusions are drawn from several randomised controlled trials with small patient numbers producing conflicting results[33,34] and do not demonstrate an improvement in symptoms or diverticulitis recurrence overall. Residue refers to any indigestible food substance that remains in the intestinal tract and contributes to stool bulk.[35] Historically, low residue diets were recommended because indigestible remnants were thought to clog in diverticula leading to diverticulitis or perforation.[36] These concerns were dismissed by conclusive evidence from the healthcare professionals follow-up study.[37]

✔ Low fibre diet has an epidemiological association with the development of diverticular disease. However, recommending fibre as a treatment for diverticulosis is largely based on outdated, poorly controlled studies.

✔ Young patients (<50 y) may be more likely to suffer from recurrent diverticulitis. There is no evidence to support aggressive surgical intervention in cases of uncomplicated diverticular disease.[31,32]

AETIOLOGY AND PATHOGENESIS

There are several theories as to the pathogenesis of diverticular disease. Aside from luminal trauma, potential aetiological factors include elevated colonic pressures, compromised colon wall integrity, and altered bacterial flora.[38–43] Colonic wall abnormalities (specifically mural thickening, increased collagen cross-linking,[44] muscle atrophy[45] and shortening of taeniae coli[9]) are thought to produce a 'stiffer' less compliant colon predisposing to diverticular herniation. In addition, abnormalities in cholinergic smooth muscle excitation and neurohumoral signalling (serotonin, nitric oxide, VIP) may contribute to disordered contractions and increased intra-luminal pressures.[46–49]

LIFESTYLE

Both the health professionals follow-up study (47 228 men) and the Swedish mammography cohort study demonstrate a positive correlation between obesity and diverticular-associated complications.[50,51] According to the American taskforce, obesity is a defined risk factor for diverticular disease.[52] This may be caused by obesity-associated, metabolically active visceral fat.[53]

SMOKING

There is evidence for an association between smoking and diverticular disease. Pathological examination suggests a higher incidence of strictures and perforation in smokers compared to non-smokers.[54] There may be a gender difference, with a higher likelihood of abscess or perforation in female smokers compared to males.[55]

NON-STEROIDAL ANTI-INFLAMMATORY DRUGS

It is hypothesised that non-steroidal anti-inflammatory drugs (NSAIDs) may cause colonic injury via direct topical injury and/or impaired prostaglandin synthesis compromising mucosal integrity, increasing permeability and enabling the influx of bacteria and other toxins.[43] Data from the health professional follow-up study showed an increased incidence of uncomplicated diverticular disease in patients who used NSAIDs compared with their asymptomatic counterparts.[55] In addition, NSAIDs are associated with diverticular complications including bleeding and perforation.[56,57]

DIVERTICULITIS

It was misquoted for many years that about 25% of patients with diverticulosis will develop an acute inflammatory condition characterised by left iliac fossa or suprapubic pain, malaise and fever (diverticulitis), a figure that was rarely challenged although the basis for it is unclear. The origin of this overestimate may have been the misquoting of the proportion represented following an episode of diverticular symptoms,[1] rather than the actual prevalence of diverticulitis. A more modern (1986–2004) population-based study found 1.7% of male healthcare professionals aged between 40–75 years developed diverticulitis giving a crude annual incidence of 1/1000 (801 events in 47 228 persons over 18 years).[37] This figure has been confirmed as an accurate representation of the USA population in whom there was an age-adjusted hospitalisation rate of 75/100 000 in 2005[58] or 1–2/1000 at the present time at the projected trajectory.[59] The population trends reflect a worldwide finding of male predominance aged under 45years but female predominance in those older, as well as an increasing incidence in the under 45 years age group. Fascinatingly, there was a large difference in the rates of diverticulitis admissions between the west (50.4/100 000) versus the other sectors of USA (>70/100 000). The west of USA also has a higher fibre intake and relatively lower colorectal cancer incidence than the rest of the country.[60] While this supports the historical assumption that high dietary fibre protects against the development of both disorders, the association is speculative until co-factors (hereditary, ethnic, socioeconomic, dietary, smoking, alcohol, etc.) are excluded.

CLASSIFICATION

It is now widely accepted that diverticulitis encompasses a wide spectrum of pathologies ranging from acute uncomplicated diverticulitis to perforation with peritonitis. Although the underlying pathophysiology may be similar in all cases, the clinical manifestation of the disease differs greatly between individuals. It is helpful to further classify patients according to those who have 'mild diverticulitis' and those with 'severe diverticulitis'.[61] The adult prevalence of perforated diverticulitis is approximately 3.5 per 100 000 and the incidence has more than doubled in recent times.[62–65] Reasons why this may be are speculative, including NSAIDs, opioids, corticosteroids and smoking (Table 9.1 and 9.2).[54,56,66]

SEGMENTAL COLITIS ASSOCIATED DIVERTICULOSIS

Segmental colitis associated with diverticulosis (SCAD) is found in less than 1% of colonoscopy procedures.[67,68] The majority of these patients have simply bleeding per rectum rather than any significant change in bowel habit or constitutional symptoms. Many resolve without therapy such that medical treatment should be reserved for those with troublesome symptoms.[69,70]

DIAGNOSIS AND IMAGING

The diagnosis of diverticulitis is largely based on clinical impression.[71] Confirmatory imaging is helpful in determining the extent, degree and local consequences of the inflammatory process as well as excluding other disorders.[72,73] Ultrasound is adequate, with reasonable sensitivity and specificity using graded compression and other tricks of waveform distortion that may not be readily available in every emergency room environment.[74,75] Although a relatively inexpensive, easily reproducible and safe modality, sonographic imaging displays reduced acoustic acuity in gas distended or obese patients. Historically, a water soluble (rather than barium-based) contrast enema with fluoroscopic images was used to confirm diverticulitis but

Table 9.1   CT classification of acute diverticulitis

Moderate diverticulitis	Severe diverticulitis
Localised sigmoid colon wall thickening (> 5 mm) Inflammation localised to pericolic fat	Moderate diverticulitis plus any of: Abdominopelvic abscess Free extraluminal gas Extraluminal contrast extravasation

Source: Ambrosetti P, Grossholz M, Becker C, et al. Computed tomography in acute left colonic diverticulitis. Br J Surg 1997;84(4):532–4.

the test was an unpleasant, messy, time-consuming endurance for patients and radiologists.[61]

Not surprisingly, computed tomography (CT) in rapid, multiple slice scanners capable of variable plane reconstruction became the gold standard in determining the diagnosis and staging of diverticulitis[75,76] (Figs. 9.1 and 9.2). Downsides include the allergic and nephrotoxic risks of intravenous contrast so assessment of relevant history and biochemistry is essential. Widespread and repeated CT exposure to radiation may harm individuals,[77] so patient age and exposure history is a factor. A pragmatic approach might be to use ultrasound initially; reserving CT for unclear cases or those in who crisp anatomical definition is required (e.g., abscess needing drainage, suspicion of malignancy, unexpected or atypical sonographic findings etc.). Note it is only with CT scanning that a classification (e.g., Hinchey) can be established clearly (Figs. 9.3 and 9.4).

Colonic imaging (either optical colonoscopy or CT colonography) is still performed routinely following an episode of diverticulitis to rule out neoplasia (either co-existent or mimicking an inflammatory process). The utility of these procedures has been questioned.[78,79] Where there has been good quality cross-sectional imaging of relatively mild diverticulitis in an otherwise asymptomatic young patient with no pre-morbid reasons to screen then diverticulitis is a soft indication for colonoscopy. Conversely, where there are atypical imaging features (i.e., localised lymphadenopathy, relative absence of diverticula, focal mass effect, more than one site of 'fat stranding') or complicated diverticulitis then early colonoscopy is very much indicated. The finding of colorectal neoplasia in the setting of complicated diverticulitis is as common as 10%.[80] While tradition considered that endoscopic insufflation would be too dangerous within 6 weeks of assumed diverticulitis,[81] there is little substance to this dogma and careful colonoscopy can be performed after an interval of 3–4 weeks where there is clinical suspicion of neoplasia (e.g., unresolved or progressive symptoms).

Magnetic resonance imaging (MRI) is of immense value in intestinal disorders because soft tissue delineation exceeds ultrasound or CT and additional benefits include fistulography, multi-phase component separation, and an absence of ionising radiation.[82–84] MRI is expensive, requires expert interpretation, and scan platforms are claustrophobic, noisy places that patients must endure for prolonged periods. Open scanners have gone a long way to address the problem, but they are few in number as yet.

Table 9.2 Classification systems for diverticulitis

	Hinchey classification	Köhler modification	Modified Hinchey	Hansen/Stock
Stage I	Pericolic abscess confined by the mesocolon	Pericolic abscess	0 Mild clinical diverticulitis I Pericolic abscess or phlegmon Ia Colonic wall thickening/confined pericolic inflammation Ib Confined small (< 5 cm) pericolic abscess	0 Diverticulosis I Acute uncomplicated diverticulitis
Stage II	Pelvic abscess, distant from area of inflammation	IIa Distant abscess amenable to percutaneous drainage IIb Complex abscess with/without associated fistula	II Pelvic, distant intra-abdominal, or retroperitoneal abscess	Acute complicated diverticulitis IIa Phlegmon, peridiverticulitis IIb Abscess, sealed perforation IIc Free perforation
Stage III	Generalised peritonitis resulting from pericolic/pelvic abscess rupture into peritoneal cavity	Generalised purulent peritonitis	III Generalised purulent peritonitis	Recurrent diverticulitis
Stage IV	Faecal peritonitis resulting from free perforation of colonic diverticulum	Faecal peritonitis	IV Generalised faecal peritonitis	N/A

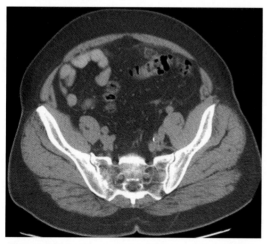

Figure 9.1 Computed tomography (CT) image of moderate sigmoid diverticulitis.

CT is the gold standard in diagnosing and staging the severity of diverticulitis.[85]

✓ Routine colonoscopy may not be warranted in asymptomatic patients after uncomplicated diverticulitis and should be determined on a case-by-case basis. Meanwhile routine colonic evaluation is advised in symptomatic patients and those who had complicated diverticulitis.[78–80]

TREATMENT

CONSERVATIVE AND MEDICAL OPTIONS

Asymptomatic patients with diverticulosis do not require treatment. There was a historical vogue (until very recently) for advising patients to avoid nuts and seeds based on the misguided assumption that they precipitated symptomatic events by local trauma or obstruction. In keeping with the folklore of diverticular management in the 20th century, this was without scientific basis or fact.[37] Furthermore, although it seems unlikely to harm and may help prevent development of diverticula, there is scant proof that changing to a higher fibre intake can change the course of symptomatic diverticular problems.[34] Even when combined with non-absorbable antibiotics (rifaxamin), any perceived benefit is small and not much better than placebo.[86] Lifestyle optimisation (i.e., high freshly sourced fibre intake, low animal fat/processed diet, smoking cessation, exercise, minimal NSAIDs intake etc.) are central to primary disease prevention and are sensible in all populations regardless of the presence of diverticula.

There are limited medical options for patients with recurrent or persistent symptoms deemed attributable to diverticulitis. There was modest benefit to a prolonged course of 5-aminosalicylates or probiotics in short-term, small trials.[87,88] There is a minimal side-effect profile to these agents because of their relatively specific intestinal drug delivery mechanism. However, the numbers needed to treat are probably high, the compliance poor, and the overall applicability of the approach is low.

✓✓ As the aetiology is unknown, diverticulitis may be an inflammatory condition rather than an infective/bacterial problem. Two randomised trials[76,89] have found antibiotic treatment for acute uncomplicated diverticulitis neither accelerates recovery nor prevents complications or recurrence. As such, observational treatment without antibiotics can be considered appropriate in non-septic patients.

✓ When antibiotics are indicated, there is currently no consensus on the most appropriate antibiotic regimen or route (oral/intravenous) for diverticulitis, however, broad-spectrum agents covering gram-negative and anaerobic organisms are advised.

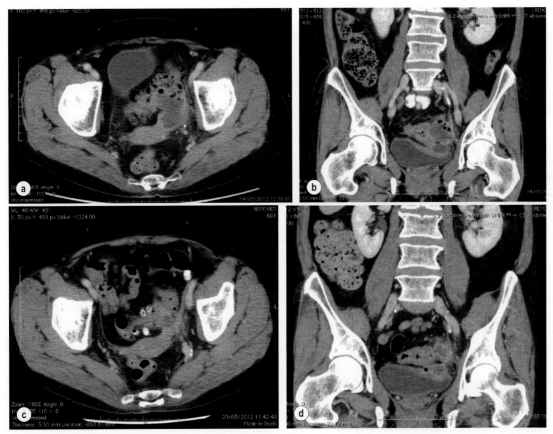

Figure 9.2   Conservative management of diverticular abscess treated with intravenous antibiotics. **(a, b)** Computed tomography (CT) abdomen on presentation demonstrates a perisigmoid abscess (Hinchey II diverticulitis). **(c, d)** CT abdomen on day 7 following treatment with IV cefuroxime, ciprofloxacin and metronidazole demonstrates resolution of abscess.

DIVERTICULAR ABSCESS

There is wide variability of practice regarding interventional radiological drainage of abscesses in this scenario. Size criteria (e.g., 5 cm) have been suggested but they lack an evidence basis. Many patients with abscesses relating to diverticulitis resolve with antibiotics alone and drainage does not obviate surgery in all cases. Where that is the case, a reasonable approach is initial intravenous antibiotic management with drainage reserved for unresolving sepsis or persistent abscess on follow-up imaging in a symptomatic patient. No firm recommendations were determined in the recent ESCP guidelines.[5]

EMERGENCY SURGERY

HISTORICAL PERSPECTIVES

Henri Albert Hartmann (1860–1952 Paris, France) first described an alternative to abdominoperineal excision of the sigmoid and rectum for carcinoma at the French Surgical Association in 1921.[90,91] The dissection extended below the peritoneal reflection with transection of the lower rectum, closure of the remaining short rectal stump and peritoneum, with formation of an end colostomy. Of course, this is not what was performed for acute diverticulitis in the last century but amazingly, the eponymous term has endured regardless of the historical inaccuracy. This was caused by

the absence of a suitable alternative to describe what was, in essence, a non-restorative subtotal sigmoid colectomy with a long, intra-peritoneal, closed rectosigmoid stump and end colostomy. This operation triumphed over previously performed three-stage procedures whereby an initial defunctioning loop colostomy was performed with subsequent resection and anastomosis (if and when the patient recovered), and eventually, colostomy closure. The mortality of this latter approach was unacceptably high and, while that of a 'Hartmann's procedure' (HP) is still 10–15% for peritonitis caused by perforated diverticulitis in the present era, a one-stage non-restorative operation was thought safer. Short-term complications include persistent sepsis (often in the residual sigmoid stump because of persistent diverticulitis or opening of the staple line), stoma problems (necrosis, retraction, stenosis etc.), and wound complications (including dehiscence). In the longer term, as many as half the patients are left with a permanent stoma because of the reluctance of the surgeon (or indeed the patient) to submit to the perils of another operation for anastomosis. Resection with anastomosis and a defunctioning stoma is advisable in stable patients with favourable anatomy and physiology (a two-stage approach).

The question of whether perforated diverticulitis requires resection in all cases was addressed by Carl Eggers (1879–1956 New York, USA), a German-American surgeon who described a series of patients with diverticulitis of whom those with generalised peritonitis he had managed with drainage alone.[92] Two randomised clinical trials (Denmark and France) in the

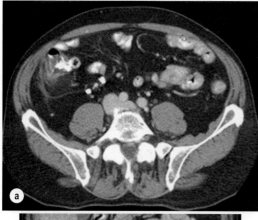

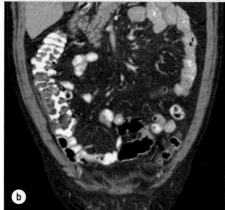

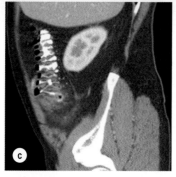

Figure 9.3 Right-sided diverticulitis. Computed tomography (CT) may be useful in patients with atypical clinical findings. The images demonstrate caecal diverticulitis as a cause for right iliac fossa pain in a 60-year-old male. **(a)** Standard cross section CT of the lower abdomen, **(b)** coronal and **(c)** sagittal plane CT of the same area.

1980s and 1990s dealt with this question. Although both were underpowered, the data did support an organ-preserving approach. Patients in whom a drainage procedure (with or without a defunctioning stoma) alone was performed for purulent peritonitis had a lower mortality than those resected.[93,94] There may have been more short-term septic issues with an organ-preserving operation but this was in an age with less broad spectrum antibiotics and widespread availability of interventional radiology drainage of abscesses than now.

LAPAROSCOPIC PERITONEAL LAVAGE FOR GENERALISED PURULENT PERITONITIS

Alas, the trials were not enough to change practice at the time. They did give food for thought to another pioneering

surgeon Gerry O'Sullivan (1946–2012 Cork, Ireland) who considered it feasible to laparoscope a patient in whom there was generalised peritonitis and pneumoperitoneum on CT or plain radiography (erect chest or abdominal x-ray) because of perforated diverticulitis. By simply performing laparoscopic peritoneal lavage (LPL), the initial results championed a stoma-free, low morbidity approach[95] (Fig. 9.5). The utility and low mortality (~5%) of the approach to generalised peritonitis because of perforated, purulent diverticulitis was confirmed in several series.

The natural selection bias inherent in non-randomised studies meant that more robust data were necessary. This led to a number of multicentre, randomised trials comparing laparoscopic lavage with colonic resection (usually with a stoma) for acute perforated non-feculent diverticulitis. To date, four randomised trials (LADIES, SCANDIV, DILALA and Lap-LAND) have been registered[96–99] (Table 9.3). Three of these trials have published results.[100–102] The SCANDIV trial randomised patients with suspected perforated diverticulitis and free air on CT scan to laparoscopic lavage ($n = 101$) or colonic resection ($n = 98$) with or without primary anastomosis, as 'determined by surgeon preference and local practices'. While the re-intervention rate was higher in the lavage group, morbidity and mortality (13.9% vs. 11.5%) were not significantly different. The LOLA arm of the Ladies trial randomised patients with Hinchey III diverticulitis to laparoscopic lavage ($n = 46$) or sigmoid resection ($n = 40$) was closed because of a higher re-intervention rate in the lavage group, although there were fewer stomas and lower mortality (9% vs. 14%). The DILALA trial randomised patients ($n = 65$) with Hinchey III (purulent peritonitis) diverticulitis at laparoscopy to laparoscopic lavage ($n = 39$) or an open resection ($n = 36$). Lavage was shorter with faster recovery and lower mortality (7.7% vs. 11.4%). Notably, the crude aggregated data from these trials show fewer stomas and lower mortality with laparoscopic lavage but possibly higher post-operative intervention (e.g., abscess drainage). Subsequent cost analyses from two of these randomised trials provide evidence that laparoscopic lavage is more cost effective than sigmoid resection.[103,104] Whilst the ESCP guidelines recommend resection, they dictate that laparoscopic lavage is also feasible (in selected patients).[5]

Shock, requirements for inotropes and infirm patients or those on immunosuppressants are contraindications to laparoscopic lavage for generalised, diverticular-related peritonitis. Furthermore, if faecal peritonitis or a visible colonic wall breach is identified at laparoscopy then resection is indicated. Many cases show features of stercoral rather than diverticular perforation (i.e., history of prolonged constipation, minimal or absent diverticula, large hole with focal necrosis, not inflammation). It should be considered routine to perform gas-leak testing during laparoscopy (transanal carbon dioxide or air insufflation of the sigmoid submerged in saline lavage) to exclude a hole before considering lavage alone. Ongoing sepsis (peritonitis should resolve within 24 hours) following seemingly successful lavage suggests source control was not achieved and re-intervention should be considered.

RESECTION WITH PRIMARY ANASTOMOSIS

Primary resection and anastomosis (PRA) with or without a defunctioning ileostomy has emerged as a worthy alternative

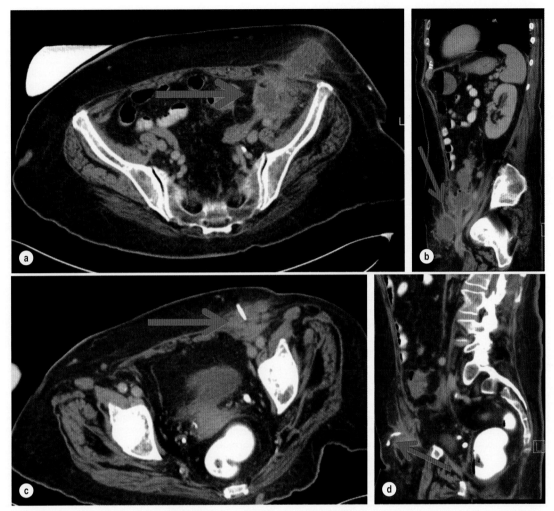

Figure 9.4   (a, b) Computed tomography (CT) abdomen demonstrating a diverticular abscess involving the abdominal wall (*red arrow*; history of right hemicolectomy and end ileostomy). **(c, d)** The abscess was drained percutaneously with resolution of symptoms. *Red arrow* demonstrates placement of drain.

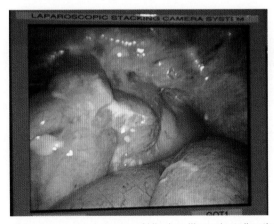

Figure 9.5   Laparoscopic image of Hinchey III purulent diverticulitis.

to HP in the setting of peritonitis secondary to diverticular perforation.[105] Indeed, some studies demonstrate superior outcomes compared to HP quoting mortality rates of 5% for PRA vs. 15% for HP.[106] Furthermore, PRA compares favourably in terms of post-operative morbidity including wound and stoma complications and sepsis. In the most recent systematic review, anastomotic leak rates were in the order of 6%,[107] notably lower than the reported anastomotic leak rate in Hartmann's reversal (8%). The DIVA arm of the LADIES trial was the first randomised trial comparing HP with sigmoid resection with anastomosis (Fig. 9.6).

✅ Aggregated data from randomised trials testing laparoscopic lavage for perforated, non-feculent diverticulitis suggests it is feasible in patients wishing to avoid a stoma. Those with ongoing sepsis caused by failure of source control may need timely re-intervention.[100–102]

ELECTIVE RESECTION – FACTS, FICTION AND FUNCTIONAL OUTCOME

Elective resection for recurrent diverticulitis was once practiced commonly after the second or third episode. However, the practice is risky with reports of 1% mortality, 30–50% morbidity, and as many as 10% receiving a stoma (at least in the short-term).[108–110] The natural history of diverticulitis is

Table 9.3   Randomised trials comparing laparoscopic lavage with resection

Name	Study	Objective	Inclusion criteria	Recruitment	Study number
LADIES The Netherlands	Multicentre two-armed randomised trial: LOLA arm – laparoscopic lavage, Hartmann's or resection and anastomosis (2:1:1); DIVA arm – for faeculent peritonitis Hartmann's or resection and anastomosis (1:1)	To assess the superiority of laparoscopic lavage compared with sigmoidectomy in patients with purulent perforated diverticulitis, with respect to overall long-term morbidity and mortality	Patients with signs of general peritonitis and suspected perforated diverticulitis. Radiological examination by radiography or a CT abdomen with diffuse-free intraperitoneal air or fluid for patients to be classified as having perforated diverticulitis	Recruitment commenced 2009	LOLA arm: 264 DIVA arm: 212
DILALA Scandinavia	Multicentre randomised trial comparing laparoscopic lavage to Hartmann's procedure as treatment for acute perforated diverticulitis (1:1)	To compare laparoscopic lavage to Hartmann's procedure as treatment for acute perforated diverticulitis	Clinical symptoms, elevated inflammatory markers, CT abdomen showing signs of free gas and/or intra-abdominal fluid. Emergency surgery decided by the attending surgeon	Recruitment commenced 2011	Laparoscopic lavage: 39 Hartmann's procedure: 36
SCANDIV Scandinavia	Multicentre randomised clinical superiority trial (centre-stratified block randomisation).	To determine whether laparoscopic lavage changes the rate of severe complications in patients with acute perforated diverticulitis who traditionally are treated with primary resection	Clinical suspicion of perforated diverticulitis with indication for urgent surgery. CT abdomen with free air and findings suggesting diverticulitis. Patients randomised after diagnostic laparoscopy	Recruitment commenced 2010	Laparoscopic lavage: 101 Hartmann's procedure: 98
LapLAND Ireland	Multicentre randomised trial comparing Hartmann's procedure or resection/anastomosis (1:1)	To compare outcomes following Hartmann's or resection with anastomosis and defunctioning stoma and laparoscopic lavage alone for the treatment of acute perforated non-faeculant diverticulitis	Clinical evidence of generalised peritonitis. Free air on erect chest X-ray or CT abdomen suggestive of perforated diverticulitis. Laparoscopy to confirm diagnosis and exclude faecal peritonitis	Recruitment commenced 2010	300 Still recruiting

such that one in six patients undergo surgery at presentation while approximately 20–25% re-present, with a similar proportion requiring surgery, such that less than 5% have more than two episodes.[111] In that series, six of the 78 patients re-admitted with diverticulitis a second time died, a proportion commented to be twice that of those presenting for the first time. Parks did not suggest elective resection to improve this statistic although many have used his data to support the premise of a 'prophylactic' operation. Indeed,

he pointed out that several patients died in their first admission from suspected diverticulitis in which radiology or necropsy tests were not performed so that they could not be classed as diverticular deaths. Had they been, the mortality was likely much higher for the first episode than reported for the second. The principles on which this outdated and flawed concept was founded pre-dated modern cross-sectional imaging such that the diagnosis was clinical and inferred from subsequent barium enema.[112–114] Some patients

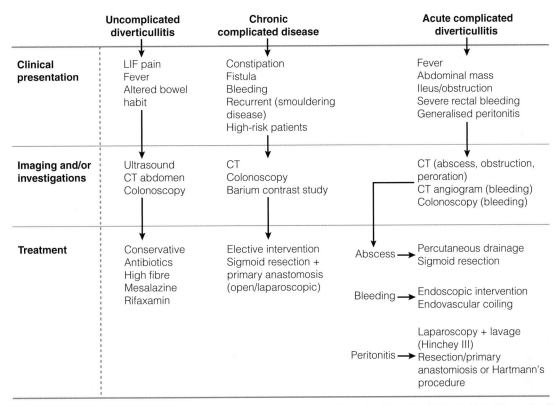

	Uncomplicated diverticullitis	Chronic complicated disease	Acute complicated diverticullitis
Clinical presentation	LIF pain Fever Altered bowel habit	Constipation Fistula Bleeding Recurrent (smouldering disease) High-risk patients	Fever Abdominal mass Ileus/obstruction Severe rectal bleeding Generalised peritonitis
Imaging and/or investigations	Ultrasound CT abdomen Colonoscopy	CT Colonoscopy Barium contrast study	CT (abscess, obstruction, peroration) CT angiogram (bleeding) Colonoscopy (bleeding)
Treatment	Conservative Antibiotics High fibre Mesalazine Rifaxamin	Elective intervention Sigmoid resection + primary anastomosis (open/laparoscopic)	Abscess → Percutaneous drainage / Sigmoid resection Bleeding → Endoscopic intervention / Endovascular coiling Peritonitis → Laparoscopy + lavage (Hinchey III) / Resection/primary anastomiosis or Hartmann's procedure

Figure 9.6   Treatment algorithm. *CT*, Computed tomography; *LIF*, left iliac fossa. (Based on Klarenbeek BR, de Korte N, van der Peet DL, et al. Review of current classifications for diverticular disease and a translation into clinical practice. Int J Colorectal Dis. 2012;27(2):207-14. With permission from Springer Science + Business Media.)

had ongoing symptoms and others came to emergency surgery for diverticulitis, so it was extrapolated that elective surgery was indicated to prevent a life-threatening event. We now know that diverticulitis follows a predictable course in the majority, such that recurrence runs at 2% per year while the risk of requiring emergency surgery following diverticulitis is calculated to be only one event in 2000 patient-years.[62] Furthermore, Mayo Clinic data suggest that diverticulitis is not a progressive disease in terms of severity or mortality risk.[115] Indeed, as it has been throughout the last century, the highest risk of extreme sepsis and death is with the first episode. The overwhelming majority of these patients have no history of diverticulitis and had no pre-morbid diagnosis of diverticulosis.[63,115–119] Successfully treated acute uncomplicated diverticulitis is no longer deemed an indication for elective surgery unless there are several recurring episodes or persistent symptoms with objective evidence of ongoing inflammation.[5]

There are certain diverticular-associated phenomena that are relative or absolute indications for elective surgery. These include fistula (e.g., colovesical, colovaginal, colocutaneous), obstruction from a stricture, and persisting diverticulitis ('smouldering diverticulitis') unresponsive to medical therapy. The latter is an uncommon event characterised by symptoms matched with a persistent subtle, tender mass in the left iliac fossa, persistently elevated markers of inflammation (e.g., C-reactive protein), and no other abnormality on colonoscopy and cross-sectional imaging.

There are specific circumstances in which surgeons should consider elective resection for recurring episodes of diverticulitis each of which resolve fully. After four defined episodes, the risk of further episodes requiring admission and surgery is particularly high in the younger (<50 years of age) population.[120] Therefore in young patients eager to avoid further morbidity and time off work in whom an elective operation can be performed with a mortality risk of <1%,[28] elective sigmoid resection is reasonable. However, the pre-operative discussion should include the fact that recurrent diverticulitis may arise, that a stoma may be required (at least in the short-term), that co-existing functional symptoms will persist and that over 20% complain of urgency and even incontinence episodes.[121] The laparoscopic approach is attractive to patient and surgeon as there are short-term advantages with smaller wounds, less morbidity, and less time dependent on supportive care.[122]

Indications for elective resection include: fistula, diverticular stricture and ongoing symptomatic disease refractory to medical management.

DIVERTICULAR HAEMORRHAGE

The proportion of patients with diverticulosis presenting with bleeding was originally thought to be as high as 3–5%.[123] However, this was based on a somewhat oversimplified quotient (number bleeding divided by number presenting to hospital with a diagnosis of diverticulosis) that would have hugely overestimated the prevalence. Modern population-based data would suggest less than one event in 2000 person-years (383 bleeds with only 70 requiring transfusion or intervention in 730 446 person-years or follow-up).[37] One group found no inflammation but non-uniform intimal thickening in the vasa recta of bleeding diverticula.[124,125] The majority of diverticular haemorrhages cease spontaneously. A requirement of more than 4 units of red cell concentrate may indicate patients at risk of ongoing bleeding.[126] Visceral angiography with embolisation[127–129] is preferable to blind colectomy with which morbidity and mortality risks are high. One of the challenges to the surgeon faced with operating on an (all too often) elderly patient with lower gastrointestinal bleeding is what to remove? Many an early career surgeon was caught out doing a left-sided colectomy on the assumption that the sigmoid was the culprit only to find ongoing bleeding –'diverticular' haemorrhage is right sided in over 50% and a proportion are caused by angiodysplasia.

Key points

- The spectrum of diverticular disease encompasses asymptomatic diverticulosis, uncomplicated diverticulitis, complicated diverticular disease (abscess, perforation, stricture, fistula), diverticular bleeding and SCAD.
- The incidence of diverticulitis is approximately 1–2/1000 in the western world.
- There is a male predominance in younger patients while females are more likely to develop diverticulitis at an older age.
- The aetiology remains unknown but genetics, geographical location, ethnicity, and lifestyle factors (smoking and obesity) play a role.
- There is a tenuous link between lack of dietary fibre and the development of diverticulosis.
- CT is the ideal investigation for symptomatic diverticular issues. A routine colonoscopy may not be necessary if CT findings are consistent with diverticulitis and there is a low clinical concern for other pathology (i.e., cancer).
- Antibiotics do not influence outcomes of uncomplicated diverticulitis in non-septic patients and can be safely omitted.
- Perforated diverticulitis with purulent (not feculent) peritonitis may be managed with laparoscopic lavage or resection depending on the clinical circumstances and patient wishes. The optimal strategy depends on the physiological status of the patient, the extent of contamination and the experience of the surgeon.
- Elective sigmoid resection after diverticulitis is unwarranted in the majority unless there are strong disease-specific (e.g., colovesical fistula) or patient-related indications (e.g., after multiple admissions in a young patient).

References available at http://ebooks.health.elsevier.com/

KEY REFERENCES

[5] Schultz JK, Azhar N, Binda GA, Barbara G, Biondo S, Boermeester MA, et al. European Society of Coloproctology: guidelines for the management of diverticular disease of the colon. Colorectal Dis 2020;22(S2):5–28.

[23] Mimura T, Emanuel A, Kamm MA. Pathophysiology of diverticular disease. Bailliere's Best Pract Res Clin Gastroenterol 2002;16(4):563–76.

[37] Strate LL, Liu YL, Syngal S, Aldoori WH, Giovannucci EL. Nut, corn, and popcorn consumption and the incidence of diverticular disease. JAMA 2008;300(8):907–14.

[61] Ambrosetti P, Jenny A, Becker C, Terrier F, Morel P. Acute left colonic diverticulitis - compared performance of computed tomography and water-soluble contrast enema: prospective evaluation of 420 patients. Dis Colon Rectum 2000;43(10):1363–7.

[76] Ünlü Ç, De Korte N, Daniels L, Consten EC, Cuesta MA, Gerhards MF, et al. A multicenter randomized clinical trial investigating the cost-effectiveness of treatment strategies with or without antibiotics for uncomplicated acute diverticulitis (DIABOLO trial). BMC Surg 2010;10.

[78] Westwood DA, Eglinton TW, Frizelle FA. Routine colonoscopy following acute uncomplicated diverticulitis. Br J Surg 2011;98(11):1630–4.

[102] Angenete E, Thornell A, Burcharth J, Pommergaard HC, Skullman S, Bisgaard T, et al. Laparoscopic lavage is feasible and safe for the treatment of perforated diverticulitis with purulent peritonitis: the first results from the randomized controlled trial DILALA. Ann Surg 2016;263(1):117–22.

[104] Vennix S, van Dieren S, Opmeer BC, Lange JF, Bemelman WA. Cost analysis of laparoscopic lavage compared with sigmoid resection for perforated diverticulitis in the Ladies trial. Br J Surg 2017;104(1):62–8.

[115] Chapman JR, Dozois EJ, Wolff BG, Gullerud RE, Larson DR. Diverticulitis: a progressive disease? Do multiple recurrences predict less favorable outcomes? Ann Surg 2006;243(6):876–80.

Ulcerative colitis

10

Scott R. Kelley | Eric J. Dozois

INTRODUCTION

Ulcerative colitis (UC) is an idiopathic relapsing inflammatory bowel disease (IBD) involving the mucosa and lamina propria of the rectum and variable extent of the proximal colon. Characterised by remissions and exacerbations, the clinical spectrum of disease can range from inactive to fulminant. Medical management is generally effective in controlling UC, but ultimately 30–40% of patients will require surgical intervention. Criteria for the management of acute and chronic disease are well established, with surgery playing a fundamental role, as removal of the colon and rectum is essentially curative.

EPIDEMIOLOGY

UC is an uncommon disease with varying incidence rates (0.5–24.5/100 000) and discernible differences are seen between different geographic and ethnic regions of the world. Less common in Asia, Africa, South America and South-eastern Europe, UC has a varied incidence of between two and 15 cases per 100 000 persons per year in developed and industrialised Western countries of North America, North-western Europe and the UK. A significant trend of increasing incidence and prevalence rates has been reported in under-developed parts of the world as they become more industrialised, thus supporting the importance of environmental factors in the development of UC.[1]

The onset of symptoms typically plateaus around the fourth decade of life, remaining fairly constant thereafter. A second peak of onset around the sixth to seventh decade has been described, though there is uncertainty as to whether this is truly a subsequent peak or merely difficulty in differentiating it from other colitides.

UC is seen with near equal frequency in males and females. Whites and blacks have a nearly equivalent incidence, while the Jewish populace experiences the highest documented rates. Hispanic, Native American, African and Asian populations have the lowest incidence.

AETIOPATHOGENESIS

The pathogenesis of UC remains enigmatic, though multiple factors have been described as potential causative or protective agents in its occurrence and include: diet, alcohol and tobacco consumption, socioeconomic status, hygiene, urban living conditions, antibiotic usage, gut flora dysbiosis,

probiotic use, non-steroidal anti-inflammatory agents, appendicectomy, breastfeeding, oral contraceptive use, stress, and familial and genetic causes.[2]

Though a significant number of dietary factors have been evaluated as potential causative agents for UC, no consensus has emerged. A decreased risk has been associated with alcohol consumption, and the risk declined as daily alcohol consumption increased.

Evidence demonstrates that smoking is protective against disease activity, and it has been shown that those who quit smoking are more likely to have a relapse. Ex-smokers are 70% more likely to develop UC when compared to those who have never smoked, though the causation remains unclear. Supplemental nicotine therapy has not consistently been shown to be more effective than placebo or conventional therapy (steroids/5-aminosalicylic acid [5-ASA]) and has a significant side-effect profile.

The hygiene hypothesis contends that cleaner living environments reduce the amount of organisms one is exposed to early in life, thus reducing the ability of the immune system to become tolerant, and subsequently causing an aberrant response when thus exposed. UC is more common among urban populations, is associated with indoor living, smaller families, and individuals of middle and upper socioeconomic status, who primarily reside in more sanitary surroundings.

Antibiotic usage and the resulting gut flora dysbiosis are commonplace in developed countries, and hypothetically a potential cause of UC when taking into consideration that higher rates of utilisation are seen in industrialised and developed nations, though this is yet to be proven. A correlation has been demonstrated in children with UC, who are more likely to have received antibiotics during their first year of life.

A predisposition for UC has been reported to be as high as 29% in those with a positive family history, and between 10% and 20% of affected individuals have a first-degree relative with IBD. Twin studies have consistently shown a higher concordant disease rate in monozygotic compared to dizygotic pairs (approximately 50% vs. nearly 0%), where the concordance among ordinary siblings was found to be around 5%.[3]

CLINICAL PRESENTATION

Colonic involvement at presentation can vary widely between different geographic regions, though proctosigmoiditis is the most common. In the USA 46% presented with proctosigmoiditis, 37% pancolitis and 17% with left-sided colitis.

Common symptoms associated with UC include urgency, diarrhoea, tenesmus and haematochezia. Constipation, a complaint in 15–20% of patients, is related to incomplete evacuation of the rectum. Symptoms correlate with severity of disease, and increasing severity leads to worsening nausea, emesis, abdominal distension and weight loss. Protein-losing enteropathy may lead to loss of lean body mass and anaemia, and growth retardation in children. Haemodynamically significant haemorrhage is an uncommon complication but is responsible for 10% of emergency colectomies. Severity can also have systemic manifestations, including tachycardia, pyrexia, leucocytosis and increased fluid requirements, indicating toxicity.

Approximately 5–15% of patients with UC develop acute severe colitis, and up to 50% present initially with fulminant disease. Intense medical treatment has a high chance of inducing remission but when unsuccessful, urgent surgery will be necessary in up to 20% of patients. Perforation is a rare but serious occurrence, with a mortality approaching 60%.

DIAGNOSIS AND EVALUATION

With an extensive differential and no one exclusive pathognomonic test, a firm diagnosis of UC is dependent on several factors, including the clinical presentation, radiological workup, endoscopic evaluation and histopathological determination of tissue biopsies. The differential diagnosis can include infectious (viral, bacterial, protozoal) as well as non-infectious causes (Crohn's disease, indeterminate colitis, collagenous colitis, ischaemic colitis, radiation colitis, diversion colitis, pharmacotherapy-induced colitis), and obtaining a detailed history and physical examination is imperative.

MICROBIOLOGY

Colitides that can mimic UC include *Clostridium difficile*, *Escherichia coli* (serotype 0157:H7), *Salmonella*, *Shigella*, *Entamoeba* and *Campylobacter* infections. Stool studies for bacteria, ova and parasites should be obtained to confirm the true diagnosis and direct appropriate treatment. An increasing incidence of *C. difficile* colitis in patients with IBD complicates their management and all patients with IBD hospitalised with an acute exacerbation should be assessed for synchronous infection.

ENDOSCOPY

Endoscopy plays a pivotal role in the evaluation and diagnosis of UC, allowing for direct mucosal visualisation as well as providing an avenue for obtaining tissue biopsies. Other important indications include evaluating the proximal extent of colonic involvement, determining severity, differentiating from Crohn's disease, as well as monitoring responsiveness to medical management and surveillance.[4]

During an acute attack, complete colonoscopy is generally avoided to decrease the risk of a potential perforation, while flexible or rigid proctoscopy is often used. Since inflammatory changes begin just above the anorectal junction and spread proximally, proctoscopy provides easy access to the lower rectum where biopsies can be obtained below the peritoneal reflection, minimising the risk of free perforation.

There is an overall lack of specific endoscopic features related to UC, though characteristic patterns of inflammation are appreciated. In the quiescent phase, the mucosa will appear relatively normal, with the exception of neovascular changes. Oedema, erythema and an abnormal mucosal vascular pattern are endoscopically observed findings with mild inflammation. Loss of the vascular pattern (the submucosal vessels seen through the transparent mucosa) is a result of mucosal oedema, which makes it appear opaque. Oedema can also cause fine granularity in which there is a delicate regular stippled appearance of the mucosal surface. As the disease activity progresses to a moderate stage, superficial erosions, ulcerations and contact bleeding secondary to scope trauma are observed. Inflamed and regenerated mucosa surrounded by ulcerations lead to the development of pseudopolyps and a cobblestone appearance, which can also be appreciated during more severe conditions. Long-standing chronic inflammatory changes can give rise to a 'featureless microcolon' with mucosal atrophy, muscular hypertrophy, a decreased luminal diameter and loss of haustral folds.

HISTOPATHOLOGY

Inflammation in UC is confined to the rectum and colon. The mucosal columnar glandular epithelium extends into the anal canal to the level of the anal transitional zone. Segmental or skip areas do not occur, rather the inflammation in the colon and rectum is diffuse without intervening normal mucosa. The rectum is always involved, although the appearance of relative rectal sparing can occur in patients receiving transanally applied anti-inflammatory agents. A spared rectum not associated with local treatment should raise the suspicion of Crohn's disease. Backwash ileitis occurs only in cases with colonic extension to the ileocaecal junction.

Microscopic examination of a biopsy in early disease will demonstrate mucosal inflammation, goblet cell depletion, crypt of Lieberkühn distortion, and vascular congestion. Mucin within goblet cells is expectorated, making them appear less evident or absent (goblet cell depletion). Branching of crypts may also be evident owing to regeneration following crypt epithelial damage. As severity progresses, the lamina propria will exhibit infiltration by neutrophils, plasma cells, lymphocytes, eosinophils and mast cells. Neutrophils present within the epithelium of crypts (cryptitis) can aggregate in the crypt lumen, forming abscesses. Mucosal destruction, ulceration and subsequent atrophy are partly the result of rupturing of crypt abscesses. In advanced or late forms of UC, crypt destruction and loss occur as a result of damage to the crypt basal epithelium. Deeper submucosal or transmural inflammation with ulceration can also be observed, leaving large areas of exposed muscularis propria covered with granulation tissue giving the appearance of pseudopolyps. In the more chronic and quiescent phase, a distorted architectural pattern with crypt distortion, branching and foreshortening can be identified.

IMAGING

Although the reference standard for the diagnosis and follow-up of patients with UC is endoscopy, multiple traditional and emerging imaging modalities can also be used to assess patients with UC.[5]

Conventional supine and upright abdominal x-rays are used to evaluate complications, including obstruction, dilatation or perforation. Dilatation of the transverse colon to greater than 6 cm is often seen in the face of toxic megacolon, and with imminent perforation is an indication for emergency surgical intervention.

There has been a movement away from contrast x-rays as endoscopic evaluation has become more commonplace. The earliest finding on double-contrast barium enema consists of a fine granular appearance in the rectosigmoid region as a result of mucosal oedema and hyperaemia. Advanced disease is characterised by the absence of haustral folds, narrowing and shortening of the colon, and diffuse ulceration. More chronic forms will present with colonic shortening, luminal narrowing, loss of haustral folds and widening of the presacral space.

In comparison to Crohn's disease, computed tomographic (CT) and magnetic resonance imaging (MRI) studies for evaluating UC are less commonly obtained. CT is a relatively poor test for detecting the mucosal abnormalities of early disease, though more advanced UC often has a hallmark finding of diffuse colonic wall thickening. The benefit of CT lies in the ability to evaluate intra-luminal and extra-luminal disease, guide and monitor response to treatment, as well as detect complications.

SEROLOGY AND MICROBIOME

Serologic markers sensitive for inflammation, but not specific, include white blood cell count, C-reactive protein (CRP) and erythrocyte sedimentation rate (ESR). Anti-saccharomyces cerevisiae antibodies (ASCS) are more specific for Crohn's disease and perinuclear anti-neutrophil cytoplasmic antibody (p-ANCA) for chronic UC. The Prometheus antigen testing panel can be used to rule out IBD but lacks the specificity to differentiate between Crohn's disease and UC.

Decreasing faecal calprotectin levels have been shown to correlate with mucosal healing when used in conjunction with ESR and CRP. Profiling the intestinal microbiome has shown promise that IBD results from alterations between the intestinal microbes and mucosal immunity, though significant research still needs to be completed.

COLORECTAL CANCER AND SURVEILLANCE

Prolonged duration, continuously active disease, severity of inflammation, primary sclerosing cholangitis (PSC) and diffuse involvement (pancolitis) are cumulative risk factors for the development of colorectal cancer in the setting of UC. Incidence rates for the development of cancer correspond to cumulative probabilities of 2% by 10 years, 8% by 20 years and 18% by 30 years.[6] As a general rule, beginning 10 years after the diagnosis of UC, the incidence of colorectal cancer increases by approximately 1% per year as long as the patient has their colon. The relative risk for cancer in relation to ulcerative proctitis has been estimated to be 1.7, left-sided colitis 2.8 and pancolitis 14.8. In relation to the general population, there is an overall eightfold higher risk of colorectal cancer, with a 19-fold higher risk in patients with extensive colitis. It has been shown that roughly 17% of all deaths in UC are a result of colorectal cancer.

Flat low-grade dysplasia (LGD) detected during colonoscopic evaluation confers a reported ninefold increased risk of developing colorectal cancer and a 12-fold risk of developing an advanced lesion (high-grade dysplasia [HGD], or cancer).[7] Progression from colitis without dysplasia to colorectal cancer does not necessarily follow a sequence of LGD, HGD and ultimately carcinoma (inflammation–dysplasia–carcinoma sequence). Rather, LGD can progress directly to colorectal cancer. LGD can present as unifocal or multifocal and treatment is to some extent controversial, with some advocating prophylactic colectomy, while others recommend intensive colonoscopic surveillance. Flat LGD has been shown to be a strong predictor of progression to advanced neoplasia (53% at 5 years) in surveillance colonoscopy, and in patients who underwent a colectomy, an unexpected advanced neoplasia (HGD or cancer) was found in nearly 24%. Other studies have shown the presence of LGD is as likely as HGD (54% vs. 67%) to be associated with an already established cancer. Repeated attempts to show LGD on endoscopic examinations should not be undertaken; rather, proctocolectomy is recommended to prevent progression to HGD or cancer.

✔✔ A large meta-analysis of 20 surveillance studies showed the risk of developing cancer in patients with LGD is high. When LGD is detected on surveillance, there is a ninefold risk of developing cancer and 12-fold risk of developing any advanced lesion.[7]

Flat HGD has been shown to have a 42–45% rate of associated colorectal cancer at the time of colectomy, thus maintaining the recommendation that colectomy is mandatory in these patients, even with completely resected HGD or with HGD found on random biopsies.

Several studies have suggested that surveillance colonoscopy in patients with UC significantly reduces the risk of developing neoplasia. To date, no randomised controlled trials have documented a reduced risk of colorectal cancer development or death by utilising surveillance colonoscopy. The American Gastroenterological Association and British Society of Gastroenterology share international guidelines recommending surveillance colonoscopy every 1–2 years starting 8–10 years after a diagnosis of pancolitis, or 15 years after left-sided colitis. Recommendations are also advocated for random non-targeted biopsies performed every 10 cm in all four quadrants, equating to 20–40 biopsies per colon. Colitis-associated cancers have been shown frequently to arise from flat mucosa, be multifocal, broadly infiltrating, anaplastic and uniformly distributed throughout the colon. It is estimated that 33 non-targeted biopsies are required to detect dysplasia with 90% confidence, though studies show this is not often achieved.[8]

Patients with PSC and UC have an increased risk of colorectal cancer in comparison to those without PSC.[9] Cumulative colorectal cancer risk has been described as 33% at 20 years and 40% at 30 years after a diagnosis of UC. Surveillance colonoscopy is recommended at the time of diagnosis of PSC and yearly thereafter. In patients without a known diagnosis of UC, diagnostic colonoscopy with random biopsies is recommended to evaluate for subclinical evidence of disease.

Flat and depressed colorectal lesions are often missed with conventional 'white light' colonoscopy and the utility of obtaining non-targeted random biopsies has been called into question. Though highly specialised, time-consuming and not universally available, the use of high-magnification chromoscopic colonoscopy (dye spraying of the mucosal surface with indigo carmine or methylene blue) has been shown to have a significantly better correlation between endoscopic and histopathological findings than conventional colonoscopy, and also increased the number of neoplastic lesions identified. Chromoendoscopy (CE) has been repeatedly shown to increase the chance of detecting dysplasia compared to standard colonoscopic surveillance, allowing the endoscopist to take fewer, but rather higher yield, biopsies.[10]

SEVERITY ASSESSMENT

Disease severity is classified as mild, moderate or severe, and is based on the original descriptions provided by Truelove and Witts. Mild disease is characterised by less than four stools daily, with or without macroscopic blood, no signs of systemic toxicity (fever, tachycardia), mild to no anaemia and a normal ESR. Severe disease results in six or more bloody bowel movements daily, signs of systemic toxicity, anaemia (less than 75% of normal value) and an increased ESR.

Unlike the Crohn's Disease Activity Index, no gold standard index exists for evaluating the severity of UC. Rather, multiple indices have been developed to measure disease severity and activity in clinical trials, many with overlapping measured variables. Some assess the clinical and biochemical aspects of disease (Truelove and Witts Severity Index, Lichtiger Index, Powel–Tuck Index, Activity Index, Rachmilewitz Index, Physician Global Assessment, Ulcerative Colitis Clinical Score), others focus on endoscopy (Truelove and Witts Sigmoidoscopic Assessment, Baron Score, Powel–Tuck Sigmoidoscopic Assessment, Rachmilewitz Endoscopic Index), while further indices evaluate a combination of clinical and endoscopic criteria (Mayo Clinic Score, Sutherland Index, Ulcerative Colitis Endoscopic Index of Severity). Common to all indices are numerical scoring systems. Scores at the elevated end of the spectrum indicate high disease activity, while lower scores signify milder or quiescent disease.[11]

EXTRA-INTESTINAL MANIFESTATIONS

Upwards of 20% of patients with UC will develop extra-alimentary (Ed: UK nomenclature describes extra-intestinal) manifestations during the course of illness including, but not limited to, musculoskeletal (the most common), hepatopancreatobiliary, dermatological, thromboembolic and ophthalmological derangements.[12] Most extra-intestinal manifestations present after an exacerbation of colonic inflammation, but they can also occur at the time of the acute flair. Colectomy is beneficial in inducing remission of peripheral arthropathy, erythema nodosum and iritis. Pyoderma gangrenosum does not universally respond, and

axial arthropathy, PSC, uveitis and episcleritis proceed independently of surgical intervention.

MUSCULOSKELETAL

Peripheral arthropathy asymmetrically involves numerous small and large joints (knees being the most common), affecting up to 20% of patients, with severity paralleling disease activity. The arthropathy is typically fleeting, rheumatoid factor negative (seronegative) and non-deforming. It disappears when medical treatment induces remission or after proctocolectomy, although it has been documented in patients with pouchitis after restorative proctocolectomy.

Axial arthropathy (ankylosing spondylitis) involving the sacroiliac joints and one or more vertebrae occurs in up to 5% of patients. The majority of cases are human leucocyte antigen (HLA)-B27 positive, unrelated to the activity of colitis and predominantly unresponsive to treatment. Asymptomatic sacroiliitis is limited to the sacroiliac joint, is HLA-B27 negative, largely unaffected by treatment and is radiographically detected in 24% of patients. Although both ankylosing spondylitis and asymptomatic sacroiliitis have an overall poor response to treatment, anti-tumour necrosis factor-α agents have shown promise.

HEPATOPANCREATOBILIARY

PSC is an idiopathic chronic and progressive disorder manifesting as stricturing, inflammation, and fibrosis of intra- and extrahepatic bile ducts. It is one of the most serious complications of UC. Patients with co-existing PSC and UC are at a markedly increased risk of colonic neoplasia (five times), necessitating close colonoscopic surveillance with extensive biopsy sampling. Around 5% of patients with UC will develop PSC, whereas upwards of 75% of patients with PSC are found to have concurrent UC. The clinical course of PSC does not parallel underlying bowel disease and may present independently of colonic symptoms. An increased risk of development has been demonstrated in patients with HLA B8, DR2, DR3 or DR6 haplotype positivity. Treatment of PSC with steroids, colectomy or antibiotics is ineffectual. Patients undergoing restorative proctocolectomy have a higher subsequent incidence of pouchitis and dysplasia in the ileal pouch mucosa.[13] Ultimately, the disease progresses to liver cirrhosis and eventual failure, which may prompt consideration for liver transplantation.

✅ The cumulative risk of pouchitis at 1, 2, 5 and 10 years after ileal pouch–anal anastomosis was 15.5%, 22.5%, 36% and 45.5% for the patients without PSC, and 22%, 43%, 61% and 79% for the patients with PSC.[13]

Cholangiocarcinoma is a rare association with UC, and PSC is the greatest risk factor for its development. The prognosis is dismal, with a median survival of 9 months after diagnosis, and 12–15% of patients transplanted for PSC have cholangiocarcinoma.

DERMATOLOGICAL

Erythema nodosum (EN) classically presents as tender, inflamed, red nodules mainly on the anterior surfaces of the lower extremities. The most common cutaneous lesion, it is seen in 10–20% of patients with UC. Exacerbations often parallel disease activity and frequently resolve after colonic disease subsides, although EN can precede bowel occurrence.

Pyoderma gangrenosum (PG) occurs in 1–10% of patients with UC and presents as plaques or pustules that break down and form painful ulcerations with undermined borders and necrotic centres. Legs are the most commonly affected area, though it can occur anywhere, including peristomally. Occurrences do not always parallel colonic disease activity.

THROMBOEMBOLIC

The incidence of deep venous thrombosis and pulmonary embolism in UC is threefold higher than the general population and associated with morbidity and mortality. Though unproven, a hypercoagulable state in UC is hypothetically related to corticosteroid usage, activation of the coagulation cascade during a systemic inflammatory state, or upregulation of acute phase reactants with flares.

Though rare, cerebral venous and dural sinus thrombosis can occur and results in a potentially devastating stroke. More commonly seen in patients with active disease, cases have been reported up to 10 years after a proctocolectomy.

OPHTHALMOLOGICAL

Manifestations of episcleritis, uveitis and scleritis can occur in up to 5% of patients. Ocular symptoms often present concurrently with peripheral arthritis and erythema nodosum. Episcleritis, the most common ophthalmopathy, presents with pain, burning and scleral injection. It usually occurs in parallel, as well as resolves with the treatment of colonic disease. Uveitis presents with pain, blurred vision, photophobia and headaches. Classically, the redness is most prominent centrally and dissipates radially. Uveitis does not typically coincide with flares, and prompt treatment is necessary to decrease the risk of visual impairment. Scleritis presents similarly to episcleritis, though it is more severe and necessitates aggressive treatment to minimise retinal detachment and optic nerve impairment. In scleritis, unlike episcleritis, the sclera will appear pink or violet between the dilated surface vessels.

MEDICAL MANAGEMENT

Inducing and maintaining clinical remission by promoting mucosal healing is the goal of medical treatment for UC. With several different medications to choose from (aminosalicylates, steroids, immunosuppressants, immunomodulators, biologics), therapy is modified in conjunction with the severity and extent of disease.

Clinical remission is characterised by symptom resolution of the inflammatory phase. This occurs with a decrease in diarrhoea, bleeding, urgency, tenesmus, the passage of mucopus and restoration of continence. Endoscopic remission will reveal regeneration of healthy mucosa, epithelial continuity, a return of a submucosal vascular pattern, and resolving ulceration, friability and granularity. Histological

remission is achieved when an absence of neutrophils in the epithelial crypts is observed.

Just as there is no standard agreement amongst scoring systems measuring disease severity and activity, there are no universally validated means of defining disease remission. Before initiating maintenance therapy, it is essential that clinical remission be achieved and verified. It has been demonstrated that high rates of relapse occur when endoscopic and histological remission has not been confirmed.[14]

✔✔ A prospective multicentre study revealed patients in clinical remission with less severe sigmoidoscopic scores (defined as normal-looking mucosa, with only mild redness and/or friability) after 6 weeks of acute treatment were less likely to relapse at 1 year than patients in clinical remission only (cumulative rate of relapse 23% vs. 80%, respectively; P < 0.0001).[14]

PROCTITIS

Disease limited to the rectum is best treated with topical therapy, including foams, enemas and suppositories. Mesalamine suppositories (1–1.5 g/day) administered nightly, or in daily divided doses, have shown superiority in comparison to oral 5-ASA compounds. Maximal response is noted within 4–6 weeks and, if unresponsive, combination therapy with topical corticosteroids has been shown to be more effective than either therapy alone. In patients unwilling to make use of, or failing to respond to, topical therapy, oral mesalamine may be given as an alternative, though higher doses are typically required. Systemic steroids are only administered in individuals refractory to topical and oral therapy, or in cases of severe disease.

MILD TO MODERATE DISTAL COLITIS

Mild to moderate distal colitis (30–40 cm) is primarily treated with a regimen of oral aminosalicylates, topical mesalamine or topical steroids. Mesalamine enemas are the treatment of choice and achieve higher rates of remission than oral 5-ASA compounds or topical steroids. Nightly administered mesalamine enemas (4 g/60 mL) have documented remission rates of between 60% and 70%, with rates increasing as the duration of therapy increases. If symptoms persist, and no response is seen within 2–4 weeks, an additional mesalamine or hydrocortisone enema can be administered each morning. Combination therapy has been shown to be superior to either therapy alone.[15] The systemic side-effects from corticosteroid enemas occur as a result of a low first-pass hepatic metabolism and can be significant in some patients. Budesonide, a corticosteroid formulation that has a high first-pass hepatic metabolism, reduces the systemic side-effect profile, and has been shown to be as effective as conventional corticosteroid enemas. Oral mesalamine can be added in combination with topical therapy for patients showing a poor response and is superior to oral or topical therapies alone. For patients not responding to or refusing topical therapy, oral mesalamine can be administered and has been shown to be a valuable alternative, though it is not as effective. Oral and intravenous corticosteroids are administered in patients refractory to topical steroids and 5-ASA compounds (oral and topical), or in cases of severe disease.

MILD TO MODERATE EXTENSIVE COLITIS

Extensive colitis involves the colon beyond the reach of topical therapy and necessitates oral pharmacotherapy. Oral sulfasalazine (2–6 g/day) is associated with remission rates of up to 80%, though with a significant systemic sulphonamide side-effect profile and high rates of intolerability (30–40%).[15] Non-sulphonamide 5-ASA formulations have been shown to be as effective as sulfasalazine, though better tolerated without dose-limiting systemic side-effects. Distal colonic and rectal disease topical therapy can also be concomitantly administered, and this combination has been shown to be more successful in inducing remission at 8 weeks than oral therapy alone. Enteral steroids are implemented in cases not responding to oral mesalamine, or when the side-effects of the 5-ASA compounds cannot be tolerated. Prednisone is typically administered, starting with doses of 40–60 mg/day until significant clinical improvement is observed. Once remission is achieved a taper of 5–10 mg/week is instituted until a daily dose of 20 mg is reached. A dose decrease of 2.5–5 mg/week is continued thereafter, while maintaining 5-ASA treatment, until completion.[15]

Thiopurines (6-mercaptopurine, azathioprine), with a primarily steroid-sparing benefit, are effective in patients who cannot be tapered off or tolerate corticosteroids. Their use is limited by a slow onset of action and prolonged duration is required to achieve optimal effectiveness (3–6 months).[15] Infliximab (Remicade) has shown effectiveness in inducing remission in patients failing corticosteroid and/or thiopurine, as well as aminosalicylate therapy. Infliximab is intravenously administered over a 2-hour period at a dose of 5 mg/kg at weeks 0, 2 and 6, and then at 8-week intervals. Those who fail to respond after the initial two doses are unlikely to respond to a third dose. Shortening the interval between doses or increasing the dose to 10 mg/kg can treat those who eventually lose responsiveness after an initial response. For those not responding to an escalated dose and decreased interval, treatment discontinuation is recommended.[16] Other biological agents include adalimumab (Humira), certolizumab (Cimzia), golimumab (Simponi) and vedolizumab (Entyvio).

✅✅ Two randomised, double-blind, placebo-controlled studies – the Active Ulcerative Colitis Trials 1 and 2 (ACT 1 and ACT 2, respectively) – showed patients with moderate to severe active UC treated with infliximab at weeks 0, 2 and 6 and every 8 weeks thereafter were more likely to have a clinical response at weeks 8, 30 and 54 than were those receiving placebo.[16]

SEVERE COLITIS

The mainstay of therapy for patients with severe/fulminant colitis is intravenous corticosteroids with a daily dose equivalent of 300 mg for hydrocortisone or 60 mg for methylprednisolone. Higher doses have not been proven to be beneficial, and 20–40% will fail to respond to therapy. Studies have been unable to confirm any incremental advantage in administering or continuing oral 5-ASA compounds and topical regimens. The utilisation of empiric broad-spectrum antibiotics, although routinely administered, has not shown benefit when treating patients with severe colitis. Intravenous ciclosporin (2–4 mg/kg/day continuous infusion) has been shown to be an effective adjuvant (82% response) in those lacking improvement while being treated with maximal medical therapy over a period of 3–5 days. Infliximab has shown short-term efficacy with approximately half of treated patients requiring a colectomy at 5 years. Patients failing to respond to maximal medical therapy or showing signs of deterioration are candidates for surgery.[15] Though published data are somewhat conflicting, several studies have shown that higher rates of anastomotic and infectious complications are seen in patients following ileal pouch–anal anastomosis when infliximab has been given within an 8-week period before surgery. Given these findings, a discussion with a surgeon to review surgical options is prudent before beginning infliximab therapy.

SURGICAL MANAGEMENT

Surgery plays a pivotal role in the management of UC. Removal of the colon and rectum is essentially curative. Indications for removal include drug intolerability or unresponsiveness, intractability, life-threatening complications (perforation, bleeding, toxicity), dysplasia or malignancy, growth impediment in children, and for the attempted improvement of some extra-intestinal manifestations refractory to medical treatment (PG, EN, peripheral arthritis, uveitis, iritis). The surgical approach depends on the presentation (emergency/urgent, elective) and can include: total abdominal colectomy with Brooke ileostomy, proctocolectomy with Brooke ileostomy, proctocolectomy with continent ileostomy, total abdominal colectomy with ileorectal anastomosis (IRA), and proctocolectomy with ileoanal reservoir/ileal pouch–anal anastomosis (IPAA). It is essential, when possible, to inform the patient, and have them site-marked pre-operatively by an enterostomal therapist.

EMERGENCY/URGENT

Toxic fulminant colitis, toxic megacolon, haemorrhage and perforation are life-threatening complications necessitating emergency colectomy. Urgent typically refers to hospitalised patients who are failing maximal medical therapy.

Historically, the Turnbull 'blow-hole' procedure was used in severely debilitated (septic, malnourished) patients with megacolon who could not withstand a major abdominal operation. A loop ileostomy, a transverse colostomy and, if needed, a sigmoid colostomy was created (Fig.10.1). This allowed for faecal diversion, minimal handling of the bowel and patient convalescence for future colectomy but did not eliminate the colitis nor the physiological impact of the inflammation on the patient. In rare circumstances (advanced pregnancy and toxic megacolon) the Turnbull approach could even now be considered.[17] Even so, recent experience in pregnant patients with fulminant disease suggests that total abdominal colectomy and Brooke ileostomy

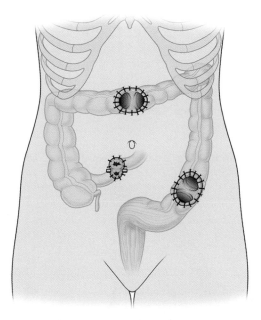

Figure 10.1 Turnbull procedure.

eliminates the systemic inflammatory consequences and can be done with low rates of maternal and foetal morbidity and mortality.[18]

✔ Subtotal colectomy and Brooke ileostomy for UC during pregnancy is safe. A multi-disciplinary team that includes a gastroenterologist, high-risk obstetrician and experienced surgeon is necessary for an optimal outcome.[18]

For patients requiring urgent or emergency intervention, total abdominal colectomy with creation of a Brooke ileostomy and preservation of the rectum for a potential future restorative procedure is most commonly performed and recommended. It eliminates most of the disease and allows for restoration of health, as well as tapering of immunosuppressant medications. When performing a total abdominal colectomy, it is imperative to dissect as close to the ileocaecal valve as possible, thus preserving all of the ileocolonic branches for a possible restorative procedure. Deferring the proctectomy will simplify a restorative procedure by maintaining pelvic and presacral tissue planes. This not only reduces the potential complications (bleeding, infection, autonomic nerve damage) in an acutely ill patient, but also permits the opportunity pathologically to exclude Crohn's disease by examining the colonic specimen. Studies evaluating the outcome of a retained rectal stump have been conflicting. Some portend that leaving a diseased, thickened rectal stump is not associated with increased rates of post-operative pelvic sepsis or complications.[19] Others encourage exteriorisation (mucous fistula or subcutaneous placement) of long stumps, having found rates of pelvic sepsis as high as 12%, increased disease activity in the retained rectum and subsequent pelvic dissection for restorative procedures more difficult with a retained short stump. If a mucous fistula is not done, the rectum should be irrigated with a rigid proctoscope to remove bloody mucous and a transanally placed rectal tube left in place for 48 hours to decrease pressure on the closed rectal stump.

ELECTIVE

Indications for elective surgery consist of medical unresponsiveness, intolerability or intractability, dysplasia or malignancy, growth retardation in children, and for the attempted improvement of some extra-intestinal manifestations. Depending on patient preference, continence, age, concerns of fertility and dysplastic changes, operative interventions include proctocolectomy with Brooke ileostomy, proctocolectomy with continent ileostomy, total abdominal colectomy with IRA, and a restorative proctocolectomy with IPAA.

PROCTOCOLECTOMY WITH END ILEOSTOMY

A proctocolectomy with end Brooke ileostomy removes all disease and has a low rate of complications but leaves the patient with an incontinent stoma. Indications for this approach are patient preference, low-rectal cancer and poor sphincter function.

The patient is placed in a modified lithotomy position. The colectomy portion of the procedure is carried out in a non-oncological approach unless neoplastic transformation has been identified. The rectal dissection and mobilisation may be done close to the perimuscular rectal wall in an attempt to minimise damage to the pelvic autonomic nerves. In the event of neoplastic changes both the colonic and rectal dissections are carried out in a standard oncological fashion. In the low anorectal region, a perineal intersphincteric dissection is carried out (except in the presence of a low-rectal cancer), preserving the external sphincter and levator ani muscles, which significantly improves wound healing. The perineum is closed in layers and the greater omentum, if present, is mobilised and placed in the pelvis. After closure of the abdomen, the ileostomy is matured in a standard evaginated Brooke fashion, with an attempted ideal projection of 2.5 cm (Fig. 10.2).

Stoma complications including retraction, peristomal skin excoriation, stenosis, prolapse and herniation can occur, with up to 30% of patients requiring operative revision. When delayed healing of the perineal wound occurs, evaluation for Crohn's disease and/or retained mucosa or foreign material (suture) should be carried out.

PROCTOCOLECTOMY WITH CONTINENT ILEOSTOMY

Initially described by Nils Kock, the continent ileostomy still remains a viable alternative for motivated patients who are not candidates for an IPAA but is only performed in a very few centres. Modifications and revisions to the original Kock continent ileostomy have been described and include the

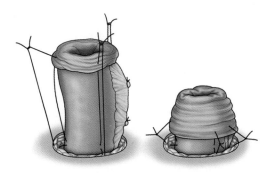

Figure 10.2 Brooke ileostomy.

Barnett continent ileostomy reservoir and T-pouch, neither of which has supporting data to suggest they are better than the Kock pouch. Contraindications to construction of a continent ileostomy include Crohn's, obesity, marginal small bowel length and anyone with a psychological or physical disability that would preclude understanding or being able to perform daily stomal intubation.

Surgical creation of a continent ileostomy is carried out by using 45–60 cm of terminal ileum and folding it into either a two-limb or S-pouch configuration. The pouch reservoir requires approximately 30 cm of ileum to construct, while a portion of the remaining distal outflow tract is intussuscepted to create a valve. As the pouch distends, it causes an increase in pressure around the valve, thus occluding the outflow tract, preventing evacuation. The end of the ileum is brought out through the abdominal wall and matured flush with the skin. A wide-bore catheter is used to intubate the pouch by inserting it through the skin level stoma, which is placed to gravity drainage for approximately 10 days. The pouch is slowly distended over time by intermittently clamping the catheter. When the catheter can be clamped for 8 hours without discomfort, it is removed and intermittent intubation is carried out three to four times per day.

Post-operative pouch complications requiring re-operation are common and include skin-level or valve strictures, volvulus, herniation, fistulisation and valve slippage. Subluxation of the nipple valve is suggested by the onset of incontinence of the stoma and difficulty in inserting the catheter. Valve slippage is the most common complication, with reported rates of nearly 30%. Contrast studies may show partial or complete prolapse of the valve. Fistulas occur in approximately 10% of patients and typically originate from the base of the nipple valve or the pouch itself. Despite the high morbidity and need for re-operative intervention with a continent ileostomy, patient satisfaction and quality of life are extremely high. It has been documented that over 90% of patients would undergo the procedure again, as well as recommend it to friends and family.[20]

ILEORECTAL ANASTOMOSIS

Colectomy with IRA should be considered only when the rectum is minimally inflamed, distensible and compliant, there is no rectal dysplasia, the patient has an intact sphincter mechanism and is willing to adhere to strict follow-up. IRA is an appealing alternative in younger patients of reproductive age to decrease the risk of impotence and reduced fecundity, as well as older patients with quiescent disease having colectomy for colonic dysplasia. Strict rectal surveillance must be adhered to because of the increased risk of future neoplastic changes. The risk of rectal carcinoma can reach up to 20% by 30 years.[21] Proctitis of the retained rectum can lead to bleeding, tenesmus, urgency, severe diarrhoea and pain. Topical, oral and systemic therapies can be used, but it has been documented that up to 45% of patients will not respond and eventually require a proctectomy. In patients who require a completion proctectomy, an end ileostomy, restorative IPAA or continent ileostomy are all options.

RESTORATIVE PROCTOCOLECTOMY/ILEAL POUCH–ANAL ANASTOMOSIS

Initially described in 1978 by Parks and Nicholls as an ileoanal ileal reservoir procedure, the restorative proctocolectomy

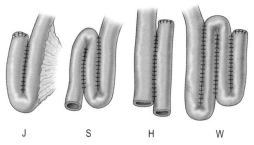

Figure 10.3 Variations of ileal pouch configurations.

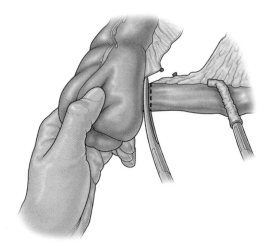

Figure 10.4 Ileal transection adjacent to caecum.

has become the most common continence-preserving procedure performed for the management of UC in patients who are appropriate candidates. The restorative pouch can be fashioned in two-limb (J), three-limb (S), four-limb (W) or isoperistaltic (H) configurations (Fig. 10.3). The J-pouch, because of its ease of construction and excellent functional outcomes, has become the most common choice for most surgeons. The S-pouch provides additional length and can reduce anastomotic tension, though the 5-cm efferent limb of ileum projecting beyond the pouch can lead to evacuation difficulties and outlet obstruction. The isoperistaltic H-pouch, with its long outlet tract, can give rise to stasis, distension and pouchitis. The W-pouch has been shown to have similar functional results when compared to the J-pouch, but it is more time-consuming and technically difficult to construct.

The patient is placed in a modified lithotomy position to allow access to the anus and abdominopelvic cavity. A total colectomy is performed, and the ileum is transected flush with the caecum (Fig. 10.4). To provide adequate perfusion to the pouch, it is imperative to preserve the ileal branches of the ileocolic and distal mesenteric arteries. At this point in the operation, if there is any doubt of the diagnosis, the colon should be removed and inspected with the pathologist. Once confident of the diagnosis of UC, evaluation for adequacy of reach of the small bowel to the deep pelvis should be undertaken. The proposed point of the pouch–anal anastomosis can be pulled down to the pubis, and if this point can be pulled 3–4 cm below the inferior edge of the pubis one can feel confident of successful reach for anastomosis. Strategies to decrease tension at the anastomosis include: complete mobilisation of the small-bowel

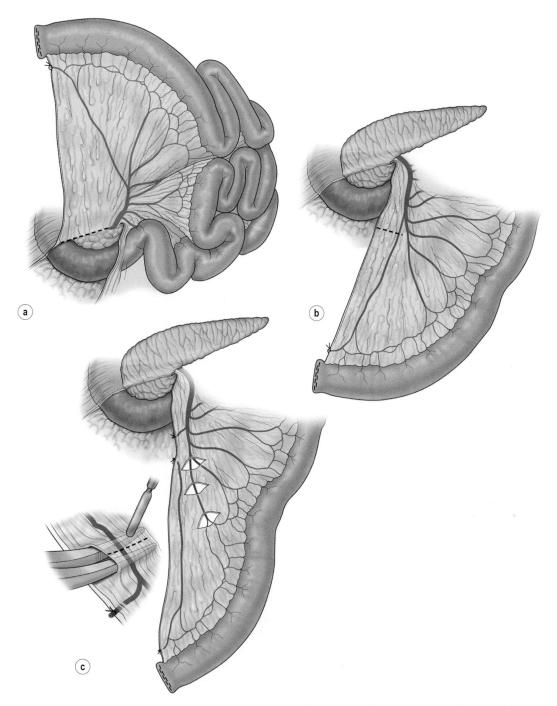

Figure 10.5 **(a)** Mobilisation of the ileal mesentery around the duodenum. **(b)** Proximal division of the ileocolic artery. **(c)** Relaxing mesenteric incisions over the terminal portion of the superior mesenteric artery.

mesentery to the root of the superior mesenteric artery cephalad to the head of the pancreas (Fig. 10.5a), proximal division of the ileocolic artery (Fig. 10.5b) and relaxing incisions of the mesentery over tension points along the superior mesenteric artery (Fig. 10.5c). Rectal dissection can be done in the total mesorectal excision plane or close to the rectal wall, depending on the concern for autonomic nerve damage and surgeon's experience with nerve-sparing proctectomy. Transection of the rectum should occur 2–3 cm above the dentate line in the anal transition zone, leaving a short rectal cuff (Fig. 10.6). After reach has been verified, a

J configuration is fashioned, with each limb measuring between 12 and 15 cm in length. The limbs are paired in an anti-mesenteric fashion and are held in position with interrupted stay sutures (Fig. 10.7).

Double-stapled technique

For a stapled technique, an enterotomy is made in the anti-mesenteric portion of the apex of the pouch and a linear cutting stapler is used to divide the walls of the two limbs, creating a common channel (Fig. 10.8). A purse-string suture is then fashioned around the enterotomy and the anvil

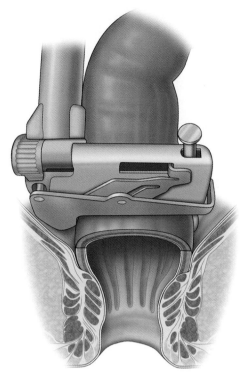

Figure 10.6   Division of the rectum with stapler.

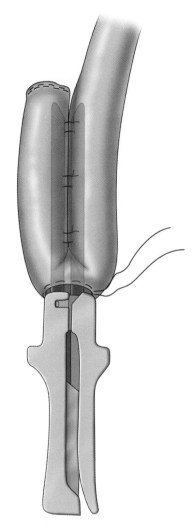

Figure 10.8   Creation of reservoir with linear stapler.

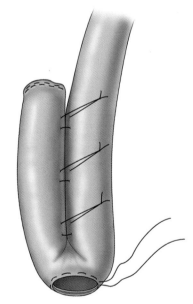

Figure 10.7   J-pouch with orientation sutures.

from a circular stapler is placed inside the pouch, where it is held in place by tightening the purse-string (Fig. 10.9). The circular stapler is then placed transanally (Fig. 10.10). After appropriate orientation, the trocar is advanced either above or below the transverse staple line and attached to the anvil. The stapler is then closed, approximating the pouch and anus (Fig. 10.11).

Hand-sewn technique

For a hand-sewn pouch–anal anastomosis, an anal canal muco-sectomy is performed, starting at the dentate line (Fig. 10.12).

Raising the mucosa with a submucosal injection of dilute saline and epinephrine (1:200 000) facilitates the dissection of the mucosa away from the internal sphincter muscle (Fig. 10.13a and b). After the circumferential mucosa and proximal rectum have been removed, the pouch is gently brought down to the level of the dentate line. An enterotomy is made in the apex of the pouch, if not already created, and it is anchored in position by placing a suture in each of the four quadrants incorporating a full-thickness bite of the pouch, internal sphincter muscle and mucosa. Sutures are placed between the anchoring stitches, in a clockface orientation, to complete a mucosally intact anastomosis (Fig. 10.14). An air insufflation leak test is performed, and a protective loop ileostomy fashioned (Fig. 10.15). The operation can be carried out without the creation of a diverting loop ileostomy in highly selected cases, with good results. However, in a meta-analysis of nearly 1500 patients, the rate of anastomotic leakage was significantly higher in patients not given a defunctioning ileostomy.[22]

✅✅ A review of 17 studies comprising 1486 patients revealed restorative proctocolectomy without a diverting ileostomy resulted in functional outcomes similar to those of surgery with proximal diversion but was associated with an increased risk of anastomotic leak. Diverting ileostomy should be omitted in carefully selected patients only.[22]

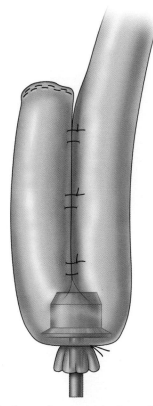

Figure 10.9 Stapler anvil secured in J-pouch with purse-string suture.

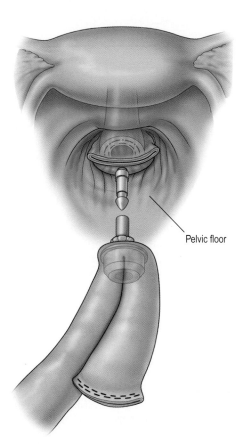

Figure 10.10 Stapler placed transanally with spike posterior to transverse staple line.

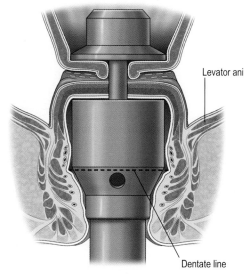

Figure 10.11 Approximation of stapler and anvil for double-stapled anastomosis.

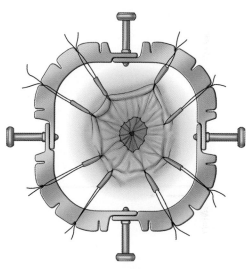

Figure 10.12 Exposure for transanal mucosectomy using Lone Star retractor.

Outcomes in stapled versus hand-sewn anastomosis

Variations exist for the creation of a J-pouch, depending on the technique (hand-sewn vs. double-stapled) chosen. A large meta-analysis demonstrated no significant differences between the two techniques. Nocturnal seepage and pad usage favoured the stapled anastomosis, in comparison to persisting symptoms because of inflammation or dysplasia in the cuff favouring the hand-sewn technique.[23] A single institution experience of over 3000 pouch procedures (474 hand-sewn and 2635 stapled) revealed patients who underwent a stapled IPAA experienced better outcomes (incontinence, seepage, pad usage) and quality of life (dietary, social and work restrictions) in comparison to the hand-sewn group.[24]

✔✔ A meta-analysis of 4183 patients demonstrated no significant differences in post-operative complications between a mucosectomy and hand-sewn versus stapled anastomosis. Nocturnal seepage and pad usage favoured the stapled anastomosis, in comparison to persisting symptoms because of inflammation or dysplasia in the cuff favouring the hand-sewn technique.[23]

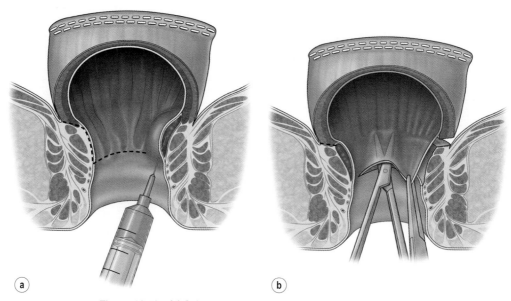

Figure 10.13   **(a)** Submucosal injection. **(b)** Transanal mucosectomy.

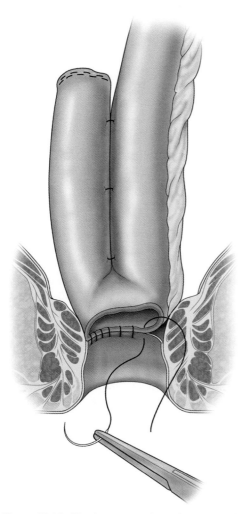

Figure 10.14   Hand-sewn pouch–anal anastomosis.

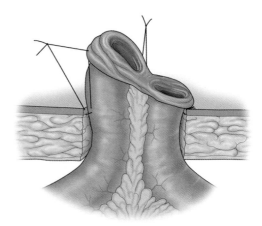

Figure 10.15   Diverting loop ileostomy.

Neoplastic changes observed in the retained anal transition zone in patients undergoing double-stapled technique are rare. The majority of reports have been associated with pathological findings of dysplasia or cancer in the initial operative specimen. A hand-sewn technique, including a completion mucosectomy, nearly eliminates the possibility of leaving columnar rectal mucosa behind, though not completely. Studies have been able to demonstrate 14–21% of excised pouches harbouring residual rectal mucosa.[25] A double-stapled technique, on the other hand, results in the retention of a small cuff of columnar mucosa. This can result in a 'cuffitis' or 'strip proctitis', which has been reported to occur in nearly 15% of stapled anastomoses and can potentially progress to dysplasia. Studies have demonstrated a 2.7–3.1% risk of developing LGD in the retained mucosa, although that has only been shown to occur when there was dysplasia or cancer in the colectomy specimen. The European Crohn's and Colitis

Organisation (ECCO) consensus on surgery for UC notes cancers are reported in patients with a stapled anastomosis as well as in those who have had a mucosectomy and that there is no data to support oncological superiority of a mucosectomy over stapled anastomosis in the presence of dysplasia or colorectal cancer. ECCO also states it is reasonable, when the indication for surgery is cancer or HGD of the lower rectum, to perform a mucosectomy and anastomosis at the dentate line.[26] For persistent or recurrent LGD, a completion mucosectomy, perineal pouch advancement and neo-ileal pouch–anal anastomosis is recommended.[27] Though studies recommending adequate pouch examination after an IPAA are lacking, long-term surveillance using annual endoscopy and biopsies is often recommended to monitor for dysplasia, although this is hard to achieve in practice.

Complications following pouch surgery

Major complications following pouch surgery include small-bowel obstruction, anastomotic stricture, pouch–vaginal or pouch perineal fistula, pouchitis and pelvic sepsis. In several series, morbidity after IPAA is a significant problem, with documented rates of over 60%.[28]

Small-bowel obstruction has been reported to occur in over 30% of patients, can present before or after loop ileostomy closure, and increases up to 10 years after operation. The cumulative risk has been shown to be 18% at 1 year, 27% at 5 years and 31% at 10 years. Adhesions are the most common cause of a small-bowel obstruction and surgical intervention is necessary in roughly 10% of patients by 10 years.[28]

Anastomotic strictures can cause pouch outlet obstruction with incomplete pouch evacuation and, depending on how stricturing is defined, have been documented with rates as high as 38%. Stricturing can often be treated with finger or sequential dilator dilatation, depending on the degree of stenosis. If excessive fibrosis and stenosis are present, stricture excision and pouch advancement or removal may be necessary.

Pouch–vaginal fistula is uncommon but is a devastating complication when it occurs. Obtaining a pouchogram prior to ileostomy closure, as well as a thorough vaginal and anal canal examination at the time of closure, can help exclude a fistula. Pouchograms may miss small leaks in low anastomoses as the delivery tube may sit above the IPAA. MRI can also be used to identify small anastomotic defects. Management depends on the level of the fistula (low vs. high) and severity. Reza and colleagues recently published a classification system based on fistula aetiology including: (1) anastomotic related, (2) IBD related with subclassifications Crohn's (Type A) and non-Crohn's (Type B), (3) cryptoglandular related and (4) malignancy related.[29] Management includes placement of a seton, diversion, pharmacotherapy and transabdominal and perineal procedures.[30] A transanal or transvaginal approach for repairing low-lying fistulas has shown success in 50–70% of patients, though often requiring repeat procedures. Healing rates for higher fistulas after abdominal advancement of the pouch also show 50–70% documented success.[31] The presence of perianal abscess or fistula-in-ano pre-operatively is associated with a 3.7- to sixfold increase in the risk of developing a pouch–vaginal fistula.[32]

The most common complication after IPAA is pouchitis, a non-specific inflammation of the pouch, which approaches 50% within 10 years. Symptoms include increased stool frequency, abdominal cramping, bleeding, urgency, tenesmus, incontinence and fevers. Diagnosis should be based on endoscopic and histological factors, rather than clinical symptoms alone. Hypothetically, pouchitis results from the overgrowth of anaerobic bacteria, local factors or ischaemia, though the exact aetiology is unknown. Extra-intestinal manifestations, specifically PSC, and high serological levels of p-ANCA, have been shown to correlate with higher levels of pouchitis and chronic pouchitis.[33] Smoking, on the other hand, has been shown to decrease rates of pouchitis and probiotics (VSL#3) have shown promise in reducing episodes of acute pouchitis as well as maintaining remission.[34] Treatment depends primarily on the administration of antibiotics (metronidazole and ciprofloxacin), with response rates documented in over 80% of patients, though topical steroid or 5-ASA therapy is occasionally required.[35] Recurrent and refractory pouchitis is difficult to manage. Diversion with a loop ileostomy does not always affect the degree of inflammation and excision with construction of a new reservoir can be followed by recurrent pouchitis. Crohn's disease should always be suspected in patients with chronic pouchitis. Pouch excision is rarely necessary.

Pelvic sepsis has been documented to occur in as many as 20% of patients and has the most clinically significant implications. Sepsis occurring in the early post-operative period confers a fivefold increased risk of subsequent failure, necessitating aggressive treatment with major or minor procedures to attempt to preserve the pouch. Pelvic sepsis can often be managed with CT-guided percutaneous drainage, but extreme cases will require operative intervention. Pouch failure and loss can occur immediately or several years following a septic complication, with estimated cumulative 3-, 5- and 10-year failure rates of 20%, 31% and 39%, respectively.[36] If pouch salvage occurs in the setting of pelvic sepsis, pelvic fibrosis leads to compromised function of the pouch.

✓ The frequencies of permanent defunctioning and excision of a pouch in 131 patients with septic complications were 24% and 6%, respectively. The 5-year pouch failure rate increased in a subgroup of patients with septic complications at the pouch–anal anastomosis when the anal sphincter was involved (50% vs. 29%). Surgery for septic complications is required in a high percentage of patients and repeated attempts are justified to decrease the risk of pouch loss.[36]

Female patients of reproductive age who undergo a proctocolectomy and creation of an IPAA have decreased post-operative fecundity, with reduced rates documented in upwards of 50%.[3]

Studies have demonstrated no difference in fertility after a diagnosis of UC compared with before a diagnosis, but higher infertility rates (38%) in females who had pelvic pouch surgery in comparison to patients managed non-operatively (13%).[38] The decreased fertility is hypothetically related to tubal occlusion secondary to adhesions and a large percentage (67%) of patients have demonstrated abnormal hysterosalpingography when evaluated post-operatively.[39] The ability to carry a foetus to term and successfully deliver vaginally has not been shown to be affected by an IPAA. Pregnancy has also not been shown to decrease pouch function or increase complications when followed long term.[40] Men report statistically improved sexual quality and function in relation to sexual desire, intercourse satisfaction, erectile function and overall satisfaction after IPAA when compared with before surgery.[41] Rare complications, particularly from pelvic surgery, include loss of or retrograde ejaculation.[42]

✅✅ A meta-analysis of eight studies revealed that an IPAA can increase the risk of infertility, defined as achieving pregnancy within 12 months of attempting conception, in women with UC by approximately threefold. Counselling female patients regarding decreased rates of fecundity following an IPAA is imperative.[37]

Risk factors found to be independent predictors of pouch survival include: prior anal pathology, abnormal anal manometry, patient comorbidity, pouch–perineal or pouch–vaginal fistulas, pelvic sepsis, anastomotic stricture and separation.[32] Pouch failure, defined as pouch excision or permanent diversion, is reported in several large series to range from 7–10% at 20 years.[28,40,43]

Removal of the pouch has a significant early and late morbidity (62%), with re-admissions and delayed healing of the perineal wound (persistent perineal sinus) in 40% of patients.[44] Thus, where failure is threatened by sepsis or poor function, it may be in the patient's interest to consider a salvage procedure that may be less traumatic and offers a chance of retaining satisfactory anal function. In general, redo pouch surgery seems to have better results when performed for mechanical than for septic complications. When performed by experienced surgeons in tertiary centres, redo pouch is a safe and effective procedure with peri-operative complication rates that range from 19–51%. Success rates for salvage surgery following restorative proctocolectomy range from 75–94%.[45,46] The outcomes after revisional surgery are also encouraging, with salvage rates ranging from 75–85% with 5-year follow-up. Quality of life after revisional pouch surgery has been assessed by several centres and the results are reported as satisfactory in 50–93% of the patients.[26]

✅ The most common indications for pouch salvage are intra-abdominal sepsis, anastomotic stricture and retained rectal stump.[46] Surgical revision using a transanal or combined abdominoperineal approach has documented success rates of 75–94%.[45,46]

Functional outcomes

The frequency of bowel movements after an ileoanal–pouch anastomosis averages six in 24 hours, with minor incontinence of 11% during the day and 21% at night when followed for 20 years.[47] Nearly half will experience nocturnal leakage and minor spotting during the first 6 months, which improves over time, with rates of 20% noted at 1 year.[48] Studies comparing quality of life before and after an IPAA procedure document greater freedom in role function, improved body image and reduced negative effects caused by colitis or life with an ileostomy. Over 90% of patients report overall satisfaction with good or excellent adjustment following

IPAA. The long-term functional and clinical outcomes of a restorative proctocolectomy are excellent, and patient satisfaction and quality of life are extremely high.[49,50]

Key points

- UC is an idiopathic relapsing IBD involving the mucosa and lamina propria of the rectum and variable segments of the proximal colon.
- The incidence is between two and 15 cases per 100 000 persons per year in more developed countries.
- The diagnosis is dependent on several factors, including the clinical presentation, radiological workup, endoscopic evaluation and histopathological examination of tissue biopsies.
- Incidence rates for the development of cancer correspond to cumulative probabilities of 2% by 10 years, 8% by 20 years and 18% by 30 years.
- Toxic fulminant colitis, toxic megacolon, haemorrhage and perforation are life-threatening complications necessitating emergency surgical intervention, of which options are limited to the most expeditious and lowest risk procedures.
- Indications for elective surgery consist of medical unresponsiveness, intolerability or intractability, dysplasia or malignancy, growth retardation in children, and for the attempted improvement of some extra-intestinal manifestations.
- IPAA has become the most common continence-preserving procedure performed in patients who are appropriate candidates. Contraindications include incontinence, poor sphincter function and low-rectal cancer.
- The foremost complication after completion of an IPAA is non-specific inflammation of the pouch (pouchitis), which approaches 50% within 10 years.
- Risk factors found to be independent predictors of pouch survival include: patient diagnosis, prior anal pathology, abnormal anal manometry, patient comorbidity, pouch–perineal or pouch–vaginal fistulas, pelvic sepsis, anastomotic stricture and separation.
- Pouch failure, defined as pouch excision or permanent diversion, is reported in several large series to range from 7–10% at 20 years.
- Success rates for salvage surgery following IPAA range from 75–94%.

 References available at http://ebooks.health.elsevier.com/

▶ RECOMMENDED VIDEOS

- Restorative proctocolectomy with formation of ileoanal pouch – https://tinyurl.com/y6vuemcc
- Technical aspects of increasing length in ileoanal pouch surgery – https://tinyurl.com/ycrago33
- Stapled ileaoanal pouch construction – https://tinyurl.com/yavo6n2v

KEY REFERENCES

[7] Thomas T, Abrams KA, Robinson RJ, et al. Meta-analysis: cancer risk of low-grade dysplasia in chronic ulcerative colitis. Aliment Pharmacol Ther 2007;25(6):657–68. PMID: 17311598.
    A large meta-analysis of 20 surveillance studies showed the risk of developing cancer in patients with LGD is high. When LGD is detected on surveillance there is a ninefold risk of developing cancer and 12-fold risk of developing any advanced lesion.
[14] Meucci G, Fasoli R, Saibeni S, et al. Prognostic significance of endoscopic remission in patients with active ulcerative colitis treated with oral and topical mesalazine: a prospective, multicenter study. Inflamm Bowel Dis 2012;18(6):1006–10. PMID: 21830282.

A prospective multicentre study revealed patients in clinical remission with less severe sigmoidoscopic scores (defined as normal-looking mucosa, with only mild redness and/or friability) after 6 weeks of acute treatment were less likely to relapse at 1 year than patients in clinical remission only (cumulative rate of relapse 23% vs. 80%, respectively; P <0.0001).

[16] Rutgeerts P, Sandborn WJ, Feagan BG, et al. Infliximab for induction and maintenance therapy for ulcerative colitis. N Engl J Med 2005;353(23):2462–76. PMID: 16339095.

Two randomised, double-blind, placebo-controlled studies – the Active Ulcerative Colitis Trials 1 and 2 (ACT 1 and ACT 2 respectively) – showed patients with moderate to severe active ulcerative colitis treated with infliximab at weeks 0, 2, and 6 and every 8 weeks thereafter were more likely to have a clinical response at weeks 8, 30 and 54 than were those receiving placebo.

[22] Weston-Petrides GK, Lovegrove RE, Tilney HS, et al. Comparison of outcomes after restorative proctocolectomy with or without defunctioning ileostomy. Arch Surg 2008;143:406–12. PMID: 18427030.

A review of 17 studies comprising 1486 patients revealed that restorative proctocolectomy without a diverting ileostomy resulted in functional outcomes similar to those of surgery with proximal diversion but was associated with an increased risk of anastomotic leak. Diverting ileostomy should be omitted in carefully selected patients only.

[23] Lovegrove RE, Constantinides VA, Heriot AG, et al. A comparison of hand-sewn versus stapled ileal pouch anal anastomosis (IPAA) following proctocolectomy: a meta-analysis of 4183 patients. Ann Surg 2006;244(1):18–26. PMID: 16794385.

A large meta-analysis demonstrated no significant differences between a mucosectomy and hand-sewn versus a stapled anastomosis. Nocturnal seepage and pad usage favoured the stapled anastomosis in comparison to persisting symptoms because of inflammation or dysplasia favouring the hand-sewn technique.

[37] Waljee A, Waljee J, Morris AM, et al. Threefold increased risk of infertility: a meta-analysis of infertility after ileal pouch anal anastomosis in ulcerative colitis. Gut 2006;55(11):1575–80. PMID: 16772310.

A meta-analysis of eight studies revealed that an IPAA can increase the risk of infertility, defined as achieving pregnancy in 12 months of attempting conception, in women with UC by approximately threefold. Counselling female patients regarding decreased rates of fecundity following an IPAA is imperative.

11 Crohn's disease

Steven R. Brown | Alan J. Lobo

INTRODUCTION

Crohn's disease is a chronic, relapsing illness of unknown cause with a transmural inflammatory process that can affect the gastrointestinal tract anywhere from mouth to anus, and which may be associated with extra-intestinal manifestations. The most frequent disease distributions include ileal, ileocolic and colonic. Perianal disease often co-exists. Classically, there are discontinuous segments of disease ('skip lesions') with areas of normal mucosa intervening. Inflammation may cause ulceration, fissures, fistulas and fibrosis with stricturing. Histology reveals a chronic inflammatory infiltrate that is typically patchy and transmural and may reveal classic granulomas with giant cell formation. Clinically, a characteristic triad of symptoms may be seen: abdominal pain, diarrhoea and weight loss. Complications include intestinal obstruction caused by stricturing disease or intestinal fistulas. A combination of clinical, macroscopic, radiological and pathological features is required to make the diagnosis. Remission of varying duration is interspersed with acute episodes or 'flares'.

EPIDEMIOLOGY

Peak age of onset is 20–30 years, with a second peak at age 50–60 years. Sex distribution is equal. The incidence has increased gradually in most regions around the world, with a higher prevalence in developed countries, particularly in urban areas.[1] The prevalence is highest in Europe and Northern America (around 200–300 per 100 000). It is notable that areas with a low incidence and prevalence have shown a steady increase in rates in parallel with their economic development. This is particularly the case in Asia where increases in incidence have been associated with rapid urbanisation suggesting that environmental factors may have a role. From genetic studies, there are some risk loci that are specific to ethnicity, but many are shared.[2]

AETIOLOGY

The aetiology involves interplay between environmental factors and genetic susceptibility, along with changes in the intestinal microflora.

ENVIRONMENTAL FACTORS

Smoking is the most studied environmental factor, doubling the relative risk of Crohn's. Antibiotic exposure in childhood may also increase risk. Other medications potentially increasing risk include oral contraception and non-steroidal anti-inflammatory drugs. Dietary factors including reduced fibre and increased saturated fat, and micronutrients such as Vitamin D, zinc and iron may be associated with a small increase in risk, but whether any of these factors are causal or simply associated is not clear.[3]

GENES

There is a genetic predisposition to Crohn's disease. About 12% of patients with Crohn's will have a family history. Ashkenazi Jews have a three- to fourfold greater risk of disease than non-Jewish populations and those of Asian and African-American descent have the lowest risk of developing the disease.[3] Relatives of patients with Crohn's disease also have an increased risk of developing ulcerative colitis. Crohn's disease and ulcerative colitis are polygenic disorders with some shared susceptibility genes.[4]

Linkage studies have identified gene associations including *NOD2* mutations, *HLA*, *MUC2* and *JAK2*. All play a role in bacterial handling in the gut, a key factor for disease. However, only a small proportion of disease hereditability is explained by genetic variation and genetics alone has so far failed to explain disease variance and phenotypes,[5] highlighting the potential importance of epigenetic and environmental factors in disease susceptibility and course.

THE MICROBIOME

Microbiome imbalance or maladaptation (dysbiosis) has been demonstrated in Crohn's patients at the time of diagnosis. This dysbiosis provides a compelling theoretical pathogenic pathway to development of disease. For instance, approximately one third of patients have an increased abundance of mucosa associated adherent-invasive *Escherichia coli*, which can cross the mucosal barrier, adhere to and invade intestinal epithelial cells and survive and replicate within macrophages provoking release of tumour necrosis factor (TNF)-α.[6] Despite significant research in this area, manipulation of the microbiome has so far mainly failed to significantly impact on treatment.

PATHOGENESIS

Normally, the gut exists in a state of tolerance to the stream of microbial, dietary and other antigens in contact with the mucosa, but this tolerance and the ability to suppress an immune-mediated inflammatory response is lost. Defects in immunoregulation are coupled with an increased mucosal permeability because of leaky paracellular pathways.

Defects in immunoregulation may include disturbed innate immune mechanisms at the epithelial barrier, problems with antigen recognition and processing by dendritic cells, and effects of psychosocial stress via a neuroimmunological interaction. In Crohn's disease, the cell-mediated response is predominant, with excessive activation of effector T cells that predominate over the regulatory T cells that turn off the process. Pro-inflammatory cytokines released by effector T cells stimulate macrophages to release TNF-α, interleukin (IL)-1 and IL-6. In addition, abnormal dendritic cell function may further drive the inflammatory response. Leucocytes then enter from the local circulation releasing further chemokines, amplifying the inflammatory process. The result is a local and systemic response, including fever, an acute-phase response, hypoalbuminaemia, weight loss, increased mucosal epithelial permeability, endothelial damage and increased collagen synthesis. Because of immune dysregulation, the inflammatory response in the intestinal mucosa proceeds unchecked, producing a chronic inflammatory state.[7]

PATHOLOGY

The macroscopic appearance and distribution are important in differentiating Crohn's disease from other forms of inflammatory bowel disease (IBD), particularly ulcerative colitis. Frequencies of regions involved are:

- small bowel alone, 30% colon alone, 25–35%;
- small bowel and colon, 30–50% (usually ileocolic);
- perianal lesions, over 50%;
- stomach and duodenum, 5% (minor subclinical mucosal abnormalities in 50%).

Skip lesions strongly suggest Crohn's disease, although occasionally, a periappendiceal or caecal patch of overt colitis may be observed with distal ulcerative colitis.

The combination of disease behaviour (stricturing, penetrating), distribution and perianal disease is captured in the Montreal classification (Table 11.1).

MACROSCOPIC APPEARANCE

The unmistakable appearance of Crohn's disease is of a stiff, thick-walled segment of bowel with fat wrapping and serosal 'corkscrew' vessels. There is creeping extension of mesenteric fat around the serosal surface of the bowel wall towards the anti-mesenteric border. This is part of the connective tissue change that affects all layers of the bowel wall. As inflammation is full thickness, there can be fibrinous exudate and adhesions on the serosal surface. Narrow linear ulcers with intervening islands of oedematous mucosa give the mucosal surface its classic cobblestone appearance. Ulceration is discrete, and serpiginous linear ulcers usually run along the mesenteric aspect of the lumen. Deep fissuring from linear ulceration may lead to formation of fistulas through the bowel wall. Closer inspection may reveal multiple aphthous ulcers that usually develop on the surface of submucosal lymphoid nodules. Aphthous ulcers are the earliest

Table 11.1   Phenotyping Crohn's disease: Montreal classification for Crohn's disease

Age at diagnosis: <17 years (A1); between 17 and 40 years (A2); or ≥40 years (A3 Location of disease:
L1: ileal
L2: colonic
L3: ileocolonic
L4: isolated upper gastrointestinal diseaseBehaviour:
B1: non-stricturing/non-penetrating
B2 stricturing
B3 penetrating

Perianal disease [p] is added if present.
The classification was modified to the Paris classification to include growth failure in a paediatric population.

macroscopic lesions in Crohn's disease and are seen before the classic appearances of more established disease. Inflammatory polyps are often found in the involved colon but are unusual in the small bowel. Enlarged lymph nodes may be present in the resected mesentery but are not caseated or matted together. Strictures can vary in length and may be stiff, like a hosepipe, with turgid oedema, or tight fibrotic strictures from burnt-out inflammation. The narrowing of the lumen may be sufficient to produce obstruction and proximal dilatation, and there may be multiple dilated segments between multiple tight strictures. Fistulas, sinuses and abscesses are often present in the ileocaecal region but may arise from any segment of active disease and can communicate with other loops of bowel, stomach, bladder, vagina, skin or intra-abdominal abscess cavities.

MICROSCOPY

The main questions asked by the histopathologist when assessing an initial biopsy for IBD are;[8]

- Is the mucosa inflamed?
- If the mucosa is inflamed: is it IBD or not?
- If it is IBD: is it ulcerative colitis, Crohn's disease, or IBD unclassified?

Inflammation involves the full thickness of the bowel wall. Early mucosal changes show neutrophils infiltrating the base of crypts, causing injury and focal crypt abscesses. The formation of mucosal lymphoid aggregates followed by overlying ulceration produces aphthous ulcers. Lymphoid follicles may be seen in the base of the mucosa in severe ulcerative colitis, but they are a prominent feature of Crohn's disease, where they are transmural, leading to the formation of a Crohn's 'rosary' on the serosal surface.

In Crohn's disease, there is relative preservation of goblet cell mucin, whereas mucin depletion is a feature of ulcerative colitis (with the exception of fulminant ulcerative colitis, where there may be surprisingly little mucin depletion).

As the disease progresses, connective tissue changes occur in all layers of the bowel wall giving the stiff, thick-walled, macroscopic appearance. There is submucosal fibrosis and muscularisation. The muscularis mucosa and muscularis propria are thickened from increased amounts of connective tissue. Typically, the chronic inflammatory infiltrate and the architectural changes in the mucosa are patchy.

The following three features are diagnostic hallmarks of Crohn's disease:

- deep non-caseating granulomas are present in 60–70% of patients and are commonly located in the bowel wall but also the mesentery, regional lymph nodes, peritoneum, liver or contiguously involved tissue;
- intra-lymphatic granulomas;
- granulomatous vasculitis.

DIFFERENTIATING CROHN'S COLITIS FROM ULCERATIVE COLITIS

Differentiation is important for planning medical and surgical treatment. Consideration of the clinical picture, radiological and endoscopic features and histological findings is essential – with the cumulative evidence informing the diagnosis.

It may be difficult even for an experienced gastrointestinal pathologist to distinguish between Crohn's colitis and ulcerative colitis on histology. No individual histological feature is diagnostic of IBD or a type of IBD but features may be more frequent in one IBD type compared to another. Considerable inter-observer variation is reported. Where the distinction between ulcerative colitis and Crohn's cannot be made, the term IBD-unclassified is used. During the course of the disease, behaviour may change, resulting in a change of diagnosis.

The following histological features favour a diagnosis of Crohn's disease over ulcerative colitis:

- Granuloma (non-cryptolytic)
- Focal or patchy lamina propria chronic inflammation (rather than continuous/diffuse)
- Focal or segmental crypt distortion (rather than continuous/diffuse)
- Ileal involvement.

Rectal sparing may be seen in ulcerative colitis, especially if topical (local) treatment has been used. Treated ulcerative colitis may also demonstrate the patchy changes listed earlier. Perianal disease is very suggestive of Crohn's, although patients with ulcerative colitis can develop cryptoglandular fistulas and abscesses. Established diversion proctitis or pouchitis may also mimic Crohn's disease.

CLINICAL

Clinical features include a typical triad of diarrhoea (70–90%), abdominal pain (45–65%) and weight loss. Perianal disease is an important and debilitating manifestation (30%).

The Crohn's disease phenotype for an individual is described using the Montreal classification – see Table 11.1.

SYSTEMIC SYMPTOMS

Weight loss is reported by 65–75% of patients. This is the result of active inflammation, anorexia, food fear and, less often, malabsorption. The latter may be caused by extensive inflammatory disease but also from bacterial overgrowth as a result of coloenteric fistulas, blind loops or stasis from chronic obstruction. With an aggressive approach to assessment and treatment, these should occur infrequently. If there is extensive small-bowel disease, there may be poor absorption of fat-soluble vitamins leading to symptoms and signs of osteomalacia (vitamin D) or a bleeding tendency (vitamin K). These are all rare. Other deficiencies are also uncommon and usually result from inadequate intake rather than increased losses. They may include deficiencies of magnesium, zinc, ascorbic acid and the B vitamins. Anaemia, however, is common and results from iron deficiency because of impaired iron utilisation or intestinal blood loss and, less commonly, from vitamin B_{12} or folate deficiency. Any fever, particularly if high and spiking, or associated with rigors, should prompt careful consideration of suppurative intra-abdominal complication being present.[9]

GASTROINTESTINAL SYMPTOMS

Clinical presentation varies depending on the site of disease. Initial presentation as an emergency is uncommon, but ileal disease can mimic acute appendicitis and colonic disease may present as a fulminating colitis.

Abdominal pain occurs because of inflammatory disease, obstructing or sub-acutely obstructing lesions. Terminal ileal disease is the most common site for obstructive lesions.

Diarrhoea results most frequently from mucosal inflammation but can also be caused by bile salt malabsorption from terminal ileal disease or resection, fistulation between loops of bowel, short bowel from previous resections or bacterial overgrowth from obstructed segments. Bile salts and vitamin B12 are absorbed from the terminal ileum. Resection of the terminal ileum – or sometimes severe disease at that site – can cause malabsorption of these. Bile salt malabsorption disrupts their enterohepatic circulation and results in a cathartic effect as the bile salts reach the colon causing diarrhoea. This is treated by bile-salt chelating agents such as cholestyramine or colesevelam. B12 replacement injections are usually advised after terminal ileal resection.

Distal colitis and proctitis, and decreased rectal compliance, produce tenesmus and frequent bowel motions. Rectal bleeding may occur in 50% of patients with colonic involvement.

Symptoms can also be those of complications – described in the Montreal classification: stricturing or perforating disease (leading to local abscess formation, internal fistula and fistulae to the skin) (Fig. 11.1).

PERIANAL DISEASE

Perianal disease varies from an asymptomatic fissure or inflamed skin tags, individual fistulas to severe disease with erythema, large fleshy skin tags, deep chronic fissures with bridges of skin and multiple fistulas creating the so-called 'watering-can perineum'. Fibrosis from chronic inflammation may produce a woody, stiff anal canal or anal/rectal stenosis. The impact of perianal disease is underestimated by clinicians and may be underreported by patients. It can present before intestinal disease is apparent.

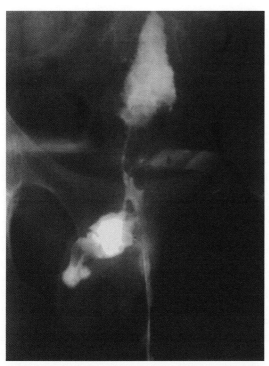

Figure 11.1 Sinogram examination demonstrating an enteroperineal fistula.

Perianal abscesses will present with local pain and swelling – with a discharge if this spontaneously leaks, particularly if there is associated fistulating disease. Perianal fistula can be complex and asymmetrically distributed when compared to idiopathic fistulas. Fistulating disease may cause local discomfort and discharge, which can by mucopurulent, bloody or faeculent. Significant perianal pain suggests undrained sepsis. Fistulas extending to the bladder can produce pneumaturia and recurrent urinary tract infection while those extending to the vagina may cause flatus or faeces vaginally. Fissures may be painful but can be large, indolent and painless.

GASTROINTESTINAL COMPLICATIONS

STRICTURING DISEASE

Chronic fibrosis results in stricturing disease – causing luminal narrowing and clinical features of obstruction. Acute inflammatory change can also contribute to the narrowing. Patients can present with complete obstruction or with milder and self-limiting episodes of sub-acute obstruction. These usually occur in patients known to have Crohn's but rarely can be the initial presenting feature. Differential diagnosis includes adhesions from previous surgery as well as other causes of obstruction, including strictures due to non-steroidal anti-inflammatory drugs.

PERFORATING DISEASE

Transmural inflammation can result in perforation with local abscess formation. Fistulation to a range of other adjacent structures may occur, for example to:

- other loops of adjacent small or large bowel: (enteroenteric, enterocolic fistulas) presenting with diarrhoea relating to reduced transit time and bacterial overgrowth
- bladder (enterovesical or colovesical) – presenting with recurrent urine infection or sterile pyuria
- skin (enterocutaneous)
- vagina (entero-, colo- or rectovaginal fistulas) – presenting with passing gas or faeces per vaginam.

Free perforation with generalised peritonitis can occur but is rare.

COLON CANCER

In Crohn's colitis, there is an increased risk of colorectal cancer similar to ulcerative colitis,[10–12] with similar risk factors: duration of disease and extensive disease. Field change in the colonic mucosa with areas of dysplasia is observed, as in ulcerative colitis.[13] Compared to the general population, the relative risk of adenocarcinoma of the colon complicating Crohn's colitis is 1.4 to 1.9 and the relative risk of small-bowel carcinoma, 21 to 27.[14] Surveillance colonoscopy should be offered, and this is probably best done with dye spray and targeted biopsies. Particular care is needed in the presence of colonic strictures, which should always be regarded as malignant until proven otherwise; this may entail a resection to make the diagnosis.

HAEMORRHAGE

Massive bleeding occurs in 1–2%.

EXTRA-INTESTINAL MANIFESTATIONS

These are outlined in Box 11.1 and are more common in association with Crohn's colitis than isolated small-bowel disease. Manifestations are similar to those that occur in ulcerative colitis, and may precede, be independent of or accompany active IBD, and can cause significant morbidity. They may be experienced by up to 50% of patients and are life-long in 25–30%.

Steatorrhoea may promote increased absorption of oxalate and increase the incidence of oxalate renal stones – though this is usually only after extensive small-bowel resection.

Primary sclerosing cholangitis may be associated with colonic disease. Patients may develop a fatty liver as a result of malnutrition or from receiving total parenteral nutrition. Mild abnormalities of liver function are common with active disease, and do not necessarily indicate significant liver disease.

Thromboembolic complications are an important association of IBD and an important source of morbidity. These are predominantly venous but can be arterial. They can be associated with active disease but there is an increased risk even without active disease. Common sites are the lower extremities and pelvic veins, and pulmonary emboli but cerebrovascular accidents have also been reported.

✔ The increased risk of thromboembolic complications is clinically important, particularly for any hospital admission or after surgery, where extended prophylaxis should be standard.[15,16]

Skin manifestations include erythema nodosum and pyoderma gangrenosum. Appearances are usually typical, but sometimes skin biopsy is needed to confirm the diagnosis. Metastatic Crohn's disease is an unusual complication in which nodular ulcerating skin lesions occur at distant sites including the vulva, sub-mammary areas and extremities, and sometimes peristomal. Biopsies show non-caseating granulomas. Clubbing is seen in some cases of extensive small-bowel disease.

Amyloidosis is reported in 25% of patients with Crohn's disease at post-mortem but only 1% have clinical manifestations. It can occur in the bowel or within other organs, including the liver, spleen and kidneys. If renal function is affected, resection of the diseased bowel may result in regression of amyloid and improvement of renal function.[9]

PHYSICAL SIGNS

Patients may appear well and have a normal physical examination. With more severe disease there may be evidence of weight loss, anaemia, iron deficiency, clubbing, cachexia, proximal myopathy, easy bruising, elevated temperature, tachycardia and peripheral oedema. Signs of extra-intestinal manifestations may be present.

Abdominal examination can be normal but tenderness in the right iliac fossa is common. An abdominal mass may be palpable because of thickened loops of matted bowel or if an abscess is present. A psoas abscess may cause fixed hip flexion (or pain on stepping down). Occasionally, there is general peritonitis. Enterocutaneous fistulas may be evident and may present through a scar.

PAEDIATRIC AGE GROUP

In children and adolescents, the gastrointestinal manifestations are similar but extra-intestinal and systemic manifestations become more important. About 15% have arthralgia and arthritis that often precedes bowel symptoms by months or years. Diagnosis may be delayed by a non-specific presentation with systemic symptoms of weight loss, growth failure, unexplained anaemia and fever. If active disease is dealt with promptly by medical or surgical treatment and adequate nutrition is maintained, retardation of growth and sexual development can usually be reversed.[9]

PREGNANCY

The disease frequently affects young adults and therefore may require management during or before pregnancy. Reduced fertility may have a number of contributing factors including reduced libido, dyspareunia and psychological morbidity. The risk of adverse outcomes in pregnancy is related to disease activity. In the absence of active disease, the outcome of pregnancy is the same as that of matched controls. With active disease at conception, there is an increase in spontaneous abortions and premature delivery, and a greater than 50% chance of relapsing disease during pregnancy. The risk of relapse is only 20–25% if disease is inactive at conception. It is therefore advisable to avoid conception during an acute flare-up. Pregnancy does not affect the long-term course of the disease.

Drug treatment during pregnancy should be discussed – taking into consideration the importance of ensuring optimum disease control. Steroids can be used if necessary. Thiopurines are normally continued during pregnancy as withdrawal may be associated with an increased risk of flare. Biological agents can be continued throughout pregnancy, but the risks and benefits need to be discussed. Withdrawal may carry a risk of poor disease control and therefore adverse pregnancy outcomes. They cross the placenta to the foetus in the third trimester, which therefore carries a risk of immunosuppression in the neonate. Live vaccines must be avoided. Detectable levels of biological drugs may still occur at 9 months. For those with inactive disease who wish to discontinue treatment, it may be reasonable to stop at the start of the third trimester. The use of methotrexate is contraindicated.[17]

INVESTIGATIONS

LABORATORY

Common laboratory findings include raised acute phase proteins (especially C-reactive protein [CRP]) a raised platelet count and anaemia. Mild episodic elevations of liver function tests are common but persistent abnormalities require further investigation. A neutrophil leucocytosis may indicate infection. CRP is used to monitor disease activity but does not necessarily correlate with endoscopic activity and in some patients with active disease is found to be normal. Erythrocyte sedimentation rate is useful in Crohn's colitis but less so in small-bowel disease.

Serum albumin is often low in active disease because of downregulation of albumin synthesis by cytokines (IL-1, IL-6, TNF).

Anti-microbial antibodies particularly anti-*Saccharomyces cervisiae* antibodies (ASCAs) may be raised and if high titres, may suggest a more aggressive phenotype. However, the sensitivity and specificity of such markers are too low for diagnostic purposes.

Stool biomarkers including faecal calprotectin are surrogate markers for intestinal inflammation and are being increasingly used as screening tests to differentiate inflammatory bowel syndrome (IBS) from IBD in primary care, monitoring disease activity and response to treatment and predicting post-operative relapse.[18–20]

Magnesium, zinc and selenium levels may be low.

ENDOSCOPY

Ileocolonoscopy is the first-line investigation for suspected Crohn's disease, particularly as it allows biopsies to support diagnosis. It provides a macroscopic view that can be recorded, enables assessment and biopsy of strictures, and can clarify the situation where significant symptoms are not backed up by clinical evidence of disease. Intubation of the ileocaecal valve allows examination and biopsy of the terminal ileum. It may not always be possible and in about 20% of cases there is isolated proximal small-bowel disease beyond the reach of the colonoscope. Endoscopic appearances are typically discontinuous and include small (<5 mm) aphthous ulcers, larger ulcers, which may be deep and linear fissuring ulcers, which may give a cobblestone appearance. Erythema and loss of vascular pattern may also occur as in ulcerative colitis but differs in usually being discontinuous.

Use of endoscopic scoring systems is essential in randomised clinical trials but could be used in clinical practice to support more consistent reporting. The simplified endoscopic score for Crohn's disease (SES-CD) evaluates ulceration, extent of inflammation and stenosis in five colonic segments.[21] The Rutgeerts score evaluates the extent of ulceration in the neoterminal ileum has proved useful in practice as more severe ulceration predicts clinical recurrence.[22]

Multiple biopsies should be taken even if the mucosa appears normal, as granulomas may be present that can confirm the diagnosis. There is not usually a role for routine follow-up endoscopy (except after surgery) and endoscopic findings correlate poorly with clinical remission. There is a cancer risk in long-standing Crohn's colitis and the same colonoscopic surveillance as for extensive ulcerative colitis is required.

Endoscopy of the upper gastrointestinal tract is indicated only if symptoms suggest upper gastrointestinal involvement from symptoms or imaging. Findings may include rugal hypertrophy, deep longitudinal ulcers and a cobblestone mucosa. Biopsies should be taken but granulomas are often absent.

Small-bowel endoscopy is now possible through video capsule endoscopy or double-balloon assisted enteroscopy.[23] The latter can be undertaken per anum or per orally. It is more invasive and uncomfortable requiring deep sedation or general anaesthetic and with risks that include perforation and pancreatitis but does allow tissue biopsy. Capsule endoscopy is sensitive but does not allow biopsy.[24] Capsule retention may occur if the procedure is undertaken in the presence of a stricture – which may then need surgical retrieval. If there is any significant concern that this may happen, a dummy dissolvable capsule should be used first, to assess luminal patency.

RADIOLOGY

Radiological imaging allows non-invasive assessment of:

- disease activity
- site of disease
- extent of disease
- complications.

Luminal barium fluoroscopic imaging was traditionally the mainstay of radiological investigation but has largely been replaced by cross-sectional imaging (magnetic resonance enterography [MRE] and computerised tomography [CT]). These techniques provide additional transmural information about inflammation or fibrosis and about extramural complications. Choice of modality depends on the clinical question, the clinical setting, local expertise and radiation exposure.[25]

MAGNETIC RESONANCE

MRE is more frequently chosen in the elective, outpatient setting. It is free of ionising radiation and not limited by poor renal function. It helps define whether changes are acute inflammatory or chronic fibrotic. It also identifies extra-luminal complications. Strictures can be identified (Fig. 11.2) aided by dynamic imaging to differentiate fixed narrowing from contractions. Abdominal abscesses can also be identified.

MR imaging (MRI) is also the investigation of choice for complicated perianal sepsis.

COMPUTERISED TOMOGRAPHY SCANNING

CT scanning is often undertaken in the emergency setting. It is frequently used to investigate acute abdominal pain when the diagnosis of Crohn's is suggested by thickened small-bowel loops, especially in the terminal ileum (Fig. 11.3). CT will also demonstrate intra-abdominal abscesses and dilatation in those presenting with obstructive features. Cumulative radiation exposure is an important consideration for people with Crohn's disease who need repeated imaging over many years. If CT enterography is used, a low-dose protocol should be considered.

OTHER IMAGING MODALITIES

High-resolution ultrasound is popular in Europe and may detect inflamed bowel and intra-abdominal abscesses but is operator-dependent.[26]

In severe acute presentations of Crohn's disease, plain abdominal films should be done initially to look for evidence of obstruction, mucosal oedema or dilatation. Plain films

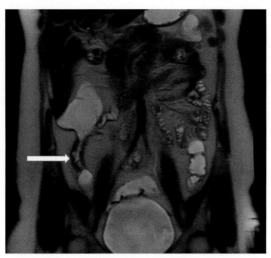

Figure 11.2   Magnetic resonance imaging (MRI) demonstrating structured terminal ileum with thickened bowel wall (*arrow*).

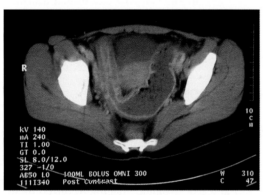

Figure 11.3   Computerised tomography (CT) scan showing thick-walled terminal ileum with proximal dilatation.

can also be useful to identify constipation proximal to a segment of colonic disease.

DISEASE ACTIVITY ASSESSMENT AND QUALITY OF LIFE

There has been a move from using symptoms alone as the measure of clinical remission to supplementing this with non-invasive markers of mucosal healing, particularly faecal calprotectin and CRP.

The IBD Control has been suggested as a patient-reported outcome measure for use in routine practice. It is an easy to use, reliable 8-item measure, which correlates well with other quality of life measures.

The Crohn's Disease Activity Index and the simpler Harvey–Bradshaw index were used to measure outcome in clinical trials, but quality of life and mucosal healing are now more widely used.

Other scoring systems used in clinical trials include the SES-CD, validated MRI scoring systems, Perianal Crohn's Disease Activity index and the Rutgeerts score used specifically to assess recurrent disease in the neo-terminal ileum after surgery.[25]

DIFFERENTIAL DIAGNOSIS

SMALL-BOWEL CROHN'S DISEASE

Box 11.2 shows the differential diagnoses of small-bowel Crohn's disease.

LARGE-BOWEL CROHN'S DISEASE

When there is no small-bowel or perineal involvement, there are two areas where the diagnosis may be difficult. An isolated segment of disease, especially if it is a short segment, has to be differentiated from diverticular disease, carcinoma, ischaemia, tuberculosis and lymphoma. Differentiating Crohn's disease from ulcerative colitis is discussed earlier.

MEDICAL TREATMENT

A summary of the typical medical treatment options for Crohn's disease is given in Box 11.3 based on NICE guidance (NG 129).[27]

Treatment comprises:

- induction of remission followed by
- maintenance of remission.

INDUCTION OF REMISSION

The most effective agents for inducing remission are systemic corticosteroids, which are effective for mild, moderate and severely active Crohn's disease regardless of site and will induce remission in 70–80% of cases. Response should be seen within 2–4 weeks. Prednisolone is usually given at a starting dose of 40 mg tapering by 5 mg weekly. Concomitant bone-protection with calcium and vitamin D should be considered. However, the benefits are accompanied by significant side-effects and prolonged treatment with steroids is considered a disutility of care. Steroid sparing strategies or the use of steroid preparations with fewer side-effects should therefore be considered – particularly in those with mild symptoms.

Oral, controlled ileal release budesonide (through its pH-dependent coating) is effective for distal ileal, ileocolic disease or right-sided colitis. Systemic bioavailability is low because of rapid first-pass metabolism in the liver. It therefore has fewer side-effects but is less effective than systemic corticosteroids. It is an option if a patient declines or cannot tolerate systemic corticosteroids. It should not be used in those with severe symptoms.

Severe disease may require hospital admission and the use of intravenous steroids.

ADDITIONAL TREATMENTS

METHOTREXATE

Methotrexate is effective for induction and maintenance of remission.[28]

Box 11.2 Differential diagnosis of small-bowel Crohn's disease

Differential diagnosis

Appendicitis
Appendix abscess
Caecal diverticulitis
Pelvic inflammatory disease
Ovarian cyst or tumour
Caecal carcinoma
Ileal carcinoid
Behçet's disease
Systemic vasculitis affecting the small bowel
Radiation enteritis
Ileocaecal tuberculosis
Yersinia enterocolitica ileitis
Eosinophilic gastroenteritis
Amyloidosis
Small-bowel lymphoma
Actinomycosis
Chronic non-granulomatous jejuno-ileitis

Useful discriminating features

History, computerised tomography (CT) scan
History, ultrasound/CT scan
Older age, colonoscopy
History
Ultrasound
CT colonography/colonoscopy
Small-bowel enema
Painful ulceration of the mouth and genitalia
Underlying systemic connective tissue disorder
History of radiotherapy
History of tuberculosis, circulating antibodies to *Mycobacterium*, stool cultures
Self-limiting, stool cultures, serology
Gastric involvement, peripheral eosinophilia
Biopsy
Radiological appearance
Microscopy of fine-needle aspirate
Clinical picture and histology

Box 11.3 Summary of medical treatment options for Crohn's disease (based on NICE guidance [NG 129][25])

Induction of remission

Mild to moderate disease

Prednisone 40 mg daily reducing by 5 mg/day each week (consider bone protecting agent)
Ileal and/or right colon: budesonide 9 mg per day
Exclusive enteral nutrition
Additional treatments
Infliximab, adalimumab
Vedolizumab,
Ustekinumab
Methotrexate

Perianal disease:

Metronidazole 400 mg t.d.s. or ciprofloxacin 500 mg b.d.
Ensure sepsis drained
Anti-tumour necrosis factor agent – infliximab preferred

Severe disease

Intravenous hydrocortisone 100 mg qds
Infliximab, adalimumab (second-line)
Maintenance of remission
Immunomodulators: azathioprine, 6-mercaptopurine, methotrexate,
Biologic agents: infliximab or adalimumab, vedolizumab, ustekinumab

AMINOSALICYLATES

Aminosalicylates are not effective in Crohn's disease.[29]

BIOLOGIC AGENTS

The term *'biological agent"* includes monoclonal antibodies targeted at mediators of the inflammatory response. Biological agents in current use are effective for both induction and maintenance of remission. They are used for disease refractory to 'conventional' treatment including steroids and immunosuppression. Costs associated with infliximab and adalimumab have been significantly reduced by the adoption of biosimilar versions – molecules that have no meaningful differences from the original therapeutic molecule in terms of quality (structure), safety and efficacy potentially making them more accessible to a wider number of patients.[30]

ANTI-TNF AGENTS

Infliximab is a mouse–human chimeric monoclonal antibody administered by intravenous infusion or subcutaneous injection. Adalimumab is a human monoclonal antibody to TNF-α administered by subcutaneous injection.

Pivotal randomised controlled trials (RCTs) have demonstrated the benefit compared to placebo for inducing remission, particularly in those with disease refractory to systemic steroids, for maintaining remission and for causing mucosal healing. The drugs reduce the need for hospitalisation and surgery during follow-up. The SONIC trial demonstrated that combined use of thiopurine and anti-TNF agents was more effective than either agent alone for people with recent onset Crohn's naïve to anti-TNF or immunomodulator treatment.[31]

The drugs are generally well tolerated but side-effects include an increased risk of infection and lymphoma, particularly if used as combination therapy. In particular, there is a risk of reactivation of latent tuberculosis. All patients starting anti-TNF medication should have investigations that include interferon gamma release assays for tuberculosis, chest x-ray and serological screening for hepatitis B and C and human immunodeficiency virus. It is essential that sepsis at any site is treated before starting this medication. Skin reactions such as a psoriasiform eruption can occur.

Biological drugs have the potential for immunogenicity potentially leading to loss of response over time. Therapeutic drug concentration monitoring of biologicals to optimise dosing, including anti-drug antibody levels, (personalised therapy) is becoming increasingly important and the addition of an immunosuppressor may have a role in lowering these antibody levels.[31]

✅✅ The ACCENT I study addressed the maintenance of remission with a year of treatment with infliximab. After an initial infusion, 58% responded. The responders were then randomised to placebo or infliximab at 2 and 6 weeks and then 8-weekly up to 54 weeks. At week 54 of initial responders, about 15% in the placebo group and 35% in the treatment group were in clinical remission.[32]

Similar results with initial moderate efficacy have been demonstrated using infliximab to treat fistulas. The ACCENT II study recruited patients with perianal (90%) and enterocutaneous draining fistulas. The primary endpoint of the study was a reduction in the number of fistulas by 50% or more. After three infusions at 0, 2 and 6 weeks, the study randomised responders at week 14 to placebo or infliximab infusions 8-weekly to week 54. The primary endpoint was loss of response, with fistulas re-activating or re-appearing. Of 306 patients enrolled, 195 (64%) responders were randomised at week 14. At week 54, about 30% of patients treated with infliximab maintained a response at 1 year, 22% having a complete response. In the placebo group after initial infliximab response, 19% had a complete response.[33] The efficacy at 1 year judged by complete response is therefore modest.

Adalimumab (a human anti-TNF monoclonal antibody) has been evaluated in the CLASSIC I and II[34,35] and CHARM studies[36] and has similar efficacy to infliximab. If an individual develops anti-drug antibodies to one of these agents, with loss of response following initial response (secondary loss of response), then treatment with the other can be tried. Following primary non-response to an anti-TNF agent, treatment would usually be switched to a different class of agent.

The CHARM study looked at maintenance therapy with adalimumab for 12 months using hospitalisation as an endpoint. After induction, all patients were randomised to adalimumab or placebo. The Crohn's-related hospitalisation rate at 12 months was 8.4% on adalimumab and 15.5% on placebo. This means 14 patients are treated to prevent one admission. The study also looked at surgery rates. Three of 517 patients who had adalimumab and 10 of 261 who had placebo required major Crohn's-related surgery in the 12 months. Rates of surgery were higher but the follow-up is short.

The SONIC trial showed infliximab as a monotherapy or in combination with azathioprine was more effective in inducing steroid-free remission and mucosal healing than azathioprine alone in those with relatively recent onset of disease who had previously been naïve to anti-TNF or thiopurines.[31] Therefore for patients with predictors of more severe disease, there is probably an advantage to a top down approach and introduction of a biological agent early, with or without azathioprine.

ANTI-INTEGRIN AGENTS: VEDOLIZUMAB

Vedolizumab is an intravenous monoclonal antibody that blocks α4β7 integrin, resulting in a gut specific effect, reducing lymphocyte traffic to the intestinal mucosa. It is indicated for those where anti-TNF therapy has been unsuccessful or who were intolerant or lost response. Because of the gut-specific effect associated with less systemic immunosuppression, it may have a particular role in the elderly or those with a contraindication to anti-TNF or thiopurines (such as

previous cancers). Benefit may not be seen until week 14 of treatment.

The GEMINI-2 trial demonstrated more patients in remission after induction with vedolizumab and at 1 year than those receiving placebo.[37] It is administered by intravenous infusion, but a subcutaneous formulation is also now available.

ANTI-IL12-23 AGENTS: USTEKINUMAB

Ustekinumab is a monoclonal antibody directed against interleukin 12 and 23 and is an option for moderately active disease where there has been an inadequate response, loss of response to or intolerance of conventional therapies including anti-TNF agents – or where they are not suitable.

In the UNITI-1 trial of patients who met the criteria for primary or secondary non-response to anti-TNF agents or had unacceptable side effects and the UNITI-2 trial of those where conventional therapy failed or unacceptable side effects occurred and follow-up maintenance in the UNITI-IM trial, there was a greater response to ustekinumab than placebo and more patients in remission at a year at 53% (for the 8 weekly dosing).[38] After an initial intravenous infusion, the drug is administered by subcutaneous injection.

MAINTENANCE THERAPY

This includes the use of biological agents described earlier.

Steroids do not have a role in maintenance of remission because of unacceptable side-effects and are ineffective. Prolonged use beyond 3 months is considered a disutility of care. Initiation of a steroid sparing strategy such as thiopurines or methotrexate is required when a patient has received two courses of steroids in 12 months and may be considered for disease with adverse prognostic features. Biological agents may be part of such a strategy.

THIOPURINES

Azathioprine and 6-mercaptopurine are purine analogues, azathioprine being metabolised non-enzymatically to 6-mercaptopurine. They inhibit cell proliferation and suppress cell-mediated events by inhibiting the activity of cytotoxic T cells and natural killer cells.

Thiopurines are used as steroid sparing agents, typically if an individual has required two or more courses of steroids in a year or following a severe episode. They should also be considered in those with features suggesting a more debilitating course (Box 11.4). The onset of therapeutic effect takes at least 6 weeks.

It is mandatory to test thiopurine methyl activity before starting a thiopurine.[25] A significant proportion of toxicity, and possibly lack of efficacy, can be caused by genetic variability in the metabolism of azathioprine. Subsequently, metabolite monitoring may help guide dosing. Toxicity occurs in 20–30%, including 3–15% of patients who develop pancreatitis. Furthermore, there is an associated increased risk of malignancy and so caution is needed in young males, patients with negative serology for Epstein Barr virus and patients over 60 years old.

More detailed guidance is available in the British Society of Gastroenterology guidelines[23] and UK National Institute for Health and Care Excellence (NICE) guidelines.[27]

EFFECT OF MEDICAL TREATMENT ON SURGICAL OUTCOMES[39]

As the majority of patients will undergo intestinal resection, there is obviously concern about the effect of drugs with immunosuppressive effect on surgical outcomes. It may be difficult to significantly alter medication, but the risks should be considered in timing of intervention and before starting drugs in a patient where surgery is inevitable or imminent.

Systemic corticosteroids are associated with an increased risk of surgical site infections, and intra-abdominal sepsis. Wound and anastomotic healing may also be impaired.

Thiopurines and methotrexate are not associated with an increased risk of infective complications after resection.

The literature for anti-TNF agents is conflicting, but confounding factors – particularly relating to disease severity and complications seem likely to influence outcomes. A pragmatic approach is to try to time surgery mid-way between doses to allow drug levels to be lower and to minimise delay of the next dose if needed.

Despite its gut selectivity, an increased risk of surgical site infection with vedolizumab has been reported,[40] but may represent the severity of the case mix in this series. Other studies have not shown an increase in risk.[41]

At present, studies do not show an increased risk in ustekinumab-treated patients following surgery.

It is well recognised that corticosteroids increase the risk of post-operative complications. Whenever possible, dose reduction should occur before surgery, certainly to below 20 mg/day for prednisolone but preferably below 10 mg/day.[42]

Where clinical circumstances permit, biological therapies should probably not be administered for 14–30 days before any planned elective surgery for Crohn's disease to reduce the incidence of infective complications and possibly anastomotic leak. However, evidence is currently poor and there is little evidence of increased post-operative complications relating to biologic agents.[39,42]

MULTI-DISCIPLINARY CARE

For the best outcomes, and for the safe and effective care of patients with IBD, multi-disciplinary care is recommended. It allows for optimal care and a personalised approach based on available expertise, infrastructure and funding. The increasing complexity of medical management combined with the need for surgical intervention at all stages of the disease process make this aspect of service delivery increasingly essential. Whilst no strong evidence base supports this recommendation, it is deemed good practice by NICE quality standards and by expert opinion.[23,43]

Meta-analyses have demonstrated the efficacy of controlled ileal release budesonide over placebo in inducing remission in Crohn's disease.[44,45] It is less effective than systemically absorbed steroids but associated with fewer side-effects.

Total parenteral nutrition is effective in inducing remission in 60–80% of patients, which matches the effect of steroids, but combining therapies gives no added benefit. Relapse rates are high after cessation. In children, exclusive enteral nutrition using elemental or polymeric formulae may have an important role as an alternative to systemic corticosteroids. The role of such diets in adults is more controversial and needs further research – including in optimising patients before surgery.[27]

OVERALL MANAGEMENT STRATEGIES IN CROHN'S DISEASE

There has been increasing attention to the overall approach to treatment – particularly medical treatment and with a focus on endpoints that go beyond symptomatic response alone. This has been prompted by the benefits that seem to derive from achieving mucosal healing. Symptoms do not correlate well with mucosal appearances, but mucosal healing is associated with reduced need for surgery and hospitalisation. Strategies have therefore been evaluated to try to maximise these benefits.

ADVERSE PROGNOSTIC FEATURES

Some clinical features may predict a more debilitating course (see Box 11.4). These features may lead to an earlier use of biological agents.

TOP-DOWN

The Step-up/top-down trial run by D'Haens[46] evaluated early combined immunosuppression (Top-down) using infliximab and azathioprine compared to azathioprine alone and additional treatment if necessary (step-up), to try to change the natural history of the disease. The benefit for top-down treatment was greatest earlier in the trial and was less evident by 104 weeks.

TREAT TO TARGET

Mucosal healing is associated with improved outcomes including quality of life, hospitalisation and need for surgery – but correlates poorly with symptoms. As a result, the concept of using this as a treatment aim has evolved.

The CALM study evaluated a strategy of treating to a target of mucosal healing – represented by faecal calprotectin47 ≥250 µg/g and/or CRP ≥5 mg/L in combination with clinical features. This approach resulted in better clinical and endoscopic outcomes than using symptoms alone.

Endoscopic recurrence after ileocaecal resection predicts future clinical relapse. This is used in a treat to target strategy in the POCER trial[48] (see later).

Box 11.4 Features of Crohn's Disease suggesting a more debilitating course

Extensive disease
Colonic disease
Perianal disease
Young age at diagnosis
Perforating disease (abscess, fistulas, involvement of adjacent structures)
Smoking
The need for steroids at presentation

USE OF CD8+ MARKERS

The ability to predict those who may run a more debilitating and aggressive course of Crohn's disease would allow targeting of more aggressive immunosuppression to such individuals. Carriage of a particular T cell signature of CD8+ cells has been associated with such a clinical course and the PROFILE trial is currently in progress to assess use of this blood profile in escalating treatment.

DRUG WITHDRAWAL

The optimum duration of anti-TNF therapy is not known. Withdrawal of anti-TNF agents has been shown to be associated with a relapse rate of about one third in the year after withdrawal. As we move into an era of early diagnosis and early aggressive intervention with complex combinations of potent and expensive drugs, de-escalation strategies will have to be developed where the risk is reduced.

EARLY SURGERY

Recent evidence points to consideration for early surgery being a good alternative to anti-TNF therapy for limited terminal ileal Crohn's.[49]

POST-OPERATIVE PROPHYLAXIS

Following ileocaecal resection, endoscopic recurrence is frequent. Symptomatic recurrence may occur in 20% at 1 year and 47% at 5 years.[50]

Smoking cessation will halve the rate of recurrence and remains the most important advice to give a patient after surgery.[51] Medical treatment may also reduce the rate of recurrence.

Currently, metronidazole for 3 months should be considered for all patients post-ileocolonic resection.[52] It is poorly tolerated (about 25% will stop therapy) but low-dose regimes may be better tolerated. Long-term treatment can be associated with neuropathic complications and patients should be warned to report symptoms of this.

The role of thiopurines remains controversial. The TOPPIC trial suggested a benefit for mercaptopurine,[53] but this was only clearly demonstrated in smokers and a previous Cochrane review showed low-quality evidence of benefit.[54]

A reduction in clinical recurrence has been less clearly demonstrated for anti-TNF agents but reduced clinical and endoscopic recurrence has been shown.[55] Adalimumab was used in thiopurine intolerant patients in the algorithm used in the POCER study (see Box 11.3). Benefit may also be less if anti-TNF use has been unsuccessful in the past.

Therefore in those considered high risk for recurrence (smoker, penetrating disease, multiple resections, perianal disease, extensive small-bowel disease, residual active disease) introduction of a thiopurine (or anti-TNF therapy if intolerant) should be considered.

The benefit of newer agents, vedolizumab and ustekinumab, compared to placebo or other agents remains to be established. Whilst in the past mesalazine was recommended, the evidence of benefit is poor and no longer recommended after ileocolonic resection.

✔✔ All patients undergoing ileocolic resection should have a colonoscopy 6–12 months after surgery with escalation of post-operative therapy for those who show evidence of endoscopic recurrence. The POCER trial compared active care using endoscopic assessment at 6 months post-operatively with standard care. All patients received metronidazole for 3 months and those at high risk of recurrence (smoker, perforating disease or previous resection) received thiopurines (or adalimumab if thiopurine intolerant). In the active group, treatment was stepped up based on endoscopic appearances at 6 months. After 18 months endoscopic recurrence was significantly lower 49% in the active group (49%) than in the standard care group (67%).[48]

OTHER DRUGS

Anti-diarrhoeal medication and anti-cholinergic agents to relieve colicky pain are useful in mild to moderate disease but should be avoided in severe exacerbations. Nonsteroidal anti-inflammatory drugs should also be avoided as they may make the disease worse, and opioids can increase bowel spasm. Bile salt chelating agents (cholestyramine, colestipol, colesevelam) are used to treat bile salt diarrhoea.

Antibiotics – most commonly metronidazole and ciprofloxacin – are used to treat perianal disease. They may reduce fistula discharge but probably have little impact on closure rates, and symptoms often return after cessation. Long-term use of metronidazole is contraindicated because of the risk of peripheral neuropathy.

The rationale for nutritional therapy is that elements of a normal diet may drive the inflammatory response and their removal will induce remission. Exclusive enteral nutrition reduces potential antigens by delivering a simplified calorific intake. Exclusive enteral nutrition is used as an alternative to conventional corticosteroids to induce remission for children or young people in whom there is concern about growth or side effects and is considered by some to be first-line treatment, improving nutrition and benefitting growth.[56] In adults, the benefits are less clear but it is occasionally used where corticosteroids are contraindicated. Patient motivation is important as the diet is difficult to sustain and mucosal healing may take up to 8 weeks.[57]

SURGERY

GENERAL PRINCIPLES

Surgery has radically changed over the last 80 years. Crohn initially described radical resection of involved segments of bowel, but high recurrence rates and the danger of short-bowel syndrome led to an era of bypassing affected segments. Frequent complications with the bypassed segments led to a return to more conservative resectional surgery. More recently, the advantages of minimal access have been recognised. Current surgery is based on these concepts along with careful discussion around the timing of surgery, pre-operative preparation, attention to surgical technique and post-operative monitoring/adjuvant medical therapy to achieve the best outcomes in terms of complications and recurrence.

OUTCOMES AFTER SURGERY

Accurate population figures about patterns of disease and complications are not easy to obtain. Many of the data are from specialist centres and may not always extrapolate to the Crohn's population at large. Often quoted data from a large Swedish cohort indicate a cumulative rate of intestinal resection of 44%, 61% and 71% at 1, 5 and 10 years, respectively, after diagnosis; the subsequent risk of recurrence was 33% and 44% at 5 and 10 years, respectively.[48] Current population based studies suggest the likelihood of bowel resection has decreased during the 21st century, with the rate of primary surgery around 50%.[58,59] It unfortunately remains the case that many patients still require multiple operations in their lifetime. Intestinal failure is the feared ultimate complication of surgery. Whilst often regarded to result from sequential bowel resection because of relapsing disease, the most common cause of this end-stage condition is in fact septic complications after surgery. The incidence from a large multicenter cohort study of 1700 patients is estimated at 0.8%, 3.6% and 8.5% at 5, 10 and 20 years after surgery, respectively.[60]

PRE-OPERATIVE OPTIMISATION

Timing of surgery is crucial in both emergency and elective settings. Patients should be optimised as much as possible. This requires resolution of sepsis using both radiological and antibiotic intervention, reversal of any nutritional compromise and reducing or eliminating immunosuppressant treatment (particularly steroids) whilst maintaining disease quiescence. Surgery should be timed to coincide with the small window when these parameters are achieved. If these goals cannot be achieved, consideration should be given to a temporary stoma rather than an anastomosis.[61] In such cases, early involvement of a stoma therapist is paramount. Stoma site marking and counselling having been shown to improve rehabilitation and adaptation of the patient and reduce post-operative complications compared with those not seen or marked.[62,63] Deep vein thrombosis prophylaxis using higher prophylactic doses of low-molecular-weight heparin, compression stockings and intermittent calf compression devices is important as patients with IBD are at higher risk of thrombotic complications.[64] Joint management in a multi-disciplinary team is an essential principle in the decision-making and hospital and post-discharge care. Psychological well-being always needs addressing because of the chronic nature of the disease.

INTRA-OPERATIVE CONSIDERATIONS

TECHNIQUE

Patients with Crohn's disease can be among the most technically difficult cases a surgeon will face. Compromise of good technique can be unforgiving. Any part of the bowel can be affected or involved with Crohn's disease. If there is any doubt, the patient should be placed in lithotomy. For laparoscopic surgery, many surgeons mobilise the bowel intracorporally, with mesenteric resection and anastomosis carried out through a small utility incision. For open surgery, a midline infra-umbilical incision gives good access, is more easily re-opened in the future and will not interfere with stomas that may be needed on either side of the abdomen. At each operation, a full examination of the bowel should be carried out to stage the disease and the length of remaining and resected bowel measured.

✔ Thick oedematous vascular mesenteric pedicles require special mention. A standard clamp and tie technique may allow a vessel to retract into the mesentery, resulting in a mesenteric haematoma with potential to compromise the blood supply to large segments of bowel. Thick pedicles should be dealt with very carefully and some recommend double-suture ligation. Spillage of gastrointestinal contents must be minimised and controlled, and meticulous haemostasis is important as there may be inevitable loss from oozing, inflamed, raw surfaces. More recent tissue sealing devices may be used but the same precaution should be taken with a low threshold for under-running the resected edges. Great care should be taken not to damage or perforate other loops of bowel or other organs in the presence of difficult adhesions and inflammation.

✔ A modern surgical concept is that of minimal access. Laparoscopy is the preferred surgical approach, particularly for primary procedures as it results in quicker recovery, earlier mobilisation, lower incidence of adhesions, incisional hernia and wound infection as well as offering better cosmesis.[65] Despite these advantages, many operations are still done through open access. This may relate to complex disease or recurrent surgery where the challenges of laparoscopy are greater and the benefits unproven. Certainly, laparoscopy in these patient groups is possible and safe in experienced hands, but there must be a low threshold for early conversion.[66,67]

EXTENT OF RESECTION

✔ Current surgery for Crohn's disease involves resecting the least amount of bowel to re-establish satisfactory intestinal function. This is based on the concept that Crohn's is a gut-wide disease and that microscopic disease at the resection margin does not influence recurrence of disease.[68,69]

A recent school of thought emphasises the mesentery as the driver of disease in Crohn's disease and that it should be an additional surgical target to reduce recurrence.[70,71] Whilst current surgical techniques either conserve the mesentery or more commonly recommend resection along the edge of the thickened mesentery, there may be a role for a more radical oncological type resection. This may not be easy if the thickening is extensive. Further research is probably required before this is considered standard practice.

ANASTOMOSIS

When considering the type of anastomosis, two outcomes are of importance; safety and recurrence of Crohn's. Several meta-analyses have assessed the different types of anastomoses according to these outcomes. The most recent data favour a stapled side-to side technique as the option that has the lowest overall rate of post-operative complications (especially anastomotic leak) as well as a decreased recurrence and re-operation rate.[72–74] However, data are conflicting and only refer to primary surgical procedures. Anastomotic technique should therefore be governed by surgical preference, using meticulous technique to achieve a well vascularised intact wide anastomosis.

The ultimate method of bowel preservation is the stricturoplasty (see later). A remarkable observation regarding stricturoplasty is the low rate of site-specific recurrence, seen in only 3% of patients in a large systematic review.[75] One underlying theory as to this low recurrence is the fact that the 'anastomosis' is carried out on the anti-mesenteric border of the bowel. This is one of the principles behind a new technique known as the Kono-S anastomosis. In addition to a totally anti-mesenteric anastomosis, the technique involves a supporting column and isolation of the join from the ligated edge of the mesentery. A recent systematic review including one RCT has demonstrated a remarkably low level of endoscopic and surgical recurrence.[76] Further evidence is required to confirm these results.

✔✔ There is insufficient evidence to suggest an association between anastomotic technique and the incidence of recurrence. Promising alternative techniques require further assessment.[40]

POST-OPERATIVE CONSIDERATIONS

Rates of post-operative thromboembolism are consistently around 2.5–3.5% in these patients and are a major reason for re-admission.[77] The need for 28 days of extended prophylaxis has already been highlighted. Patients on high doses of pre-operative steroids will often be at risk of adrenal suppression and the need for steroid cover should be considered. Smoking cessation should be encouraged, and use of metronidazole has been covered earlier. Involvement of a gastroenterologist in the follow-up period should be standard, with additional medical therapy dictated by endoscopic assessment at 6–12 months.

✔ Continuing to smoke after a surgical resection doubles the risk of recurrence and patients must be urged to stop smoking.[52] As mentioned earlier, prophylactic treatment should be discussed with patients, especially if still smoking.

OTHER FACTORS THAT MAY REDUCE RECURRENCE

Many studies have looked at risk factors for recurrence. Recurrence can be defined by radiological findings, endoscopic findings, the return of symptoms or the need for further surgery. Most studies have been retrospective, and although some claim to identify risk factors, others report no association for the same risk factor. There is no consistently robust evidence that age of onset of disease, gender, site of disease, number of resections, length of small-bowel resection, proximal margin length, microscopic disease at the resection margin, fistulising versus stricturing disease, number of sites of disease, presence of granulomas, blood transfusion or genetic markers have an important impact on recurrence.[78,79]

SITE SPECIFIC CONSIDERATIONS

GASTRODUODENAL DISEASE

Symptomatic gastroduodenal disease is present in 0.5–4% of patients and is usually associated with disease in other sites. The first and second parts of the duodenum are most commonly involved, leading to stricturing, bleeding and pain from ulceration. Often it is difficult at endoscopy to differentiate Crohn's from peptic ulcer disease, but a trial of medical ulcer therapy may help. A common presentation is obstruction related to stricturing. Strictures are often short and therefore amenable to balloon dilatation. Most series describe 60–80% success rates but repeat dilatation is often required and there is a 1–2% risk of perforation. Nevertheless, this remains the first-line treatment.[80] If balloon dilatation fails gastrojejunostomy is indicated. Whilst historically vagotomy was often added to reduce stomal ulceration, proton pump inhibitors allow the potential side-effects of vagotomy to be avoided.

In selected cases, stricturoplasty may be considered, leading to better function but results are variable and complications can be significant.[81,82] Massive acute upper gastrointestinal bleeding is rare, but if endoscopic methods are unsuccessful, bleeding should be controlled by underrunning. Fistulas involving the duodenum occur in 0.5% of patients with Crohn's disease and generally arise from other diseased segments fistulating into the duodenum. Surgical therapy is usually successful, and prognosis relates to the severity of disease in the primary segment. Closure of secondary duodenal defects with a jejunal serosal patch or Roux-en-Y limb may be preferable to primary suture.

SMALL BOWEL AND ILEOCAECAL DISEASE

INDICATIONS FOR SURGERY

The commonest indication for surgery in this group is failure of medical management. This can be caused by primary non-response or subsequent loss of response. Surgery may also be indicated in medical non-compliance or when complications arise. There are caveats to the concept of initial medical management. In a patient with obstructive symptoms and signs with underlying fibrosis, medical therapy is less likely to work, and surgery should be considered earlier. Some argue that early surgery is indicated before escalation of medical therapy regardless. They point to the fact that up to 80% of patients treated medically will need surgery within 5 years[83] and the morbidity of protracted medical therapy is not insignificant. Often, patients who come to surgery, having received protracted medical therapy have more complex disease and are more likely to suffer with surgical complications. In contrast, whilst some patients who undergo primary surgery may develop recurrent disease, 50% will be symptom free at 10 years and two-thirds will avoid further surgery.[84] Clearly the decision to opt for medical or surgical therapy requires a shared decision-making process between the gstaroenterologist, the surgeon and the patient. Whilst one might consider patients always opt for medication initially, this may not necessarily be the case. A survey of patients who had undergone ileocaecal resection revealed that about three-quarters wished they had had surgery earlier.[85]

✔ The LIRIC trial randomised patients who developed recurrent disease after initial medical treatment (steroids +/- azathioprine) into either receiving infliximab therapy or undergoing laparoscopic ileocaecal resection.[86] Quality of life was similar between the two groups at 12 months. After a median of 63 months follow-up, 26% of the surgical group had started anti-TNF therapy and no patient required a second resection. In the infliximab group, 48% underwent resection and the remainder maintained, switched or escalated their medical therapy.[50]

Growth retardation is the commonest extra-intestinal manifestation of Crohn's disease in children and adolescents. Whilst medical management includes nutritional support and immunomodulators, surgery may be indicated, with catch up growth usually occurring within 6 months of surgery.[87]

ENDOSCOPIC BALLOON DILATATION

Balloon dilatation is an alternative to surgery in some patients with stricturing disease.[72] Suitable patients are determined by the characteristics of the stricture; it should be accessible to the endoscope, short (<5 cm) and not angulated. There are risks associated with this intervention, including failure to completely dilate, perforation and bleeding in the short term, and recurrence in the longer term.

✔ A recent meta-analysis suggests that the therapeutic response to endoscopic balloon dilatation is up to 70% with a 5–8% complication rate. However, it should be emphasised that endoscopic dilatation is essentially a short-term solution to symptoms with 75% of patients undergoing surgery within 5 years.[80]

SURGICAL MANAGEMENT OF STRICTURING DISEASE

If there is isolated small-bowel disease, it is most commonly in the terminal ileum and is usually suited to a limited resection. More extensive disease can produce strictures throughout the small bowel. In the past, patients requiring surgery had multiple resections, with a risk of short-bowel syndrome. In an endeavour to maximise conservation of bowel length, the concept of stricturoplasty was introduced. It is ideally suited to short fibrotic strictures, but it may be used for strictures up to 25-cm long. Long strictures with active inflammation are usually better managed with resection unless there is concern about bowel length because of previous resections. In most series, half the patients having a stricturoplasty will also have a segmental resection.

The Heineke–Mikulicz technique is usually used for strictures <10 cm. In cases with longer strictures (10–25 cm) where bowel conservation is required, a Finney or Jaboulay stricturoplasty may be used. For even longer narrowed segments (>25 cm) a side-to-side isoperistaltic technique described by Michelassi may be used.[88] Here the diseased bowel is divided at its midpoint and opened on the antimesenteric border, the ends spatulated, the proximal and distal ends advanced so that the diseased segments lie side by side, where they are anastomosed to each other, trying to ensure stenotic segments are complemented with dilated segments. Despite often long suture lines, results are similar to other stricturoplasty techniques.

To ensure no significant strictures have been missed, a Foley catheter or ball should be passed along the small bowel through an enterotomy. Using a catheter, the balloon is inflated with a measured amount of saline to a diameter of 25 mm and pulled back through the bowel, allowing occult strictures to be identified. Alternatively, a 25-mm marble or stainless-steel ball can be traced through the bowel to identify strictures. The ball technique perhaps enables better control of spillage of bowel content, but a stricture cannot be passed until it has been corrected, whereas a balloon can be deflated.

Results of stricturoplasty have proved it to be safe and effective. Overall morbidity is 10–20%. Post-operative abdominal septic complications occur in 5–10%, and overall, 98–99% gain symptomatic relief. Post-operative bleeding occurs in about 3% of patients, but usually resolves with conservative measures. Recurrence requiring re-operation is about 30% at 5 years and rates are similar whether or not a limited resection is included. The re-operation rates are similar after first, second and third recurrences requiring surgery. Fewer than 10% of stricturoplasties themselves re-stricture, most of the recurrent disease instead occurring at new sites.[89]

CROHN'S RELATED ABSCESSES

Crohn's disease results in transmural inflammation with deep fissuring. In some this may result in abscess formation. Whilst surgical drainage may be indicated, there is an increasing trend to manage such patients medically at least initially. Percutaneous drainage and antibiotics forms part of the optimisation principle mentioned earlier, allowing safer surgery with an increased likelihood of restoration of bowel continuity at initial surgery. In 30% the abscess completely resolves[88,90] and the question becomes whether subsequent resection should occur or whether medical therapy is continued. Currently, there is insufficient evidence to guide which management is best. In this situation, a shared decision approach is indicated with the risks of immunosuppression and the benefits of avoiding surgery discussed with each patient.

ENTERIC FISTULAS

The transmural inflammation may, in 30% of patients with certain disease phenotypes, result in fistulation. Often fistulation is to other organs including other small bowel loops, colon (especially sigmoid colon) bladder and duodenum. Some fistulas are asymptomatic, but others may result in diarrhoea, abdominal pain, weight loss and in the case of bladder fistulation, urinary tract infections. The principal target for surgery is the diseased bowel. Often the recipient organ can simply be repaired rather than resected.

Enterocutaneous fistulas may occur as a primary manifestation of disease, especially after percutaneous abscess drainage. Whilst medical management can be considered,[33] many patients require surgery to resect the diseased bowel and debride the fistula tract. Around a quarter of enterocutaneous fistulas result from anastomotic failure.[91] Many such patients require aggressive and coordinated multidisciplinary management with drainage of sepsis, correction of electrolyte abnormalities, nutritional support and wound care followed by surgical resection once the patient is optimised. It is very important not to operate too soon. A wait of at least 6 weeks is imperative and, on occasions spontaneous closure may occur especially if low output. Before surgery carry out careful radiological workup to define the extent of intestinal disease, exclude any obstructing lesions and delineate the fistula tracts. The management of these patients can be summarised with the useful acronym 'SNAP' (Sepsis and Skin care, Nutrition, intestinal Anatomy and surgical Procedure). Enterocutaneous fistulation is considered in more detail in Chapter 12.

✔ There has been a vogue for using somatostatin analogues to decrease fistula output but it has shown no benefit.[92] Some may still argue to use it for very high volume proximal fistulas, which were not part of this trial.

SURGERY FOR COLONIC AND RECTAL CROHN'S DISEASE

INDICATIONS

The most common indication for colonic surgery is intractable disease that is not controlled with medical therapy. The need for surgery and the choice of operation depends on extent of the disease. About one-third of patients will have segmental disease, a third left-sided disease and a third total colitis. Overall, a third will have associated perianal disease. After 10 years about half will have had surgery and a quarter will have an ileostomy.[93] Many of those with severe colitis will settle with medical treatment. However, half of these patients will require colectomy within 1–2 years.[92]

EMERGENCY COLECTOMY AND COLECTOMY AND ILEOSTOMY

Acute colectomy for Crohn's disease constitutes a small portion of operations for acute Crohn's disease. Indications include toxic dilatation, haemorrhage, perforation and severe colitis not responding to medical therapy. If medical treatment for acute severe colitis brings a response in 48–72

hours and urgent surgery is avoided, early elective colectomy should be considered as the chance of recurrent toxic colitis in the following years is significant and symptomatic control is often poor. Severe haemorrhage and perforation both occur in about 1% of patients with colitis. Urgent surgery is again a total colectomy and ileostomy.

Subsequent preservation of the rectum is more likely in Crohn's colitis than in ulcerative colitis as there may be rectal sparing or rectal disease may respond to medical therapy. This may allow for restoration of bowel continuity with an ileorectal anastomosis. However, a completion proctectomy is required if there is significant associated perianal fistulating disease, or stricturing or active proctitis not responding to treatment. In addition, many recommend resection if there has been associated colonic or rectal dysplasia.[42] Completion proctectomy is usually left until the patient is in good health. If the rectum is retained long term, there is a risk of cancer and surveillance is required.

For those that undergo ileorectal anastomosis, clinical recurrence is reported in 50% at 10 years. Of those who lose their ileorectal anastomosis, many will still have obtained 4–5 years of useful function, particularly important if a stoma is deferred for teenage and young adult years. At 10 years, over half will retain their rectum. The development of perianal disease usually leads to proctectomy.

In exceptional cases of Crohn's colitis, a loop ileostomy may be used to defunction the bowel, allowing clinical improvement in over 80%. Half will be able to have the stoma closed initially, but only 20% continue without relapse after medium-term follow-up.[94]

SEGMENTAL COLECTOMY AND PANPROCTOCOLECTOMY

Unlike ulcerative colitis, the options for Crohn's colitis in the non-emergency setting are complex. The pattern of disease may allow less extensive resection than removal of the colon, rectum and anus. Clearly extensive disease or cancer/high-grade dysplasia warrant a radical option. However, where there is isolated disease, a segmental resection or colectomy and ileorectal anastomosis may be considered. Indeed, in cases with isolated rectal disease a proctectomy may be indicated. The best option requires clinical judgement and careful patient counselling. Proctocolectomy results in lower rates of recurrence but at the cost of potential perineal wound issues and a permanent stoma. Less radical resection may reduce complications and avoid a stoma but at the price of higher recurrence.

✔✔ A recent meta-analysis concluded that segmental colectomy, subtotal colectomy and panproctocolectomy were equally effective treatment options for patients with colonic Crohn's, the choice of operation depending on extent of disease as well as patient choice regarding a lower recurrence with panproctocolectomy but a higher risk of complications.[95]

TECHNIQUE OF PROCTECTOMY IN CROHN''S DISEASE

Two steps in the technique of proctectomy for Crohn's require discussion. Firstly, the plane of rectal dissection. Most colorectal surgeons are familiar with total mesorectal excision, and this is certainly indicated when there is dysplastic or cancerous change. An alternative approach is the close rectal dissection resulting in excision of the rectal muscle tube and preservation of the mesorectum. Advocates point to the reduced risk of nerve damage and the smaller dead space remaining in the pelvis, which may reduce infection and subsequent perineal herniation. However, this technique is more technically challenging and there is an increased risk of intra-operative bleeding. A modified 'total mesorectal excisio' technique is favoured by others, moving the dissection into the mesorectum at areas where the nerves may be deemed at risk. The concept of the mesentery driving further disease has been suggested as a contraindication to leaving the mesorectum in situ but the evidence is weak.[96]

The second step is the technique of anal resection. Many recommend an inter-sphincteric excision to preserve the external sphincter and minimise the skin excision, potentially allowing better healing. This technique may not be possible if there is extensive perianal disease.

Whichever of these steps is preferred, the surgeon has to be prepared to modify technique to account for severe perineal or perirectal disease that can make dissection very difficult. The perineal wound is best treated with primary closure and suction drainage from above. Delayed wound healing is a problem in up to 40% and it may take 4–6 months to heal completely. Vacuum-assisted closure systems may reduce this in many cases. About 10% will have longer-term problems with perineal sinuses, most of which settle with further surgery including repeated debridement, and exclusion of an enteroperineal fistula or cutaneous Crohn's disease. Some cases eventually need local excision of the sinus. In extreme cases, there is a role for wide excision and some form of musculocutaneous flap reconstruction.

PERIANAL DISEASE

Perianal manifestations of Crohn's disease are common with up to one third of patients developing disease within their lifetime. Surgical therapy has essentially two roles. The primary role is draining sepsis, stabilising disease and preventing tissue destruction. This allows for symptom relief but also acts as a bridge to medical therapy. The second role of surgery is aimed at definitive repair. The chronic relapsing nature of perianal Crohn's disease, and the current less than perfect definitive surgical options dictate the need for careful counselling of the patient to define their needs and goals. Many will accept a more palliative approach to surgical intervention.[97]

PERIANAL FISTULATING DISEASE

INITIAL SURGERY

Fistulating disease presents with abscess formation, purulent or faecal discharge or incontinence. Surgery is required to treat sepsis (Fig. 11.4). In the emergency setting, this requires adequate drainage. If fistulae are readily identifiable a loose seton should be placed. As surgery is associated with poor wound healing, care should be taken to preserve tissue. The tendency to loose motions emphasises the need to preserve the sphincter and fistulae should not be laid open.

After acute sepsis has been drained, the surgical goal is to confirm disease control by effective seton drainage if setons

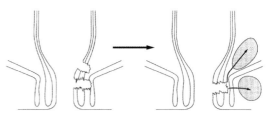

Figure 11.4 Pathogenesis of anal suppurative disease. Deep cavitating ulcers give rise to extra-sphincteric and supra-levator abscesses.

have not already been placed. The utilisation of an MRI may be helpful to both guide seton placement and confirm resolution of associated sepsis after seton insertion (Fig. 11.5). The use of antibiotics (metronidazole and ciprofloxacillin) is unlikely to heal fistulating disease but may reduce symptoms for instance whilst awaiting investigation or surgical drainage.

MEDICAL MANAGEMENT

Current best practice in the management of fistulating perianal Crohn's disease is multimodal therapy with initial effective surgical drainage followed by anti-TNF and/or immunomodulators. The surgeon's role is to ensure adequate resolution of sepsis and advise on the timing of seton removal (which has to occur if healing of the fistula is the desired outcome). Most would remove the seton just before or after the second dose of biological therapy. However, variations may occur based on the number and size of the fistulating tracks and patient perception of optimal outcome. There is no evidence base to guide these decisions, but trial data would suggest about 55% will achieve healing with multimodal therapy compared with 25% receiving either medical or surgical therapy alone.[98]

DEFINITIVE SURGERY

If medical management is contraindicated or fails and the patient wishes to achieve healing as opposed to symptom control, various surgical options are available to try to close the fistula. A fistula plug has the advantage of causing minimal tissue disruption, avoiding wound healing problems and worsening incontinence. Analysis of the data available suggests there is weak evidence to support use with successful healing occurring in up to one third of patients.[99]

Other surgical options include the LIFT procedure, advancement flaps, glue, biomaterials, clipping devices, laser ablation and video-assisted anal fistula treatment. Although there is some evidence for the use of an advancement flap in the absence of proctitis and anorectal structuring, there is a high failure rate and an associated risk of incontinence.[42] There is currently insufficient evidence to guide recommendations for the use of the other techniques.

> Recent evidence is emerging for the use of allogenic adipose-derived mesenchymal stem cells. A large multicenter trial suggested a greater proportion of patients treated with these cells in combination with curettage of the fistula tract and suture closure of the internal opening achieved remission compared with those undergoing the same surgical 'conditioning' (intention to treat 51% vs. 34%).[100] It is interesting to note the high remission rate in the control arm. Given this factor, the current high cost of producing the stem cells, the difficulties in logistical delivery (stem cells must be used within 72 hours of development) and the unknown long-term efficacy, further evidence is required before routine use can be recommended.

SKIN TAGS, FISSURES, ANAL STRICTURES AND ULCERS

Profuse and atypical skin tags are often pathognomonic of perianal Crohn's disease. Whilst patients may request removal, conservative management is the key as excision frequently leads to deterioration in symptoms. A Crohn's fissure may occur at any position on the anal circumference. Sometimes the atypical position is the first alert to the suspicion of Crohn's disease. The fissure tends to be painless. Again, treatment tends to be conservative. Anal and low-rectal strictures occur in about 10% of patients with perianal Crohn's disease. If symptoms occur, simple dilatation is often effective. Refractory cases usually require proctectomy. Anal ulceration is usually treated medically with the surgeon required to exclude an underlying abscess. Occasionally, especially in children, a severe variant termed 'high-destructive perianal Crohn's' may be observed.[101] Again, the mainstay of treatment is medical with really severe cases requiring a defunctioning stoma.

MANAGEMENT OF THE FAILED PERINEUM

Pain, persistent discharge and incontinence define the failed perineum. There is a point when the patient decides the effect on quality of life is so severe that therapy aimed at local treatment is futile. The surgeon can only guide the patient to this conclusion, being realistic as to what can be offered. If the patient reaches this conclusion, a defunctioning stoma may be considered. The type of stoma will depend on the pattern of disease. Whilst a loop ileostomy is easier to construct and more commonly used, a colostomy may be more appropriate for isolated anorectal disease. It is important for the patient to realise that a stoma is highly likely to be permanent, with just 10% of patients eventually undergoing reversal.[102]

In many, persistent symptoms result in the need for subsequent proctectomy. Proctectomy in the context of perianal Crohn's disease is associated with poor healing in up to 40% of patients. Extensive disease may require reconstruction using myocutaneous flaps.

RECTOVAGINAL FISTULAS

Rectovaginal fistulae occur in 5–10% of women presenting with Crohn's disease. Principles of management are similar to perianal Crohn's fistulae, namely control of sepsis followed by multimodal therapy. In this way, a small proportion of fistulae may heal. For those that do not, definitive surgical therapy may be attempted using a variety of surgical approaches including advancement flaps and tissue interposition techniques (e.g., gracilis, Martius). With persistence and possibly more than one procedure, closure rates of over 50% may be possible.[42] A temporary stoma may be considered for complex repairs and proctectomy is required in up to 20% of patients.

PROGNOSIS

Standardised mortality rates are slightly higher for patients with Crohn's disease (odds ratio 1.4). This particularly relates to patients who have the onset of their disease before the age of 20 years, and the risk is particularly high early in the disease course, although the absolute mortality is low. Causes of death include sepsis, peri-operative complications, electrolyte disturbances and gastrointestinal tract cancer.[9]

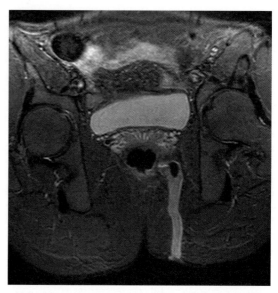

Figure 11.5   Magnetic resonance imaging (MRI) demonstrating wide fistulous tract associated with perianal Crohn's disease.

Quality-of-life issues are important to these patients, and they express concerns over energy levels, fear of surgery and body image. Often, loss of energy and malaise contribute more to functional disability than specific gastrointestinal symptoms. In terms of academic success and advancement, patients are not hampered by the disease, and employment rates are the same as matched healthy controls. However, patients frequently express impairment of employment, recreation, and interpersonal and sexual relationships. Most continue to function optimistically and adapt successfully. Nevertheless, Crohn's patients are twice as likely to suffer anxiety and depression disorders and are more likely to require treatment with psychotropic drugs. Disease relapse produces considerable stress, and psychological support from counsellors, psychiatrists, non-medical and patient support groups should be utilised.

> **Key points**
>
> - Patients with Crohn's disease usually enjoy reasonable health punctuated by periods of increased disease activity, initially managed medically.
> - Many patients will require surgery at some stage.
> - Multi-disciplinary management is essential now that biological treatments are well established. Surgical input into medical treatment decisions is important so that all options are considered.
> - Surgery for small-bowel disease is usually necessary because of failure of medical therapy or complications of disease such as strictures and fistulas.
> - There may be a role for consideration of surgery before escalation of medical therapy
> - Surgery for large-bowel disease is usually necessary because of inability of medical treatment to control symptoms.
> - Severe disease in young people can be life-threatening and expert surgical care is required.

 References available at http://ebooks.health.elsevier.com/

ACKNOWLEDGEMENT

This chapter in the sixth edition was written by Mark Thompson-Fawcett and we are grateful to him for those parts of the chapter, which we have kept in this edition.

KEY REFERENCES

[25] Kennedy NA, Jones G-R, Lamb CA, et al. British Society of Gastroenterology consensus guidelines on the management of inflammatory bowel disease in adults. Gut 2020;69:984–90.
   British Society of Gastroenterology UK guidelines summarising medical treatment of IBD.

[32] Hanauer SB, Feagan BG, Lichtenstein GR, et al. Maintenance infliximab for Crohn's disease: the ACCENT I randomised trial. Lancet 2002;359:1541–9.
   Many centres took part with small numbers from each. There is drug company representation on the writing committee. Infliximab is moderately effective at inducing remission but at 12 months is only a little better than placebo. The data need to be interpreted carefully, infliximab is very expensive, has a poor cost–benefit ratio and there are concerns about serious long-term side-effects. On the other hand, there are many anecdotes of dramatic clinical responses when other measures have failed. It has a role to induce remission in refractory cases.

[33] Sands BE, Anderson FH, Bernstein CN, et al. Infliximab maintenance therapy for fistulizing Crohn's disease. N Engl J Med 2004;350:876–85.
   This study looks at the role of infliximab for fistulating Crohn's disease and is a similar design to ACCENT I. Similar comments apply as for ACCENT I earlier.

[34] Hanauer SB, Sandborn WJ, Rutgeerts P, et al. Human anti-tumor necrosis factor monoclonal antibody (adalimumab) in Crohn's disease: the CLASSIC-I trial. Gastroenterology 2006;130:323–33.
   First RCT to establish the efficacy of induction therapy with adalimumab.

[35] Sandborn WJ, Hanauer SB, Rutgeerts P, et al. Adalimumab for maintenance treatment of Crohn's disease: results of the CLASSIC II trial. Gut 2007;56:1232–9.
   First RCT to demonstrate the efficacy of adalimumab for maintenance of remission out to 56 weeks after successful induction therapy with adalimumab in CLASSIC I.

[36] Colombel JF, Sandborn WJ, Rutgeerts P, et al. Adalimumab for maintenance of clinical response and remission in patients with Crohn's disease: the CHARM trial. Gastroenterology 2007;132:52–65.
   This RCT looked at the frequency of dosing for maintenance of remission, every other week (40%) versus every week (47%) versus placebo (17%) at 56 weeks.

[42] Brown SR, Fearnhead NS, Faiz OD, et al. The Association of Coloproctology of Great Britain and Ireland consensus guidelines in surgery for inflammatory bowel disease. Colorectal Dis 2018;20:3–117.
   UK guidelines summarising the surgical treatment of IBD.

[46] D'Haens G, Baert F, van Assche G, et al. Early combined immunosuppression or conventional management in patients with newly diagnosed Crohn's Disease: an open randomized trial. Lancet 2008;371:660–7.
   Study introducing the concept of 'top down' therapy for Crohn's disease.

[48] De Cruz P, Kamm MA, Hamilton AL, et al. Crohn's disease management after intestinal resection: a randomised trial. Lancet 2015;385:1406–17.
   Study indicating Crohn's patients undergoing resection should have endoscopic follow-up within 6–12 months with step up therapy if evidence of recurrence.

[49] Stevens TW, Haasnoot ML, D'Haens GR, et al. Laparoscopic ileocaecal resection versus infliximab for terminal ileitis in Crohn's disease: retrospective long-term follow-up of the LIR!C trial. Lancet. Gastroenterol Hepatol 2020;5:900–7.
   Study suggesting the early surgery for recurrent ileocaecal Crohn's may be more effective than escalation of medical therapy.

[65] Dasari BVM, McKay D, Gardiner K. Laparoscopic versus open surgery for small bowel Crohn's Disease. Cochrane Database Syst Rev 2011:CD006956.
   Meta-analysis of RCTs suggesting laparoscopic surgery for Crohn's Disease is as safe as open surgery with many potential advantages.

[72] Gionchetti P, Dignass A, Danese S, et al. 3rd European evidence based consensus on the diagnosis and management of Crohn's Disease 2016: part 2: surgical management and special situations. J Crohn's Colitis 2017;11:135–49.
   European guidelines for management of Crohn's disease.

[86] Ponsioen CY, de Groof EJ, Eshuis EJ, et al. Laparoscopic ileocaecal resection versus infliximab for terminal ileitis in Crohn's disease: a randomised controlled, open-label, multicentre trial. Lancet Gastroenterol Hepatol 2017;2:785–92.
   Original LIRIC trial comparing quality of life after surgery versus infliximab for ileocaecal Crohn's.

[95] Angriman I, Pirozzolo G, Bardini R, et al. A systematic review of segmental vs subtotal colectomy and subtotal colectomy vs total proctocolectomy for colonic Crohn's disease. Colorectal Dis 2017;19:e279–87.
   Meta-analysis concluding that segmental, subtotal and panproctocolectomy were equally effective treatment options for patients with colonic Crohn's.

12 Intestinal failure

Carolynne Vaizey | Akash Mehta

INTRODUCTION

Intestinal failure (IF) is defined as the reduction of gut function below the minimum necessary for the absorption of macronutrients and/or fluid and electrolytes, such that intravenous supplementation is required to maintain health and/or growth.[1,2]

IF can be classified on the basis of onset, metabolic and expected outcome criteria:[2,3]

- Type 1: acute, short-term, without significant intestinal pathology and usually self-limiting. The vast majority of IF cases are type 1 and frequently occur secondary to post-operative ileus. They are routinely managed in general surgical units.
- Type 2: prolonged acute condition requiring artificial nutrition for more than 28 days, often in metabolically unstable patients, requiring complex multi-disciplinary care and intravenous supplementation over periods of weeks or months. This type is considered potentially reversible.
- Type 3: chronic, in metabolically stable patients, requiring intravenous supplementation over months or years and, in a subset of patients, permanently.

Types 2 and 3 are distinguished by loss of functional gut due to massive intestinal loss following surgery, or loss of functioning intestine available for absorption, as can occur after development of enterocutaneous fistula (ECF).

Patients with Type 1 and a subset of patient with Type 2 IF would be expected to return to full enteral autonomy in time.

Management of these cases may be complex, prolonged and expensive, in terms of financial cost and clinical input. The care of these patients should therefore be in a specialist IF unit. Such a unit should include a nutrition support team with the capacity to facilitate transition of the patient's care from a hospital environment to a home environment. The care of patients with IF is prolonged and involves specialist gastroenterological, surgical, nursing, pharmacy, dietetic and psychological input. Surgical treatment is generally the last of many steps in the management but accounts for an important part of the workload of specialised IF units.[1]

The nursing staff on the ward and in clinic, specialist nutrition nurses and the home parenteral nutrition (PN) team are the backbone of delivery of care to these patients and their families. The different functions of each of these groups and their separate locations make it imperative that all are coordinated in their approach to each patient. Failure to achieve this results in confusion and demoralisation of this psychologically vulnerable group of patients, who are faced with prolonged hospital admission, debilitating illness, the prospect of no longer being able to eat normally (or at all) and the likelihood of incomplete functional recovery. Those who survive find it difficult to accept the major limitations to their opportunities in life, especially in the case of young adults who constitute a significant proportion of these patients. A high level of technical training of patient and family (where necessary) is required, which necessitates a specialist centre to maintain the technical base to these skills.

Guidelines on surgical management have been published by the Association of Surgeons of Great Britain and Ireland and the European Society of Coloproctology.[2,4] The National Health Service has set up and funded two national reference centres in England through the National Specialist Commissioning Advisory Body. One is at St Mark's Hospital in London, the other is at Salford Royal Hospital in Salford. Currently, a national procurement process for severe IF is underway, aiming to set up and fund home PN centres, integrated care centres (for the joint medical and surgical management of IF) and national reference centres (the two existing national units).

EPIDEMIOLOGY

The prevalence of IF is unknown, but estimates can be made by considering those who require home PN. The incidence of home PN in Europe is estimated to be 3 per million population and the prevalence at 4 per million population, of whom 35% have short-bowel syndrome (SBS).[5,6] In the USA the use of home PN is estimated to be 120 per million population, of whom approximately 25% have SBS.[7] Such data do not include the patients who have not required home PN or those who have been successfully weaned off home PN. In the UK the estimated incidence of IF requiring treatment at a specialised unit is 5.5 per million population.[1]

As SBS is an uncommon condition, specialised centres with expertise in SBS have been created.[1,8,9] A recent study showed an overall survival rate of 86% in patients undergoing autologous surgical reconstruction in a specialised unit at a median follow-up period of 2 years.[10] Similar results have been achieved in other units and highlight the importance of multi-disciplinary care.[1,11]

CAUSES

IF can be caused by the following major pathophysiological conditions, which may originate from various gastrointestinal or systemic diseases:[2]

128

1. Loss of intestinal length: SBS.
2. Loss of functional intestinal length: intestinal fistula.
3. Loss of intestinal function: intestinal dysmotility and mechanical obstruction.
4. Loss of intestinal absorptive capacity: extensive small-bowel mucosal disease.

LOSS OF INTESTINAL LENGTH

In the adult population, IF is most commonly related to a loss of intestinal length as a result of multiple resections or one massive intestinal resection.[12,13] Multiple resections are most common in recurrent Crohn's disease; an isolated massive enterectomy usually follows a vascular catastrophe, such as mesenteric arterial thrombosis or embolism or a venous thrombosis. Massive resection can also be necessary in cases of volvulus, trauma or, in the case of children, necrotising enterocolitis or gastroschisis.

The relation between the amount of bowel removed and the degree of IF is variable, influenced by the age of the patient, the site of resection and the presence or absence of colon. The normal small bowel is around 600 cm in length but may range between 300 and 800 cm. The important figure is not how much small bowel is removed but how much remains.

Post-operative small bowel anatomy can broadly speaking be categorised in three different groups for which the prognosis differs according to the surgical anatomy and the length of remaining small bowel:[2]

- Group 1: small bowel ending in an end jejunostomy; long-term IF mostly associated with <100 cm residual small bowel
- Group 2: jejunocolic anastomosis; long-term IF mostly associated with <50 cm residual small bowel anastomosed to complete colon; more small bowel is required where there is less colon
- Group 3: jejuno-ileal anastomosis with preservation of the ileocaecal junction: long-term IF mostly associated with <30–50cm residual small bowel.

Children may function with shorter bowel as small bowel adaptation (see later) can be more dramatic. The function of the remaining bowel may also be influenced by the presence of active Crohn's disease as well as the presence or absence of colon, as this may have a significant absorptive function.

LOSS OF FUNCTIONAL ABSORPTIVE CAPACITY

ECF or entero-atmospheric fistula (EAF) is the commonest cause of IF where the mechanism is loss of functional absorptive capacity. Fistulous disease commonly bypasses otherwise normal functional small intestine. This is usually the result of an ECF, but entero-enteric or enterocolic fistulae (such as those seen in certain Crohn's phenotypes) may also be responsible.

At a specialised IF unit, 42% of patients had Crohn's disease and the commonest complication necessitating admission was formation of ECFs (in 44% of patients).[1] The second most common cause of fistulae is abdominal surgery: in non-Crohn's patients, ECFs most commonly result as a post-operative complication from either partial breakdown of an intestinal anastomosis or inadvertent bowel injury.[14,15] Risk factors for this include the age of the patient, the state of the bowel undergoing anastomosis, pre-operative nutritional status and the site of anastomosis.[15] When associated with malignancy, factors including tumour fixity, presence of obstruction, previous radiotherapy, associated abscess and surgical technique all affect the risk. Non-absorbable mesh can erode into the bowel and cause fistula, particularly where there is fragile post-operative or diseased bowel. The use of vacuum-assisted closure (VAC) systems in the open abdomen can result in fistula when applied next to the bowel wall. In patients with intestinal or peritoneal inflammation and/or multi-organ failure, there is a 20% rate of intestinal fistulisation associated with the use of a VAC system.[16] Irrespective of VAC dressings or mesh, the inappropriate formation of a laparostomy (i.e., leaving the abdomen open without a plan for short-term primary fascial closure) is in itself fistulogenic.[17,18]

Other causes of fistula formation include colorectal cancer, diverticular disease and radiation. Fistulae resulting from radiation damage are usually complex and carry a high mortality. Rarer conditions include trauma and congenital fistulae, such as a patent vitellointestinal tract. Tuberculosis may fistulate as a complication of an ileal mass, and actinomycosis is an alternative possibility. Ulcerative colitis may fistulate, but this is more common post-operatively, and occasionally, the diagnosis needs reviewing with regard to the possibility of Crohn's disease.

LOSS OF INTESTINAL FUNCTION

In the acute setting, post-operative ileus is the commonest reason for loss of intestinal function, but this is usually self-limiting and does not require more than short-term supportive treatment. More chronic conditions, such as pseudo-obstruction, gastroparesis, visceral myopathy or autonomic neuropathy, can result in functional disability and present a significant challenge for management.

LOSS OF INTESTINAL ABSORPTIVE CAPACITY

Inflammatory conditions of the small bowel can result in non-functioning enterocytes that reduce absorptive capacity. Such conditions include inflammatory bowel disease, scleroderma, amyloid, coeliac disease and radiation enteritis.

PATHOPHYSIOLOGY

THE THREE STAGES OF INTESTINAL FAILURE

Following the initiating event, intestinal 'recovery' results in three recognisable phases that have implications for management.

STAGE I: HYPERSECRETORY PHASE

Of the 7 litres secreted daily by the duodenum, stomach, small intestine, pancreas and liver, about 6 litres are reabsorbed proximal to the ileocaecal valve and a further 800 mL are reabsorbed in the colon, leaving just 200 mL of water in the faeces.

Lack of absorption results in large volume losses. This phase can last 1–2 months and is characterised by copious diarrhoea and/or high stoma or fistula outputs. The main focus of treatment is on fluid and electrolyte replacement, while PN may be required to maintain nutrition.

STAGE II: ADAPTATION PHASE

The process of intestinal adaptation involves a series of histological changes in the intestinal mucosa that permit enhanced mucosal absorption within the residual intestine. The triggers for adaptation are the maintenance of fluid and electrolyte balance and the gradual introduction of enteral feeding. The process of adaptation takes 3–12 months and the degree of adaptation varies with age (more adaptation occurs in the paediatric population), underlying disease extent, and the site of resection (ileum has better capacity for adaptation than jejunum).

STAGE III: STABILISATION PHASE

Maximum intestinal adaptation may take up to 1–2 years and the extent and route of nutritional support will vary. The overall goal for the patient is to achieve as normal a lifestyle as possible, which means achieving stability at home.

Normal physiological functioning of the intestine involves complex fluid, electrolyte and nutrient exchanges to maintain homeostasis. Interruption of this can result in gross imbalances that require supplementation enterally or parenterally. The normal physiology of the intestine is discussed later.

FLUID AND ELECTROLYTES

Sodium absorption in the small bowel is actively linked to the absorption of glucose and certain amino acids. Water absorption is passive and follows the sodium. The jejunum is freely permeable to water, so the contents remain isotonic.

✔ Movement of sodium into the lumen occurs if luminal sodium concentration is low, and absorption of sodium, and hence water, occurs only when the concentration is greater than 100 mmol/L.[19]

Sodium absorption normally occurs in the ileum and colon. In the absence of the absorptive capacity of the ileum and colon, the net sodium losses are expectedly high. This occurs in the presence of a high fistula or jejunostomy; the daily net loss of sodium and net loss of water from the body will be approximately 300–400 mmol and 3–4 L, respectively. This highlights the importance of sodium replacement when there is a high jejunostomy or fistula. Oral fluid concentrated in sodium will help reduce enteric fluid losses. The minimum required daily oral sodium replacement is 100 mmol. The sodium concentration that is absorbable is limited by palatability.[20]

The colon has a significant absorptive capacity, amounting to 6–7 L of water, up to 700 mmol of sodium and 40 mmol of potassium per day. Connection of colon in continuity with the residual small bowel will significantly reduce water and sodium losses.

Potassium absorption is usually adequate unless there is less than 60 cm of small bowel. In this scenario, standard daily intravenous requirements of potassium are 60–100

mmol. Magnesium is usually absorbed in the distal jejunum and ileum. Loss of these will result in significant magnesium loss and deficiency. Magnesium deficiency may precipitate calcium deficiency because hypomagnesaemia impairs the release of parathyroid hormone.

NUTRIENTS

CARBOHYDRATES, PROTEINS AND WATER-SOLUBLE VITAMINS

The upper 200 cm of jejunum absorbs most carbohydrates, protein and water-soluble vitamins. Nitrogen is the macronutrient least affected by a decrease in the absorptive surface and utilisation of peptide-based diets rather than protein-based ones has demonstrated no benefit.[20] Water-soluble vitamin deficiencies are rare in patients with SBS, although thiamine deficiency has been reported.[21]

FAT, BILE SALTS AND FAT-SOLUBLE VITAMINS

Fat and the fat-soluble vitamins (A, D, E and K) are absorbed over the length of the small intestine,[21] hence loss of ileum will impair absorption. Bile salts are also reabsorbed in the ileum and bile salt deficiency will contribute to reduced fat absorption. However, bile salt sequestrants such as cholestyramine have shown no benefit and may worsen steatorrhoea due to binding of dietary lipid and may also worsen fat-soluble vitamin deficiency.[22] In view of multifactorial metabolic bone disease, vitamin D_2 supplements are often given empirically along with calcium supplements. Vitamin A and E deficiencies have been reported, but usually an awareness that visual or neurological symptoms may indicate deficiency, combined with infrequent monitoring of serum levels, are all that is necessary. If the patient is wholly dependent on PN, then replacement along with vitamin K injections is required. Most patients have lost their terminal ileum and so require vitamin B_{12} replacement. Trace elements appear not to be a problem, with normal levels being found in patients on long-term PN.

Loss of bowel results not only in decreased absorptive capacity but also rapid transit. Reduced time for absorption will exacerbate nutritional deficiencies.

ADAPTATION

Following massive small-bowel resection, there are changes in the mucosal surface of the remaining small intestine. Most experimental work has been in small animals such as rats. It appears that adaptation will occur only if there is enteral feeding. Patients who are wholly dependent on PN have mucosal atrophy, which is reversed on re-feeding enterally. The mechanism for this is at present unknown, but various trophic factors have been proposed. Current theory is that increased crypt cell proliferation leads to lengthening of villi and deepening of crypts, so resulting in increased surface area. Because the ileum has shorter villi, it is able to adapt further, but is unfortunately more frequently resected. The stimulation to adapt appears to be threefold: (i) direct absorption of enteral nutrients leading to local mucosal hyperplasia; (ii) enteral nutrition resulting in the release of trophic hormones and a paracrine effect; and (iii) increased fluid and protein secretion with subsequent resorption, leading to increased enterocyte workload and adaptation.[23]

Another form of adaptation occurs in neonates, infants and young children, where continued developmental growth of the small intestine may make the difference between dependence on PN and managing with an enteral diet.[24]

ROLE OF THE COLON IN SHORT-BOWEL SYNDROME

The colon has significant absorptive capacity, not only for fluid and electrolytes as described earlier, but also for short-chain fatty acids.[25,26] These are an energy substrate and in the region of 500 kcal may be derived in this way. It is estimated that having a colon is the equivalent of approximately 50 cm of small bowel for energy purposes.[27] The colon will also slow intestinal transit, particularly if the ileocaecal valve is present, which will improve absorption.

Having overcome the immediate problems of fluid balance and nutritional replacement, a frequent problem for those patients who still have their large bowel in continuity is diarrhoea. Excessive carbohydrate entry into the colon may result in osmotic diarrhoea.[28,29] Alternatively, choleric diarrhoea may be brought on by failure to reabsorb bile salts completely. Colonic bacteria deconjugate and dehydroxylate these into bile acids, which stimulate water and electrolyte secretion. In more extreme cases of SBS, bile salt depletion may occur that will give rise to steatorrhoea from incompletely digested long-chain fatty acids. Bile salts increase colonic permeability to oxalate. As the undigested fatty acids bind calcium in preference to oxalate, there is a resultant increase in enteric oxalate uptake and hence increased renal stone formation.[28]

✔ There is an increased frequency of mixed gallstones, possibly because of interruption of the enterohepatic circulation.[30]

Lastly, D-lactate acidosis is a rare syndrome that comprises headache, drowsiness, stupor, confusion, behavioural disturbance, ataxia, blurred vision, ophthalmoplegia and/or nystagmus.[31] It only occurs in patients with a short bowel and a preserved colon. Colonic bacteria may degrade a surplus of fermentable carbohydrate to form D-lactate, which is absorbed but not easily metabolised. In addition to a metabolic acidosis with a large anion gap, increased concentrations of D-lactate are found in blood and urine. Treatment involves restricting mono and oligosaccharides and encouraging the more slowly digestible polysaccharides (starch), thiamine supplements, and broad spectrum antibiotics. In rare cases, the patient may need to fast while receiving PN.[22]

INTESTINAL FAILURE: CRITERIA FOR REFERRAL

The following criteria are an indication of the type of cases that warrant referral to a nationally designated IF unit:[4,32]

1. Short bowel especially if less than 30 cm remaining jejunum or a stoma output greater than 4 L/24 hours on treatment.
2. Recurrent intestinal fistulation after failed surgical treatment for Type 2 IF.
3. Multiple intestinal fistulae within a dehisced abdominal wound.
4. Persistent abdominal sepsis.
5. Small-bowel obstruction not relieved by or not appropriate for surgery.
6. Small-bowel dysfunction.
7. Persistent nutritional or metabolic problems associated with a high stoma or fistula output.
8. Other:
   a. Venous access – difficult access or central vein thrombosis
   b. Recurrent catheter-related sepsis
   c. Associated or co-existing liver or renal disease
   d. Psychosocial problems.
9. Any nutritional or fluid problem that relates to the gut and is outside the expertise of the referring hospital.

MANAGEMENT OF INTESTINAL FAILURE AND SURGICAL CATASTROPHE

GENERAL CONSIDERATIONS

The management of IF and ECF can present a paradigm of multi-disciplinary care. In patients who do not heal spontaneously, surgical treatment is generally one of the last of many steps in treatment. Owing to the heterogeneity of this condition, randomised controlled trials have not been performed and most recommendations are based on expert opinion. The multi-disciplinary approach to management involves initial source and sepsis control and medical management followed by definitive surgical management. It is vitally important to initiate wound and psychological management early to prevent and reduce effluent-associated excoriation and prepare the patient mentally for what may be at least a few months of therapy.

RESUSCITATION

The scenarios in which patients usually develop IF are often acute catastrophes, and the very nature of IF is such that patients are often severely fluid- and electrolyte-depleted. In light of this, urgent fluid and electrolyte replacement is vital. This will often have been undertaken when the patient was first admitted to hospital, before transfer to a specialist IF centre.

RESTITUTION

The key components of restitution may be summarised by the acronym SNAPP, representing sepsis, nutrition, anatomy, protection of skin and planned surgery. Regardless of the mnemonic, the management strategy for patients with intestinal and concomitant abdominal wall failure should address the management of sepsis, wound care, nutritional support and optimisation (including the management of high fistula/stoma outputs), intestinal mapping, prehabilitation and surgical planning.

SEPSIS

Sepsis is often present in patients who have developed IF and adversely influences outcome. There is evidence that intestinal function is impaired in sepsis, as a consequence of mucosal oedema, defective enterocyte maturation and downregulation of nutrient transporters.[33] When combined with the increased metabolic demand and impaired fuel utilisation associated with sepsis, the presence of impaired intestinal function may lead rapidly to a state of cachexia not unlike that observed in advanced malignant disease. In addition, nutritional support, however aggressive, is unlikely to be successful in the restoration of lean body mass in the presence of sepsis.[34]

Moreover, inadequately treated sepsis is the most common cause of death in patients with acute IF; in the management of enteric fistulae, control of sepsis has been shown to be the major determinant of a successful outcome.[35]

✅ In a study of patients with ECFs, Reber et al. reported an overall mortality of 11%, with 65% of these associated with sepsis. In patients who had their sepsis controlled within 1 month, the mortality was 8%, with spontaneous closure of the fistula in 48%. In those where sepsis remained uncontrolled, the mortality was 85%, with a spontaneous closure rate of 6%.[15]

The diagnosis of sepsis should be entertained in any patient with a history of gastrointestinal surgery who is failing to make satisfactory progress. The classic features of sepsis (swinging pyrexia, leucocytosis and abdominal signs) are not invariably present, especially in malnourished patients. Failure to respond to adequate nutritional support is a classical sign of sepsis. The classical haematological and biochemical hallmarks of sepsis, such as a high white cell count and high C-reactive protein may not be present but more subtle signs of raised platelets and low ferritin and B12 should be heeded. Hypoalbuminaemia, hyponatraemia, hypophosphataemia or unexplained jaundice may be more subtle signs of abdominal sepsis and should lead to a careful search for a septic focus.

Awareness of the high probability of associated sepsis is vital, and if the suspicion arises patients should be thoroughly investigated. Currently, the optimal tool to identify collections is intravenous contrast-enhanced computed tomography (CT). When combined with oral contrast, CT will be able to distinguish collections from immobile and fluid-filled bowel loops.[33]

Especially when IF first becomes apparent, patients may be profoundly septic. The compulsion to 'jump in' in an attempt to surgically address the underlying issue (especially in cases of iatrogenic IF) mostly leads to further enteric injuries and hardly ever achieves its goal. The goal in these patients is source control, which is virtually always achievable with a combination of anti-microbial treatment and targeted percutaneous (radiological) drainage procedures, with due consideration given to targeted and careful surgical drainage procedures for clinically significant collections not amenable to radiological drainage.

NUTRITION

Sepsis and inflammatory bowel disease can add to patients' state of malnutrition. Replacement of fluid, electrolytes and nutrients, including carbohydrate, protein, fat and vitamins, is vital. Monitoring fluid and electrolyte replacement is a key part of nutritional support and involves serum electrolyte measurements and regular weight measurements. Hiram Studley in 1936 commented that 'weight loss is a basic indicator of surgical risk' and this still remains true today.

Fluid and electrolytes

Following resuscitation, fluid and electrolyte requirements will depend on the patient's losses. As described earlier, the first stage of IF is a hypersecretory phase, with high outputs and gastric hypersecretion. Fluid and electrolyte replacement should be by the intravenous route, with the following daily requirements:

- Water: losses + 1 L
- Na^+: losses (100 mmol/L effluent) + 80 mmol
- K^+: 80 mmol
- Mg^{2+}: 10 mmol.

Nutritional support

Early return to enteral nutrition should be the aim as soon as the patient is haemodynamically stable and fluid and electrolyte replacement complete. PN should be regarded as a support mechanism rather than the main source of calories. Overall energy requirements depend on the size and weight of the patient, activity levels and metabolic status, with sepsis increasing demand. In general, males require 25–30 kcal/kg/day and females 20–25 kcal/kg/day of non-protein energy. For research purposes, more exact estimates can be made using the Harris–Benedict equation:

$$\text{Male energy expenditure} = [66 + (13.7 + W) + (5 + H) \\ - (6.8 + A)] + SF$$
$$\text{Female energy expenditure} = [665 + (9.6 + W) + (1.7 + H) \\ - (4.7 + A)] + SF$$

where W represents weight (kg), H height (cm), A age (years) and SF stress factor.

However, the Harris–Benedict equation is inconvenient for daily use. Replacement should also include 1.0–1.5 g/kg/day of protein.

Daily requirements from the American Gastroenterological Association for patients with SBS are recorded in Table 12.1.[36]

PN will provide calories (carbohydrate and fat), protein (amino acids), vitamins and trace elements. The volume should also be considered as part of the daily fluid requirement, with additional fluid given as normal saline.

The decision regarding the optimal route of nutritional support (enteral vs. parenteral) depends on the developmental 'stage' of a given ECF and the length of proximal small bowel. In general, whilst a fistula is still developing (in the absence of a direct tract from the intestinal lumen to the skin), parenteral support (often combined with a period of 'nil by mouth') is often necessary to 'rest' the bowel and either reverse the fistulating process or prevent further sepsis due to ongoing leakage of enteric contents in the absence of adequate drainage (spontaneous or otherwise). When the fistula tract matures, usually after 7–10 days, the

Table 12.1 Dietary macronutrient recommendations for short-bowel syndrome

	Colon present	Colon absent
Carbohydrate	Complex carbohydrate, 30–35 kcal/kg daily soluble fibre	Variable, 30–35 kcal/kg daily
Fat	MCT/LCT, 20–30% of caloric intake, with or without low fat/high fat	LCT, 20–30% of caloric intake, with or without low fat/high fat
Protein	Intact protein, 1.0–1.5 g/kg daily, with or without peptide-based formula	Intact protein, 1.0–1.5 g/kg daily, with or without peptide-based formula

LCT, Long-chain triglyceride; *MCT*, medium-chain triglyceride.
Reproduced from Buchman AL, Scolapio J, Fryer J. AGA technical review on short bowel syndrome and intestinal transplantation. Gastroenterology 2003;124:1111–34. With permission from Elsevier.

risks of rupture of the tract, with diffuse peritoneal soilage, becomes minimal, and oral (full liquid) or nasoenteric enteral feeding can be begun (except in those patient with a proximal fistula, where there is simply not enough bowel in circuit for adequate nutritional absorption). Especially in patients with a degree of intestinal obstruction/stricturing distal to the fistula, a low-fibre enteral support option would be appropriate. In patients without distal obstruction, serious consideration should be given to the possibility of distal limb feeding by enteroclysis or fistuloclysis.

The decision regarding the optimal route of nutritional support also depends on the length of small bowel still in circuit. In patients with an estimated small-bowel length of <50 cm upstream of a fistula or stoma, PN will be necessary to ensure adequate nutritional support; in patients with >100 cm, enteral support will often be sufficient, although this may need to be supplemented by intravenous fluid/electrolyte supplementation.

Therefore the traditional treatment of ECF of almost exclusive mid-to long-term total PN (TPN) + nothing by mouth (NBM) may no longer be appropriate in a substantial proportion of patients; in the early stages of fistulation, TPN may be appropriate but may be replaced by enteral nutrition once a fistula tract has been firmly established.

Reduction of output

The common strategies used to address high stoma/fistula output (commonly known as '*high output regimens*') are listed in Fig. 12.1.

Losses from stomas, fistulae or the anus may be very substantial, making replacement and simple management difficult. A number of strategies should be introduced to reduce these losses. Although they should be allowed to eat solids, patients should be restricted to around 1 L of water orally per day, as hypotonic drinks will increase output in patients with SBS. They should be cautioned against consumption of plain water and be given electrolyte solution, which will reduce intestinal fluid and electrolyte losses. There are several commercially available formulas. The St Mark's electrolyte solution is made from 1 L of water to which is added 20 g of glucose (six tablespoons), 3.5 g of sodium chloride (one level 5-mL teaspoon) and 2.5 g of sodium bicarbonate (one heaped 2.5-mL half teaspoon). This provides 100 mmol of sodium per litre. The problem is palatability, although this may be improved by the addition of orange squash or similar flavourings. Patients at home can make up this solution themselves. The World Health Organisation solutions are similar but also contain 20 mmol of potassium chloride.[37]

Loperamide and codeine are the anti-motility agents of choice in high output regimens. Loperamide is not readily absorbed from the bowel and therefore has no addictive or sedative side effects; it should therefore be considered first-line treatment.[38] Codeine is used for a similar effect to loperamide, but should be used in conjunction with rather than instead of loperamide. This is caused by the systemic side effects of codeine, such as drowsiness and dependence.[6]

Anti-secretory medications are used to reduce gastric secretions and are effective at reducing outputs without consequences for energy or micronutrient absorption.[39] Proton-pump inhibitors (e.g., omeprazole) and H2-receptor blockers (e.g., ranitidine) are commonly used anti-secretory drugs. It is important to note that proton-pump inhibitors are often associated with hypomagnesemia, in which case a trial of H2-receptor blockers should be considered before parenteral magnesium replacement.

Octreotide and somatostatin analogues are often prescribed to achieve the same goal as the more traditional anti-secretory drugs. However, there are several disadvantages to these drugs: possible negative effect on post-resectional intestinal adaptation, predisposition to cholelithiasis, high financial cost, and discomfort associated with the administration.[6] Moreover, the role of these drugs in non-pancreatic intestinal fistulae is paradoxical at best. On balance, it seems unlikely that octreotide will help fistula closure where local factors are in favour of continued fistula patency. The European Society of Coloproctology consensus statement on the surgical management of IF in adults does not support the routine use of somatostatin and its analogues in patients with ECFs.[2]

Bulking agents have shown no benefit in reducing stomal effluent. Cholestyramine may be used to treat hyperoxaluria, but it has no place in those with a jejunostomy, and in

Drink little hypotonic fluid		Maximum 1L/day
Drink a glucose-saline solution		Maximum 1L/day
Drug therapy	Antimotility	Loperamide (up to 40mg QDS)
		Codeine phosphate (up to 60mg QDS)
	Antisecretory	Omeprazole (40mg BD)
		Octreotide (50μg BD)
Magnesium supplements		Magnesium oxide Vitamin D
Nutrition		Low residue diet

Figure 12.1 High output regimens to address high stoma/fistula output.

those with a colon in continuity, it may reduce jejunal bile salt concentration to a level below the minimal micellar concentration for absorption of fat, resulting in steatorrhoea.

A review of long-term medication is always useful, paying particular heed to site of uptake. Enteric-coated tablets are unlikely to be useful.

Dietary modification

Oral feeding should be introduced gradually with additions made one at a time and assessed. A low-fibre diet is usually recommended; although limited evidence exists, the theoretical advantage of low fibre is an increased intestinal transit time and thereby a longer contact time with the gut lumen, allowing more absorption of macronutrients.

Patients should remain fluid-restricted and continue on oral rehydration solution, gastric anti-secretory drugs and anti-motility medication, the latter taken 30 minutes before meals. Drinking should be avoided during meals as this increases losses. It is important to continue intravenous maintenance therapy during this time as this will reduce the pressure on the patient to drink. In the early part of the second clinical stage, it may be necessary to feed the patient wholly using PN, as gastric hypersecretion in response to even the smallest volume of enteral feeding can prejudice newly stabilised fluid balance.

A change of eating pattern to one of 'grazing' or 'little and often' increases the absorption window for the small intestine.

Oral magnesium oxide capsules, 12–16 mmol daily, are started and intravenous therapy is gradually withdrawn. Magnesium replacement may need to remain intravenous, albeit intermittent.

The precise balance between oral and parenteral requirements will vary between patients. In general, daily stoma/fistula losses below 1500 mL may be managed with oral replacement alone; losses between 1500 and 2000 mL require sodium and water replacement, usually as subcutaneous or intravenous fluids, but no PN; and losses of more than 2000 mL per day require PN. Requirements will change over time as adaptation occurs; this can continue for up to 2 years and in the case of children can be very dramatic.

Outcome aims and monitoring

Clinically, the aim is for the patient to have no thirst or signs of dehydration, with acceptable strength, energy and appearance. Biochemical targets should include the following:

- Gut loss: <2 L/day
- Urine: >1 L/day
- Urine Na^+: >20 mmol/L
- Serum Mg^{2+}: >0.7 mmol/L
- Body weight within 10% of normal.

The mainstays of monitoring in the first stage are those used in the normal post-operative patient (temperature, pulse, lying and standing blood pressure, urine output, and daily urea and electrolytes), combined with random estimations of urinary sodium osmolality. If urinary sodium content falls below 20 mmol/L, then deficiency is likely. As the patient stabilises, fluid balance is monitored with daily weight measurement and the observations are reduced in frequency. A meticulous watch is kept on the input/output volumes, with specifically designed charts for ease and clarity of recording. With the fluid balance under control and the eradication of any associated sepsis, re-assessment of the underlying trend in the patient's nutritional status is performed. This is done by calculating body mass indices, skinfold thickness and serum albumin, and by making an estimate of likely return to normal activities. As the patient moves into the third stage of maximum adaptation, the common nutrient deficiencies are assessed (Table 12.2) and the rarer complications are clinically sought (Box 12.1).

Table 12.2   Supplementation required in patients with intestinal failure depending on whether the patient needs partly enteral or wholly parenteral feeding

Nutrient	Parenteral	Partly enteral	Route
Potassium	Yes	If <60 cm and a jejunostomy	In PN or oral supplement
Magnesium	Common with a jejunostomy Uncommon with a colon		Magnesium oxide 12–24 mmol daily
Calcium	Uncertain	Vitamin D_2 400–900 IU daily	
Vitamin D	Uncertain		
Vitamin A	Uncommon		Watch for visual and neurological symptoms and monitor levels 3-yearly
Vitamin E	Uncommon		
Vitamin K	Yes	Normal	Monthly injections
Vitamin B complex	Yes	Normal	In PN
Vitamin C	Yes	Normal	In PN
Vitamin B_{12}	If terminal ileum lost (most patients)	Bimonthly hydroxycobalamin 1000 μg	
Iron	Yes	Normal	In PN
Zinc	Yes	Normal	In PN
Copper	Yes	Normal	In PN

PN, Parenteral nutrition.

Parenteral nutrition

PN is used either as a temporary measure to maintain fluid and energy intake while the remaining small bowel undergoes adaptation, or as definitive treatment in itself. The advantages of maintaining some enteral nutrition, even if not totally sufficient in terms of energy needs, include maintenance of normal gut flora, increased gastrointestinal adaptation and prevention of biliary sludge accumulation.

Central venous TPN is recommended in patients with large fluid requirements or acutely ill adult patients, who may have energy requirements greater than 2000 kcal/day. Central venous TPN is also necessary where it is evident that a prolonged period of parenteral feeding is likely to be required. For expected relatively short periods of TPN (months rather than years), peripherally inserted central venous catheters may be used, whilst for patients requiring prolonged (years rather than months) TPN, true central vascular access (e.g., Hickmann catheters) will be more appropriate.

With better understanding has come a willingness to maintain patients at home on PN. This is a great advantage for those who are dependent on PN and who have not otherwise responded to medical therapy. The benefits of the home environment cannot be overestimated in terms of morale and psychological well-being in an otherwise chronically hospitalised patient.[40]

Home PN depends upon a stable physiological condition, a suitable social set-up and good patient education, coupled with a dedicated PN team providing technical support and advice. Even then, it is not without complications, the chief among them being catheter-related bloodstream infections.[41] Meticulous aseptic technique on the part of the team and patient is essential if this is to be avoided. It takes about 3 weeks as an inpatient for the nursing staff to teach sufficiently rigorous self-care of the feeding line. It has clearly been established that catheter-related sepsis rates are negligible if the whole team adheres to the strictest of aseptic techniques.[1] Other complications, such as catheter occlusion, hepatic dysfunction, gallstones and bone disease, may occur.[42] Guidelines to its use are well established.[43]

Distal limb feeding

Enteroclysis (the term *fistuloclysis* is used in relation to enteroclysis via a fistula) or distal limb feeding involves cannulating the distal limb of a fistula or stoma and providing feeding to the distal non-functioning part of the bowel. This can be performed either with a commercially available enteral feeding solution or alternatively by chyme re-infusion (feeding the fistula/stoma effluent into the distal bowel). Before enteroclysis is carried out, it is essential to ensure that there is no obstruction in the distal bowel and the efferent limb of the fistula/stoma can be cannulated easily. As shown in Fig. 12.2, the catheters can often be left in the bowel and covered by the stoma appliance. In specialist centres, chyme re-infusion has been shown to reduce the need for PN and parenteral hydration support.[44–47] The initial setup of distal limb feeding is a truly multi-disciplinary process, involving dedicated stoma therapy nurses, nutrition nurses and dietitians.

> ### Box 12.1 Complications of intestinal failure
>
> **Early**
> - Dehydration
> - Hyponatraemia
> - Shock
> - Hypokalaemia
>
> **Intermediate**
> - Low morale
> - Weight loss
> - Immune compromise
> - Peptic ulcers
> - Gastro-oesophageal reflux disease
> - Proximal small-bowel inflammation
> - Diarrhoea
> - Bacterial overgrowth
> - Peristomal excoriation
>
> **Late**
> - Vitamin deficiency syndromes
> - Growth retardation in children
> - Depression
> - Parenteral nutrition–induced liver disease
> - Recurrent sepsis
> - Intravenous line-related complications
> - Cholelithiasis
> - D-Lactate acidosis
> - Urolithiasis

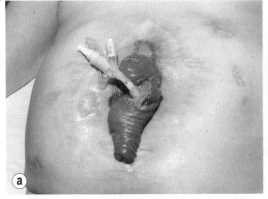 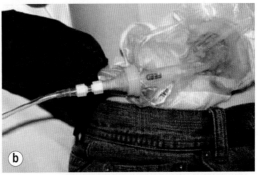

Figure 12.2   The distal feeding catheter placed in the distal limb and subsequently covered by a stoma appliance.

ANATOMY (MAPPING)

The anatomy of the digestive tract and abdominal wall is often significantly disrupted in patients with IF. These changes will often affect decisions regarding nutritional support, the likelihood of spontaneous fistula closure and, ultimately, the proposed strategy for definitive surgical procedures. Crucial information regarding the current anatomy of the digestive tract may often be gained by meticulous perusal of operative records. However, definitive mapping of the intestinal anatomy is based on imaging; in most centres, the mainstay of this mapping is a CT of the abdomen and pelvis with intravenous and positive oral contrast (supplemented with arterial phase scans for patients with a history of mesenteric ischemia). Although fluoroscopic investigations such as barium follow-through studies will yield sufficient information regarding the length and patency of small bowel proximal to a stoma or fistula, cross-sectional imaging modalities such as aforementioned CT, or alternatively CT-/magnetic resonance enteroclysis,[48–50] yield valuable additional information on the condition of the abdominal wall, the best site to gain safe surgical access to the abdomen, any remaining foci of sepsis and involvement of other structures (such as ureters or gynaecological organs). In addition to imaging of the proximal small bowel, contrast-enhanced studies of those sections of the digestive tract, which are out of circuit and not amenable to oral contrast enhancement, are often warranted, especially to assess the patency and length of distal bowel when distal limb feeding is being considered and to rule out any distal obstruction, which might need to be addressed before or during definitive surgical management; these modalities include loopograms, tubograms and fistulograms. In Crohn's disease, full restaging of the disease (both of the small bowel and the colorectum) should be considered. Intravenous urography, endoscopic retrograde cholangiopancreatography, CT-mesenteric angiography and other mapping modalities may also be required, depending upon the anatomy of the fistula.

Active discussion between the IF team and specialist gastrointestinal radiologists is essential as each case is unique and poses different questions.

Taken together, the information gathered from these various sources forms a comprehensive map of the patient's anatomy, which can be used to guide further management and optimisation, as well as to enable adequate planning of the definitive surgical procedure(s). Most clinicians have found it helpful to amalgamate all the information from different sources and schematically represent these in one single anatomical diagram, which has been useful for other healthcare professionals involved in the care of the patient, in determining the challenges to enteral nutrition and to inform patients about their own anatomy and what further surgery would involve. It has also proved useful in planning surgical procedures. An example of this is provided in Fig. 12.3, which offers a schematic representation of the anatomy of a patient who, after undergoing an abdominoperineal excision of the rectum, underwent a repeat laparotomy due to stoma necrosis and full thickness dehiscence; his abdominal wall defect was bridged with an absorbable mesh and unfortunately, he developed multiple EAFs (Fig. 12.4). A CT of the abdomen and pelvis with intravenous and positive oral contrast was performed, followed by a series of fistulograms to assess the segments of small bowel between the various ECFs as well as the distal small bowel, and a water-soluble contrast enema study via his end colostomy to assess the colon.

PROTECTION OF SKIN

Protection of the skin is an essential component of management of patients with IF. Small-bowel output is caustic and excoriation of skin around a stoma or fistula is a painful, demoralising and highly visible immediate complication. The extent of the problem will vary, ranging from a standard end ileostomy/jejunostomy, through patients with an ECF, to those with a laparostomy and multiple open loops of small bowel visible in the wound (Fig. 12.5).

This requires specialist stoma care from highly skilled nurses who use a wide variety of shaped appliances, wide-necked bags and protective dressings and pastes to protect the skin and contain the small-bowel contents. In exceptional situations, expedited surgery is indicated to either refashion a stoma or construct a controlled proximal stoma in the presence of a more distal fistula. An example of the need for this may be an enterovaginal fistula, where a proximal stoma is the only means of control possible.

The resolution of wounds over time may be very significant. This is usually a result of time, nutrition and skin protection. In the case of patients with laparostomy, there is usually significant reduction in the diameter of the wound and bowel loops become indistinguishable following growth of granulation tissue over them.

PLANNED SURGERY

Surgical intervention should be planned and is usually delayed. In the case of IF associated with ECF, early operative intervention to close the fistula is contraindicated by the associated high mortality due to re-fistulisation, sepsis, malnutrition and difficulties with fluid balance.[51]

Delaying surgery for 6–12 months after the last operation has been shown to reduce both the mortality and fistula recurrence rates at subsequent definitive surgery (Table 12.3).[52–55]

Early surgery should be avoided if at all possible. Rarely the surgeon is forced to intervene for:

1. excision of ischaemic bowel;
2. laying open of abscess cavities or removal of abdominal wall mesh;
3. construction of a controlled proximal stoma, for example, in high output enterovaginal fistula.

These are usually the most septic patients and there is an associated high mortality with these procedures. Only in life-threatening situations should surgery be undertaken early in these patients and the decision should not be taken lightly as early surgery can result directly in multiple complications.

Patients managed with an open abdomen have a higher mortality and ECF rate when compared with historical case-matched controls with a closed abdomen, patients with an open abdomen having a mortality rate of 25% and fistula formation rate of 14.8%.[56] When leaving an abdomen deliberately open at the index laparotomy, a plan must be in place aimed at achieving early fascial closure, rather than establishing a long-term laparostomy; a systematic review of early vs. delayed abdominal closure in patients with an open

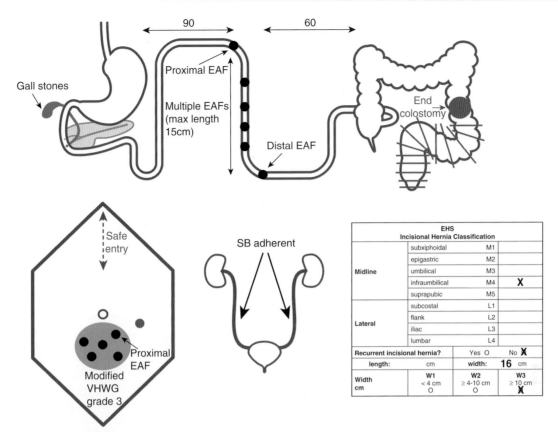

Figure 12.3 Worked example of standardised, editable template allowing for graphical representation of the intestinal tract, the anterior aspect of the abdominal wall and the genito-urinary tract. *EAF*, entero-atmospheric fistula; *SB*, small bowel; *VHWG*, Ventral Hernia Working Group; all measurements in cm.

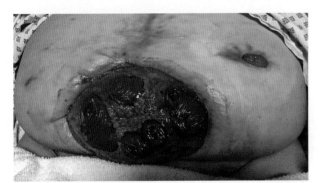

Figure 12.4 Multiple entero-atmospheric fistulae in granulating infra-umbilical laparostomy wound; end colostomy is visible in the left-iliac fossa.

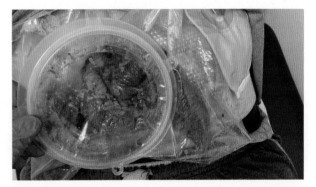

Figure 12.5 Granulating laparostomy wound with multiple fistulating entero-atmospheric fistulae, managed with a custom-made wound manager system.

abdomen demonstrated significantly lower mortality rates in patients where early fascial closure (within 2–3 weeks after the index laparotomy) was achieved (12.3% vs. 24.8% for early vs. delayed fascial closure, respectively), with lower rates of post-operative complications (including fistula development).[57]

PREHABILITATION

Prehabilitation encompasses all of the aforementioned considerations regarding nutrition and wound care, but goes beyond these principles in formulating a pathway (quite often personalised) to enable the team and the patient to

work towards their common goal of offering the patient a definitive procedure with the highest possible chance of success with the lowest possible risk of complications. Although very patient-specific, basic components of such a prehabilitation 'programme' should include the following:

- Exercise and cardiovascular fitness
- Smoking cessation
- Nutritional assessment and optimisation including micronutrient status and consideration of distal limb feeding (also as a trial of integrity of downstream bowel over and above radiology)
- Controlled weight loss (ideally to a BMI of less than 30 kg/m²)

Table 12.3 The risk of mortality and ECF recurrence according to the delay to definitive surgery after the initial insult/surgery

	Early	3–12 weeks	6–12 months	>12 months
Mortality	30–100%	7–20%	3–9%	0–3%
ECF recurrence	40–60%	17–31%	10–14%	3%

ECF, Enterocutaneous fistula.

- Acceptable diabetic control (measured by HbA1C levels with a cut-off point frequently agreed at 7.3% or 56.3 mmol/mol)
- Anaemia correction
- Psychological well-being and preparation, expectation management, shared decision making on priorities and what the patient considers a good outcome
- Assessment of superficial abdominal lipocutaneous tissues if significant weight loss from when catabolic and what to do with pannus
- Analgesics and opiate weaning pre-op to provide headroom for post-operative analgesia

RECONSTRUCTION

When considering reconstructive surgery, the aim is to have a well patient, with no signs of dehydration or evidence of sepsis and with good nutritional status. The aim of the management described earlier is to produce this scenario, such that surgery can be undertaken as safely as possible. The decisions then concern when to operate and what to do.

The decision about when to operate is vital. In the 1960s, Edmunds et al. proposed that early intervention using a conservative approach was associated with 80% mortality compared with 6% mortality for an operative approach. Supportive care has changed significantly since that time, however, particularly the use of PN. In 1978 Reber et al. proposed planned intervention following eradication of sepsis. In the case of ECF, they reported a proportion of spontaneous closures, of which 90% occurred within 1 month, 10% within the next 2 months and none thereafter.[15]

Early surgery is made extremely difficult by the severity of adhesions. It is important to delay surgery until these adhesions have softened, thereby reducing the risk of iatrogenic complications. This will often necessitate a delay of 5–6 months following the patient's previous surgical intervention. Clinically, this may be indicated by the identification of prolapse of stomas or fistulas, and by the impression, on examination that the abdominal wall is moving separately from the underlying bowel (Fig. 12.6).[2]

The second decision is what definitive reconstruction to undertake and this must be individualised. It may range from connecting an end stoma to the remaining colon, with the aim of bringing the colon into continuity, to closure of multiple complex fistulae in a hostile abdomen full of severe adhesions. Clearly, the exact nature of surgery required will depend upon the intestinal anatomy and aetiology of IF in the individual patient. Regardless of the exact surgical strategy, re-operative surgery of this nature is extremely technically demanding and adequate amounts of time should be set aside. Sharp, rather than blunt dissection is required to avoid tearing the bowel at the site of adhesions

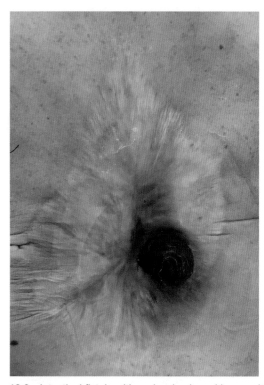

Figure 12.6 Intestinal fistula with prolapsing bowel in an epithelialised laparostomy wound, indicating correct time for surgery.

and segments of bowel with fistulae should be resected rather than bypassed. Intestinal anastomosis should only be attempted if the patient is free from sepsis, well-nourished and local conditions are entirely favourable. It is particularly important to avoid leaving an anastomosis within an old abscess cavity as this will inevitably lead to re-fistulation. In the latter type of case, consideration should be given to exteriorising a fistula as a double barreled or loop stoma, ensuring sufficient washout and drainage of any abscess cavities, and closing the stoma months later as a staged approach.

Surgery to increase nutrient and fluid absorption by either slowing intestinal transit or increasing intestinal surface area is not commonly undertaken in the adult population. The operations include reversed small-bowel segments,[58,59] colonic interposition and tapering with small-bowel lengthening.[60,61] The first two attempt to slow the transit of luminal contents by anti-peristaltic activity or interposition of colonic tissue. They have achieved some clinical success but run the risk of further sacrifice of small bowel, obstruction or anastomotic leakage. Tapering with small-bowel lengthening (the Bianchi technique) has been applied in children with some success.[62] It involves dividing the dilated adapted bowel in two longitudinally, while maintaining mesenteric blood supply via careful dissection in the axis of the mesentery, allocating vessels to either segment. The bowel is then tubularised and joined sequentially.[63,64] However, no new mucosa is formed and there are risks of multiple adhesions and leakage or stenosis from the long anastomotic line.

The serial transverse enteroplasty (STEP) procedure involves serially stapling the dilated short bowel, leaving a lumen of 1–2 cm. The staple direction is alternated between the mesenteric and anti-mesenteric borders and the bowel length (but not overall surface area) is increased. Sudan et al. describe their experience with both the Bianchi and STEP procedures. In a combined analysis incorporating both children and adults, 69% of patients were off PN after intestinal lengthening. The exact benefit of intestinal lengthening procedures in the adult population is unclear in this analysis.[65]

Artificial valves, re-circulation loops, electrical pacing,[66,67] tapering and plication, growth of neomucosa and mechanical tissue expansion[68] are all experimental techniques that are either untried in clinical practice or limited to case reports only.

ENTEROCUTANEOUS FISTULA

High-output proximal small-bowel fistulae are associated with IF by producing functionally short bowel, and are often associated with significant problems with sepsis, malnutrition and difficulties with fluid balance. Initial management is as described earlier in this chapter.

Natural resolution of the fistula depends on the underlying pathology. Possibly up to 60% of fistulae will close spontaneously within 4–6 weeks of supportive treatment. One major IF unit has reported 46.4% spontaneous closure rate with conservative management alone after a median follow-up of nearly 2 years, with borderline significant difference in fistula closure rates between low versus high output fistulas (58.8% vs. 18.2%, respectively).[55] In general, the time range for closure is an estimated 3–90 days and, although closure can still occur beyond 90 days, the chances of this are quite small. Factors preventing healing may be specific to the fistula itself, as indicated in Table 12.4,[33] or general, including ongoing sepsis, nutritional deficiency, or infiltration of the tract by underlying disease such as malignancy, Crohn's or tuberculosis.

Surgical intervention tends to be somewhat 'freestyle' as, despite detailed investigations, findings at surgery may be unexpected. General principles are well described.[2] The

abdominal cavity is entered and the small bowel mobilised carefully as the adhesions are usually considerable. The fistula-bearing segment(s) of bowel is resected en bloc and the remaining ends of bowel re-anastomosed. This includes resection of any cutaneous abdominal wall component of the fistulous tract. If an anastomosis is likely to be in an area of residual sepsis, a stoma is usually advisable.

Abdominal wall closure may be problematic and may necessitate a component separation to obtain fascial closure due to tissue loss from the abdominal wall, or the use of a bridging non-cross–linked biological mesh. In some circumstances where the loss of domain is quite significant, tissue flaps may be required to treat the abdominal wall defects. The risk of re-fistulation is particularly high if abdominal wall reconstruction (AWR) is carried out with cross-linked porcine collagen mesh or synthetic non-absorbable mesh.[69]

Serious consideration needs to be given to whether or not it is actually appropriate to perform a formal AWR at the time of the definitive restoration of intestinal continuity. It may be more appropriate to bridge the abdominal wall defect with a synthetic absorbable or non- cross–linked biological mesh without disruption of the retrorectus and retromuscular planes; and perform the definitive AWR (possibly with a synthetic mesh) as a staged procedure rather than as part of the restoration of intestinal continuity. This staged approach would allow for 'downstaging' of the modified Ventral Hernia Working Group classification from a grade III to a grade I/II defect,[70,71] and does not 'burn any bridges' by avoiding disruption of the retrorectus and retromuscular planes. Moreover, in some patients undergoing restoration of continuity, a temporary stoma may be formed, which will need to be reversed at a later stage, and a case could be made to postpone the AWR till that time. Finally, the very nature of these procedures entails a relatively high risk of enteric leak, either from anastomoses or from enterotomies, which could necessitate further surgery, and thereby a re-opening of the reconstructed abdominal wall. Conversely, bridging the abdominal wall defect almost guarantees development of a ventral hernia and, with it, the need for future surgery, which could have been avoided by a single-stage approach.

The decision regarding whether to stage or combine the restoration of intestinal continuity and AWR is based on numerous factors,[72] which will be different for every clinical situation and therefore a purely algorithmic, 'one size fits all' approach would be inappropriate. In essence, the decision-making will come down to a consideration of the complexity of the intestinal procedure versus the complexity of the AWR.

In general, a patient undergoing a low-complexity 'simple' restoration of continuity (e.g., reversal of a proximal jejunostomy) and requiring a simple AWR (e.g., a Rives-Stoppa repair without the need for additional component separation) would not likely stand to gain much from a staged approach and it would be considered appropriate to perform the AWR at the same time as the restoration of continuity. In contrast, a patient with multiple complex ECFs in a previously fully dehisced abdominal wall will be undergoing a high-risk intestinal procedure with a complex AWR, and simply bridging the abdominal wall defect with a synthetic absorbable or non-cross–linked biological mesh and performing a deferred formal AWR with a synthetic mesh would be considered appropriate. However, even this decision is not straightforward and different surgeons would come to different, and equally

Table 12.4 Factors influencing spontaneous fistula closure

	Unfavourable	Favourable
Anatomy	Jejunum	Ileum
	Short and wide fistula	Long and narrow fistula
	Mucocutaneous continuity	Mucocutaneous discontinuity
	Discontinuity of bowel ends	Continuity of bowel ends
Small bowel	Active disease (e.g., Crohn's, irradiated bowel, malignancy), foreign body or continuing sepsis/abscess in/around fistula origin	No active disease, foreign body or continuing sepsis/abscess
	Distal obstruction	No distal obstruction

justified decisions. In general, it must be borne in mind that a patient with an ECF or more particularly an EAF who ends up with intestinal continuity and nutritional autonomy is a success story regardless of the recurrence/occurrence of an incisional hernia, as long as the abdomen is closed and does not dehisce at/after reconstructive surgery.

REHABILITATION

The goal of therapy is for the patient to resume work and a normal lifestyle, or as normal as possible. This can be a considerable undertaking as the patient will generally have spent a prolonged period of time in hospital. Sending patients home on PN whilst they await surgery reduces the time to long-term rehabilitation.

Rehabilitation must be multi-disciplinary, involving stoma care, physiotherapy, dietetics and occupational health. There needs to be detailed stoma care for patients with high-output stomas and referral to a community continence service for patients with intestinal continuity and incontinence due to liquid stools. Referral to a medical social worker for assistance with social security benefits is important. A proportion of patients will need to remain on intravenous therapy, either saline or PN. Patients must be taught how to manage their tunnelled feeding lines appropriately to allow them to move from a hospital environment to home.

Considerable psychological support may be required and patients should be put in contact with supporting organisations. Long-term sequelae must also be considered. This may involve long-term home PN or recurrence of the underlying disease. Long-term care will include regular monitoring and review of therapy, vitamin B_{12} replacement if more than 1 m of terminal ileum has been resected, and review of other nutrients such as zinc, iron, folic acid and fat-soluble vitamins.

TRANSPLANTATION

Around two patients per million commence home PN and 50% are suitable for consideration of small-bowel transplantation. In the UK this results in a possible 50 cases per year (50% children). A study of 124 consecutive adult SBS patients with non-malignant disease at two centres in France reported survival of 86% at 2 years and 75% at 5 years.[73] Dependence on PN was 49% at 2 years and 45% at 5 years.

The latest update of the international intestinal transplant registry showed that 2887 transplants were carried out in 2699 patients since 1985. These procedures were carried out in 82 centres and individual centre volumes were low. It was difficult to determine specific reasons for graft failure from the registry data. Actuarial survival rates of 76%, 56% and 43% at 1, 5 and 10 years have been described. When a segment of colon was involved the function was better. Patients with a transplanted liver component, those with induction immune suppression and those who were not hospitalised in the period before transplantation were more likely to have better graft survival.[74]

A recent review of the adults in the Scientific Registry of Transplant Recipients showed that the risk of rejection is approximately 40% and before the year 2000, Crohn's disease was associated with a higher risk of rejection but after 2000, there has been no difference based on aetiology.[75] Five-year survival rates for intestine-only transplants of 100% and multivisceral transplants of up to 70% have been reported in individual centres in recent years, indicating the potential

benefits of experience and potentially more effective immunosuppressive medications.[2,76]

The most recent evaluation has reported 1-year patient and graft survival of 79% and 64%, respectively, for intestine-only transplants, and 50% and 49%, respectively, for intestine/liver transplants. Long-term patient and graft survival for intestine-only transplants is 62% and 49%, respectively, at 3 years, and 50% and 38% at 5 years.

Because survival is poorer than that of patients on home PN, the indication for transplantation is SBS not maintainable on dietary supplements, and in whom PN is no longer possible due to severe complications. These usually include lack of access sites because of central venous occlusion, or cholestatic liver disease progressing to fibrosis and cirrhosis. The possibility of gut-lengthening operations must be considered first. The portal vein must be patent and should be checked by Doppler studies, as should the other great veins, in a search for vascular access for the peri-operative period.

Complications are chiefly due to graft rejection and immunosuppression. Rejection leads to bacterial translocation and sepsis in an immunosuppressed patient who is often already malnourished. Current immunosuppressives such as tacrolimus have been paramount in reducing graft sepsis but have adverse effects of neurotoxicity, nephrotoxicity and glucose intolerance. The anti-proliferative agents may cause bone marrow suppression. The consequences of chronic steroid use are osteoporosis, cataracts and diabetes, and growth retardation in children. Opportunistic infections are a major problem, particularly cytomegalovirus.[77]

SUPPORTING ORGANISATIONS

Like most chronic conditions, a supporting structure has evolved to assist in overall management. The patient support group is Patients on Intravenous and Nasogastric Nutrition Therapy (PINNT). The paediatric version is called half-PINNT. Apart from the functions of providing advice and understanding from patients in a similar condition, the association also enables the borrowing of portable equipment to allow holidays away from home.

The professional supporting body is the British Association of Parenteral and Enteral Nutrition. Keeping an overall view of IF is the British Artificial Nutritional Survey, which maintains a census of patients on long-term nutritional support. Most importantly, the pharmaceutical firms that supply the various nutritional preparations are also involved in providing and delivering the bags to patients at home; this includes maintenance contracts that ensure continued functioning of the necessary fridges and emergency back-up in case of failure.

The Association of Coloproctologists of Great Britain and Ireland set up an Intestinal Failure Subcommittee in 2021.

SUMMARY

Recent developments in IF, including home PN and a greater understanding of the pathophysiology of massive intestinal resection, have allowed clinicians to treat and maintain such patients, resulting in long-term survival. The complex medical and surgical management is prolonged and multidisciplinary. It is summarised in Box 12.2.

Box 12.2 St Mark's intestinal failure protocol

Stage 1: Establish stability

Restrict oral fluids to 1000 mL daily

Achieve and maintain reliable venous access

Administer intravenous sodium chloride 0.9% until the concentration of sodium in the urine is greater than 20 mmol/L

Maintain equilibrium by infusing:

1. Fluid: calculated from the previous day's losses and daily body weight records
2. Sodium: 100 mmol/L for every litre of previous day's intestinal loss plus 80 mmol (more if the intestinal loss is excessive)
3. Potassium: 60–80 mmol daily
4. Magnesium: 8–14 mmol daily
5. Calories, protein, vitamins, trace elements: only if enteral absorption is inadequate

Stage 2: Transfer to oral intake

1. Continue intravenous maintenance therapy
2. Start low-fibre meals
3. Start anti-motility agents (loperamide and codeine) 30 minutes before meals
4. Start gastric anti-secretory drugs (proton-pump inhibitor or H2-receptor blocker)
5. Start oral rehydration solution. Discourage drinking around meal times
6. Restrict the intake of non-electrolyte drinks to 1 L daily
7. Encourage snacks and supplementary nourishing drinks, within above limits

Consider the need for enteral tube feeding

1. Confirm access to and patency of small bowel distal to stoma/fistula
2. Start oral magnesium oxide capsules 12–16 mmol daily
3. If intestinal losses remain high, consider octreotide 50–100 mg s.c. t.d.s.
4. Gradually withdraw intravenous therapy

Stage 3: Rehabilitation

1. The patient and family should by now understand the physiological changes that have occurred and the rationale for treatment
2. There needs to be detailed stoma care for patients with high-output stomas
3. Referral to community continence service for patients with intestinal continuity and incontinence due to liquid stools
4. Referral to medical social worker for assistance with social security benefits
5. If intravenous therapy cannot be withdrawn because of continuing intestinal losses (>2 L/day), teach the patient to perform intravenous therapy at home

Stage 4: Long-term care

1. Regular monitoring and review of therapy
2. Vitamin B_{12} replacement if more than 1 m of terminal ileum resected
3. Review other nutrients such as zinc, iron and folic acid and also fat-soluble vitamins

Key points

- Intestinal failure is a multifactorial entity with improved long-term outcome with developments in nutritional and specialised care.
- A clear understanding of normal intestinal physiology is required to understand the pathophysiology of IF.
- Prevention of IF is important and involves meticulous attention to anastomotic technique and techniques to preserve intestinal length in conditions such as Crohn's disease. The use of definitive laparostomies, non-absorbable mesh and VAC dressings should be avoided in the setting of intestinal inflammation.
- Nutritional requirements will vary according to phase of IF. In the hypersecretory phase, the aim is to maintain fluid balance and reduce stoma output, and PN may be required. In the adaptation and stabilisation phases, enteral nutrition is encouraged and TPN requirements may be reduced or weaned.
- A staged approach to management will ensure good long-term outcome. Nutritional management, defining the anatomy by radiological means and skin protection should be the initial steps in management. Any definitive surgery should be deferred until nutritional optimisation has been achieved, all sepsis is eradicated and maturation of adhesions has occurred.
- The multi-disciplinary team approach to management of IF is the standard of care and consideration should be given to referring these patients to a centre dedicated to the management of IF.
- Intestinal transplantation is a valuable addition to the armamentarium of treatments available for IF.

KEY REFERENCES

[19] Spiller RC, Jones BJ, Silk DB. Jejunal water and electrolyte absorption from two proprietary enteral feeds in man: importance of sodium content. Gut 1987;28:681–7. PMID: 3114056.
   Highlights the importance of sodium concentration in water reabsorption in the intestinal lumen.
[30] Nightingale JM, Lennard-Jones JE, Gertner DJ, et al. Colonic preservation reduces need for parenteral therapy, increases incidence of renal stones, but does not change high prevalence of gall stones in patients with a short bowel. Gut 1992;33:1493–7. PMID: 1452074.
   Seminal paper on the role of the colon in reducing extra-intestinal manifestations of IF.

References available at http://ebooks.health.elsevier.com/

13 Faecal incontinence

Gregory P. Thomas | Paul-Antoine Lehur

INTRODUCTION

Faecal incontinence (FI), the involuntary loss of solid or liquid stool, is a debilitating condition with potentially devastating consequences for both physical and psychosocial well-being. Although surveys of the adult population have estimated the prevalence of FI to be between 1% and 19%, the majority of sufferers do not seek medical help because of embarrassment and social stigmatisation.[1,2] As a result, the condition remains largely undiagnosed.

It is estimated that FI affects over half a million adults in the UK. This symptom/functional disorder has very profound negative consequences for the patient. Fear of embarrassment or public humiliation can impose major restrictions on individuals and their families.

✔ Faecal incontinence (FI) occurs when a person loses the ability to control their anal sphincter and bowel movements, resulting in leakage of faeces.

ANATOMY AND PHYSIOLOGY OF THE ANAL CANAL

The adult anal canal is approximately 4 cm long and begins as the rectum narrows, passing backwards between the levator ani muscles. There is in fact wide variation in length between the sexes, particularly anteriorly, and between individuals of the same sex. The canal has an upper limit at the pelvic floor and a lower limit at the anal opening. The proximal canal is lined by simple columnar epithelium, changing to stratified squamous epithelium lower in the canal via an intermediate transition zone just above the dentate line. Beneath the mucosa is the sub-epithelial tissue, composed of connective tissue and smooth muscle. This layer increases in thickness throughout life and forms the basis of the vascular cushions thought to aid continence.

Outside the sub-epithelial layer, the caudal continuation of the circular smooth muscle of the rectum forms the internal anal sphincter, which terminates distally with a well-defined border at a variable distance from the anal verge. Continuous with the outer layer of the rectum, the longitudinal muscle of the anal canal lies between the internal and external anal sphincters and forms the medial edge of the inter-sphincteric space. The longitudinal muscle comprises smooth muscle cells from the rectal wall, augmented with striated muscle from a variety of sources, including the levator ani, puborectalis and pubococcygeus muscles. Fibres from this layer traverse the external anal sphincter forming septa that insert into the skin of the lower anal canal and adjacent perineum as the corrugator cutis ani muscle.

The striated muscle of the external sphincter surrounds the longitudinal muscle and between these lies the inter-sphincteric space. The external sphincter is arranged as a tripartite structure, classically described by Holl and Thompson and later adopted by Gorsch and by Milligan and Morgan. In this system, the external sphincter is divided into deep, superficial and subcutaneous portions, with the deep and subcutaneous sphincter forming rings of muscle and, between them, the elliptical fibres of the superficial sphincter running anteriorly from the perineal body to the coccyx posteriorly. Some consider the external sphincter to be a single muscle contiguous with the puborectalis muscle, while others have adopted a two-part model. The latter proposes a deep anal sphincter and a superficial anal sphincter, corresponding to the puborectalis and deep external anal sphincter combined, as well as the fused superficial and subcutaneous sphincter of the tripartite model. Anal endosonography and magnetic resonance imaging (MRI) have not resolved the dilemma, although most authors report a three-part sphincter where the puborectalis muscle is fused with the deep sphincter. The external anal sphincter is innervated by the pudendal nerve (S2–S4), which leaves the pelvis through the lower part of the greater sciatic notch, where it passes under the pyriformis muscle. It then crosses the ischial spine and sacrospinous ligament to enter the ischiorectal fossa through the lesser sciatic notch or foramen via the pudendal (or Alcock's) canal.

The pudendal nerve has two branches: the inferior rectal nerve, which supplies the external anal sphincter and sensation to the perianal skin; and the perineal nerve, which innervates the anterior perineal muscles together with the sphincter urethrae and forms the dorsal nerve of the clitoris (or penis). Although the puborectalis receives its main innervation from a direct branch of the fourth sacral nerve root, it may derive some innervation from the pudendal nerve.

The autonomic supply to the anal canal and pelvic floor comes from two sources. The fifth lumbar nerve root sends sympathetic fibres to the superior and inferior hypogastric plexuses, and the parasympathetic supply is from the second to fourth sacral nerve roots through the nervi erigentes. Fibres of both systems pass obliquely across the lateral surface of the lower rectum to reach the region of the perineal body.

The internal anal sphincter has an intrinsic nerve supply from the myenteric plexus together with an additional supply from both the sympathetic and parasympathetic nervous systems. Sympathetic nervous activity is thought to enhance and parasympathetic activity to reduce internal sphincter contraction. Relaxation of the internal anal sphincter may be mediated by non-adrenergic, non-cholinergic nerve activity via the neural transmitter nitric oxide.

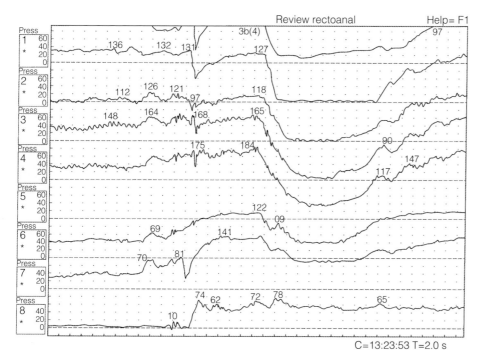

C=13:23:53 T=2.0 s

Figure 13.1 Normal rectoanal inhibitory reflex.

Anorectal physiological studies alone cannot separate the different structures of the anal canal; instead, they provide measurements of the resting and squeeze pressures along the canal. Between 60% and 85% of resting anal pressure can be attributed to the action of the internal anal sphincter.[3] The external anal sphincter and the puborectalis muscle generate the maximal squeeze pressure. Symptoms of passive anal leakage (where the patient is unaware that episodes are happening) are attributed to internal sphincter dysfunction, whereas urge symptoms and frank incontinence of faeces are caused by external sphincter problems.

Faecal continence is maintained by the complex interaction of many different variables. Stool must be delivered at a manageable rate from the colon into a compliant rectum of adequate volume. The consistency of this stool should be appropriate and accurately sensed by the sampling mechanism. Sphincters should be intact and able to contract adequately to produce pressures sufficient to prevent leakage of flatus, liquid and solid stool. For effective defecation, there needs to be coordinated relaxation of the striated muscle components with an increase in intra-abdominal pressure to expel the rectal contents. The structure of the anorectal region should prevent herniation or prolapse of elements of the anal canal and rectum during defecation.

Because of the complex interplay between the factors involved in continence and faecal evacuation, a wide range of investigations is needed for full assessment. A defect in any one element of the system in isolation is unlikely to have great functional significance and so in most clinical situations, there is more than one contributing factor.

RECTOANAL INHIBITORY REFLEX

Increasing rectal distension is associated with transient reflex relaxation of the internal anal sphincter and contraction of the external anal sphincter, known as the *rectoanal inhibitory reflex* (Fig. 13.1). The exact neurological pathway for this reflex is unknown, although it may be mediated via the myenteric plexus and stretch receptors in the pelvic floor. Patients with rectal hyposensitivity have higher thresholds for rectoanal inhibitory reflex; it is absent in patients with Hirschsprung's disease, progressive systemic sclerosis, Chagas' disease, and initially absent after a coloanal anastomosis, although it rapidly recovers.

The rectoanal inhibitory reflex may enable rectal contents to be sampled by the transition zone mucosa to allow discrimination between solid, liquid and flatus. The rate of recovery of sphincter tone after this relaxation differs between the proximal and distal canal, which may be important in maintaining continence.[4]

Further studies investigating the role of the rectoanal inhibitory reflex in incontinent patients show that as rectal volume increases, greater sphincter relaxation is seen, whereas constipated patients have a greater recovery velocity of the resting anal pressure in the proximal anal canal. There is a longer recovery time back to resting pressure in patients with FI.

AETIOLOGY OF FAECAL INCONTINENCE

The ability to maintain continence to stool relies on a coordinated interplay of several factors, including stool consistency, rectal capacity and compliance, intact neural pathways, normal anal sphincter and pelvic floor function, and normal anorectal sensation. Deficiencies or failures in any component can lead to incontinence. In many cases, the aetiology of FI is multifactorial and it is impossible to ascertain the relative contribution of each factor, adding to the complexity of managing this condition.[5]

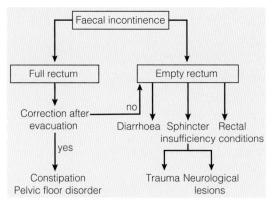

Figure 13.2 The various mechanisms responsible for faecal incontinence: a guide to identifying a cause.

FI is most commonly an acquired disorder, so finding a cause is the first step to adequate management (Fig. 13.2). Faecal loading or impaction is a major contributor to FI in an elderly, frail population. A rectum impacted with faeces can result in 'overflow incontinence'. It is easily diagnosed on digital examination. A rectally administered treatment is required to clear the bowel, followed by regular checks to avoid recurrence. When 'empty' on digital examination or when there is no relief from incontinence after evacuation of the rectum, the three main mechanisms (sometimes acting in combination) contributing to FI are: anatomical/functional injuries to the anal sphincter complex, rectal volume/compliance reduction and diarrhoea or loose stool (see Fig. 13.2).

SPHINCTER INJURY

In adult females, the most common cause of sphincter injury is obstetrical trauma. After vaginal delivery, up to 10% of primiparous women have a clinically recognised sphincter disruption (Fig. 13.3a), and the incidence of occult injuries diagnosed sonographically can be as high as 30% after normal delivery.[6,7] More complicated deliveries, such as those involving instruments (forceps/vacuum-assisted), a large birth weight or a prolonged second stage of labour increase the risk of FI, and an episiotomy has not been shown consistently to protect against sphincter injury.[6–10]

Anorectal surgical procedures responsible for direct trauma to the anal sphincters with resultant incontinence include haemorrhoidectomy and fistulotomy.[11–13] With the former, some patients report minor degrees of incontinence to flatus and/or faecal soiling due to loss of the normal anal cushions allied to sensory impairment in the anal canal. Risk factors for incontinence following fistula-in-ano surgery include high or complex fistulas or repeated procedures for recurrence or persistence (Fig. 13.3b). Manual anal dilatation for anal fissures has been associated with incontinence rates of up to 20% (in contrast, the use of lateral internal sphincterotomy has resulted in much lower rates). Incontinence may also arise following major colorectal resections, such as low anterior resection with colorectal or colo-anal anastomosis, due to the reduction in or loss of the rectal reservoir capacity and also to the disruption of intra-mural nerve pathways. Function can be further adversely affected by chemotherapy and/or radiation. This forms part of what is referred to today as low anterior resection syndrome

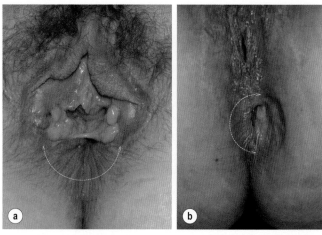

Figure 13.3   (a) Examination in lithotomy (gynaecological) position: anterior anal sphincter defect, a sequela of fourth-degree tear following vaginal delivery. Obstetric injury of the perineum is classified as a first-degree tear if confined to vaginal mucosa and perineal skin, second-degree if the perineal muscles are torn, third-degree if the anal sphincter is torn, and fourth degree if both sphincter and ano-rectal mucosa are torn. In the illustrated situation, the anal sphincter muscles and perineal body have separated, leaving a large anterior hemi-circumferential defect splaying open the anal sphincters in a horseshoe-type configuration (*arrows*). Here the defect was such that the anal and vaginal mucosa have healed to form a cloacal defect. **(b)** Examination in lithotomy (gynaecological) position: left lateral anal sphincter defect, sequela of an extensive fistulotomy for complex anal fistula, resulting in a gaping anus (*arrows*).

Trauma to the perineum or pelvis, such as pelvic fractures or impalement injuries, can be associated with significant damage to both the anal sphincter and its nerve supply,[8,12] along with collateral damage to other pelvic floor structures, such as the bladder and urethra. Occasionally, injuries associated with a sexual assault may result in FI.

Neurological diseases, such as multiple sclerosis, muscular dystrophies or congenital myelomeningocele (spina bifida), can cause incontinence, frequently coupled with constipation and evacuation problems.

The sequelae of congenital abnormalities, like anal agenesis or Hirschsprung's disease treated in childhood, can also be responsible for later FI, with their own specific management.

RECTAL COMPLIANCE

The rectum can become stiff and uncompliant, so that it will not adapt to filling, due to conditions such as inflammatory bowel disease (Crohn's disease, ulcerative colitis), radiation proctopathy and irritable bowel syndrome.[13]

'IDIOPATHIC' FAECAL INCONTINENCE

Often, the precise aetiology is unclear, and the incontinence is termed '*idiopathic*'. Pudendal neuropathy, conceptually demonstrated by delayed pudendal nerve terminal motor latency and an increase in mean nerve fibre density (which can be hard to show in practice), is considered to be present in the majority of these patients.[14] Low squeeze pressures and decreased anal canal sensation are usually found. Idiopathic FI may result from chronic straining during defecation and perineal descent, as first described by Parks.[15] Perineal descent also appears to be related to the number of vaginal deliveries, thereby leading to another way in which the pudendal nerves can be damaged. Indeed, a majority of cases of FI secondary to obstetrical damage is due to a combination of traumatic injury to the anal sphincters and the associated trauma to the pelvic floor nerve supply, the latter only becoming evident many years later at the onset of menopause. To make matters worse, these patients present frequently with associated urinary incontinence (double incontinence), which should be identified and managed accordingly.

This multifactorial aetiology results in a wide variation in clinical presentation and much overlap between the aforementioned groups. Clinically, patients may present with either a pattern of 'urge incontinence', where they are unable to actively defer a bowel movement, 'passive incontinence', with the patient unaware of stool leakage, or a 'mixed pattern'. While a patient presentation with urge incontinence may suggest external anal sphincter pathology, this may also be a feature of rectal pathology, such as proctitis or carcinoma. Conversely, passive incontinence and soiling are more suggestive of a deficient internal anal sphincter or an anatomical deformity from a fistula-in-ano or post-surgical scarring.

Added to the complexity is the frequent co-existence of other pelvic floor pathologies, such as rectal intussusception, which can itself result in patients presenting with varying combinations and severity of urge and passive incontinence or post-defecatory leakage. Indeed, up to 75% of patients with rectal intussusception have incontinence, with some presenting only with this symptom.[16] Although the exact mechanism remains unclear, it is postulated that rectal intussusception stretches the internal anal sphincter and inappropriately triggers the rectoanal inhibitory reflex, leading to temporary reversal of the pressure gradient in the anal canal and soiling. The accompanying incomplete rectal emptying of this defecatory disorder can also contribute to post-defecatory leakage.

✔ Faecal incontinence is a symptom, not a diagnosis. This symptom should not be ignored as something can be done. It is important to identify the underlying causes for each individual and this is often multifactorial.

PRESENTATION

HISTORY

Clinical assessment starts with a detailed history. The frequency and severity of incontinence episodes (also called *accidental bowel leakage – ABL*) are best quantified using a 2–3-week stool diary completed by the patient. It is an essential and simple tool to ascertain a baseline of incontinence episodes. It will serve as a useful comparator when referred back to during treatment. Standardised scoring systems are a useful complement and provide an objective assessment tool (Table 13.1).[17] In the near future, recording using electronic devices would allow easier and accurate reporting on the occurrence of leakage episodes. It is also important to assess stool consistency using the Bristol stool chart, which rates it on a seven-point scale from hard to liquid. Finally, a quality-of-life assessment is provided by the Faecal Incontinence Quality of Life instrument that attempts to measure any impairment in quality of life 'caused by ABL' in four different domains: lifestyle, coping and behaviour, depression and embarrassment.[18]

The history offers clues to the possible aetiology of incontinence. In women, an obstetrical history is mandatory, including number of pregnancies, mode of delivery, birth weight and type of presentation. The hormonal status is recorded, as well as the presence of any concomitant urinary incontinence, which could suggest a more global pelvic floor deficiency. A history of anal surgery is important, particularly in men, because up to 25% of male patients with FI have an iatrogenic sphincter injury.

It is too simplistic to attribute all patients with urge incontinence and all patients with passive incontinence as having external and internal sphincter weakness, respectively. The scenario is often more complex, with patients presenting with an overlap of symptoms. Some may even present with mixed symptoms of FI and obstructed defecation, which should make the clinician consider a possible rectal intussusception.[19]

EXAMINATION

A general examination (abdomen and neurological examination of the back and lower limbs) should be performed.

Table 13.1   St Mark's incontinence score

	Never	Rarely	Sometimes	Weekly	Daily
Incontinence for solid stool	0	1	2	3	4
Incontinence for liquid stool	0	1	2	3	4
Incontinence for gas	0	1	2	3	4
Alteration in lifestyle	0	1	2	3	4
			No	Yes	
Need to wear a pad or plug			0	2	
Taking constipating medicines			0	2	
Lack of ability to defer defecation for 15 minutes			0	4	

Definitions: *Never*: no episodes in the past 4 weeks. *Rarely*: one episode in the past 4 weeks. *Sometimes*: more than one episode in the past 4 weeks but less than one a week. *Weekly*: one or more episodes a week but less than one per day. *Daily*: one or more episodes a day. Add one score from each row: minimum score = 0 (perfect continence); maximum score = 24 (totally incontinent).

Next, the perianal skin should be inspected for any scars of trauma or surgery (see Fig. 13.3), as well as skin excoriation that might suggest long-term seepage of stool. The pelvic floor should be examined for evidence of a descended perineum (perineal descent at rest). A gaping anal orifice when pulling apart the buttocks suggests decreased resting tone, absent or weak voluntary contraction and pudendal neuropathy. The patient should be asked to strain to accentuate a descending perineum (perineal descent during a Valsava effort) or exteriorise any rectal prolapse or rectocele. An external prolapse may become more evident if the patient is examined on the lavatory. In addition, when examining the patient in the gynaecological position, any mid- or anterior compartment deficiencies should be visible, to identify an associated utero-vaginal prolapse and/or cystocoele, respectively.

Sensory perception at the anal margin must be checked and a digital rectal examination performed to assess resting and squeeze anal pressures and contraction of the puborectalis muscle, as well as to confirm the presence of a rectocele. With an educated finger, the so-called 'bioprobe', defects in the sphincter muscles can be felt, and straining can also reveal subtle cases of rectal intussusception and enterocele. Finding impacted stool suggests overflow as a possible mechanism for incontinence.

INVESTIGATIONS

The indications for and extent of diagnostic workup are guided by duration and severity of symptoms, response to initial conservative management, and ultimately fitness for surgery (Box 13.1). It is also imperative to exclude any co-existing organic pathology that could lead to symptoms of FI and warrant urgent attention.

Box 13.1 Workup for faecal incontinence: a summary

A. Symptom assessment
- Careful history-taking
- Three-week stool diary
- Faecal Incontinence Score
- Bristol stool chart
- Faecal Incontinence Quality of Life instrument
- Urinary incontinence
- Constipation

B. Clinical assessment
- General examination (including neurological)
- Anorectal examination
- Assessment of the anterior compartment
- Cognitive assessment (if needed)

C. Investigations
- Exclude organic pathology
- Colonoscopy – or flexible sigmoidoscopy
- Pelvic ultrasound – cervical smears
- Anorectal physiology tests
- Endoanal ultrasonography
- Standard or magnetic resonance imaging dynamic defecography

---

Anorectal physiology studies are essential in providing an objective assessment of anal sphincter pressures, rectal sensation, rectoanal reflexes and rectal compliance, all of which guide management.[8] Although the findings of anorectal physiology studies do not consistently correlate with symptom severity, they may influence the treatment options and guide biofeedback (BFB) training modalities.

Anorectal physiological assessment is essential as an objective measure in patients with FI and for the diagnosis of Hirschsprung's disease and may help select those patients who will have acceptable function after coloanal anastomosis or an ileoanal pouch.

Endoanal imaging is the gold standard in the pre-operative determination of sphincter integrity and defines those patients most likely to benefit from surgical intervention.

ANAL MANOMETRY

Up until recently, water-perfused catheters were typically used for anal manometry. These may be hand-held or automated. Hand-held systems are withdrawn in a measured stepwise fashion with recordings made after each step (usually of 0.5–1.0-cm intervals); this is called a *station pull-through*. Water-perfused catheters use hydraulic capillary infusers to perfuse catheter channels, which are arranged either radially or obliquely staggered. Each catheter channel is then linked to a pressure transducer (Fig. 13.4). Infusion rates of perfusate (sterile water) vary between 0.25 and 0.5 mL/min per channel. Systems need to be free from air bubbles, which may lead to inaccurate recordings, and must avoid leakage of perfusate onto the perianal skin, which may lead to falsely high resting pressures because of reflex external sphincter action. Perfusion rates should remain constant, because faster rates are associated with higher resting pressures, while larger diameter catheters lead to greater recorded pressure.

High-resolution anal manometry (Fig. 13.5) uses the same catheters as standard manometry, but updated software presents the information in a new way that may

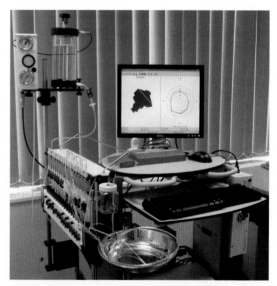

Figure 13.4 Perfusion system used for anorectal manometry. Standard water perfusion set-up plus computer interface for anorectal manometry. The screen shows a vector volume profile.

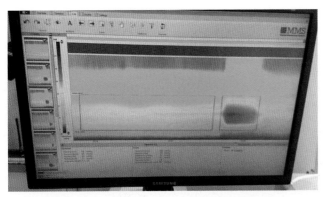

Figure 13.5 High-resolution anorectal manometry.

increase its clinical utility, especially when used to produce a three-dimensional picture of the anal canal. High-definition manometry may use newer closely spaced sensors on solid state catheters. These allow simultaneous measurement of circumferential pressures in the rectum and throughout the anal canal, so there is no need to perform a station pull-through manoeuvre.

A randomised trial to compare the measurement obtained in a series of patients with both water-perfused and solid-state catheters suggested that the solid-state catheter enabled a greater sensitivity during dynamic manoeuvres, such as squeeze and cough pressure measurements.[20]

Significant variation exists in the results of anorectal manometry in normal asymptomatic subjects. Men have higher mean resting and squeeze pressures.[21] Pressures decline after the age of 60 years, changes most marked in women.[22] These facts must be considered when selecting appropriate control subjects for clinical studies. Normal mean anal canal resting tone in healthy adults is 50–100 mmHg. Resting tone increases in a cranial to caudal direction along the canal such that the maximal resting pressure is found 5–20 mm from the anal verge. The high-pressure zone (the part of the anal canal where the resting pressure is >50% of the maximum resting or squeeze pressure) is similar at rest between men and women (20 mm in length) but longer in men than women when squeezing (31 mm vs. 23 mm). In a normal individual, the rise in pressure on maximal squeezing should be at least 50–100% of the resting pressure (usually 100–180 mmHg). Reflex contraction of the external sphincter should occur when the rectum is distended, on coughing, or with any rise in intra-abdominal pressure.

A recent consensus paper has attempted to standardise which manoeuvres should be applied during anorectal physiology testing to determine anorectal function. Standardised terminology has also been introduced.[23]

In the assessment of patients with FI, both resting and maximal squeeze pressures are significantly lower in patients with incontinence than in matched controls,[24] but there is considerable overlap between the pressures recorded in patients and controls.[25]

ANAL AND RECTAL SENSATION TESTING

The anal canal is rich in sensory receptors, including those for pain, temperature and movement, with the somatic sensation of the anal transitional mucosa being more sensitive than that of the perianal skin. In contrast, the rectum is relatively insensitive to pain, although crude sensation may be transmitted by the nervi erigentes of the parasympathetic nervous system.

A variety of methods have been used to measure anal sensation. Currently, electrical sensitivity is most commonly used. The ability of the mucosa to detect a small electrical current can be assessed by the use of a double platinum electrode and a signal generator providing a square wave impulse at 5 Hz of 100 μs duration. The lowest recorded current of three readings at the point at which the subject feels a tingling or pricking sensation in the anal canal is noted as the sensation threshold. Normal electrical sensation for the most sensitive area of the anal canal (the transition zone) is 4 mA (2–7 mA). Rectal mucosal electrical sensation may also be measured using the same technique as that used for anal mucosal electrical sensation measurement, with slight modification of the stimulus (500 μs duration at a frequency of 10 Hz).[26]

The sensation of rectal filling is measured by progressively inflating a balloon placed within the rectum or by intra-rectal saline infusion. Normal perception of rectal filling occurs after inflation of 10–20 mL, the sensation of the urge to defecate occurs after 60 mL, and normally up to 230 mL is tolerated in total before discomfort occurs.

Anal mucosal electrical sensation threshold increases with age and thickness of the sub-epithelial layer of the anal canal. Anal canal electrical sensation is reduced in idiopathic FI, diabetic neuropathy, descending perineum syndrome and haemorrhoids. There are differing reports on whether there is any correlation between electrical sensation and measurement of motor function of the sphincters (pudendal terminal motor latency and single-fibre electromyography). The sampling mechanism and maintenance of faecal continence are complex multifactorial processes, as seen by the fact that the application of local anaesthetic to the sensitive anal mucosa does not lead to incontinence and in some individuals actually improves continence.

PUDENDAL NERVE TERMINAL LATENCY

Pudendal nerve terminal latency (PNTL) was a method of assessment of pudendal nerve function. PNTL is measured with a finger mounted St Mark's electrode, which stimulates the pudendal nerve at the level of the ischial spine. The conduction time to sphincter contraction was measured. Normal PNTL was 2.2 milliseconds. Prolongation of this, may reflect pudendal neuropathy. It is not certain how this would influence treatment choice. Unfortunately, significant inter- and intra-observer differences were also noted. This unreliability means that PNTL is now of historical interest only.

RECTAL COMPLIANCE

The relationship between changes in rectal volume and the associated pressure changes is termed *compliance*, which is calculated by dividing the change in volume by the change in pressure. Compliance is measured by inflating a rectal balloon with saline or air or by directly infusing saline at physiological temperature into the rectum. The use of the barostat to measure rectal compliance has been shown to be reproducible at pressures of between 36 and 48 mmHg. The compliance of the rectum does not differ between men and women up to the age of 60 years, but after this age, women have more compliant rectums. Compliance is reduced in Behçet's disease and Crohn's disease and after radiotherapy in a dose-related fashion. It is also reduced in irritable bowel syndrome.

ENDOANAL ULTRASONOGRAPHY

Endoanal ultrasonography (EAUS) is the procedure of choice to diagnose sphincter defects in patients with suspected sphincter injury.

Three-dimensional endoluminal ultrasound uses a double-crystal design with 6–16 MHz frequency range encased in a cylindrical transducer shaft. The anal canal mucosa is generally not seen on EAUS; the sub-epithelial tissue is highly reflective and surrounded by the low reflection from the internal anal sphincter. The thickness of the internal sphincter increases with age: the normal width for a patient aged 55 years or younger is 2.4–2.7 mm, whereas in an older patient the normal range is 2.8–3.4 mm. As the width of the sphincter increases, it becomes progressively more reflective and indistinct; this may be because of a relative increase in the fibroelastic content of this muscle as a consequence of ageing. Both the external anal sphincter and the longitudinal muscle are of moderate reflectivity. The inter-sphincteric space often returns a bright reflection (Fig. 13.6).

The development of high-resolution three-dimensional EAUS constructed from a synthesis of standard two-dimensional cross-sectional images produces a digital volume that may be reviewed and can be used to perform measurements in any plane, yielding more information on the anal sphincter complex. This provides more reliable measurements, and volume measurements can also be performed. Another development is the use of volume rendering in three-dimensional EAUS, allowing the analysis of information inside a three-dimensional volume by digitally enhancing individual voxels. The volume-rendered image provides better visualisation performance when there are no large differences in the signal levels of pathological structures compared with surrounding tissues.

EAUS has revealed that some patients who were previously thought to have idiopathic FI in fact have a surgically remediable sphincter defect. It has also been shown that a much higher proportion of women sustain sphincter damage during childbirth than is suspected by clinical assessment alone. While the true incidence of sphincter tears may be lower than initially thought, many women sustain important morphological changes to the sphincter following delivery.[27] The ability of EAUS to diagnose and correctly assess the extent of external sphincter damage has been validated by comparison with electromyography studies and findings at surgery. Three-dimensional EAUS has led to a better understanding of sphincter injury. A direct correlation exists between the length of a defect and the arc of displacement of the two ends of the sphincter.[28]

When performed by an experienced clinician, EAUS approaches 100% sensitivity and specificity in identifying internal and external sphincter defects.[29] However, the presence of a sphincter defect does not necessarily correlate with incontinence. In a study of 335 patients with incontinence, 115 patients who were continent and 18 asymptomatic female volunteers, EAUS detected sphincter defects in 65%, 43% and 22%, respectively.[30]

Dynamic standard or MRI defecography is useful in selected cases when there are mixed symptoms – including obstructed defecation, where an occult prolapse may be responsible for the incontinence – particularly when other tests have failed to identify a clear cause (e.g., normal or near-normal anal pressures and intact anal sphincters).

✔ Baseline assessment in faecal incontinence relies on a structured evaluation, including patient reporting of symptoms, careful and sensible clinical examination, and investigations that arise from this focused history-taking and examination.

MANAGEMENT OF FAECAL INCONTINENCE IN ADULTS

The treatment of FI is mainly guided by the severity of symptoms, the aetiology and the structural integrity of the sphincter muscles. Despite a number of publications on the topic, it has to be borne in mind that current recommendations are based more on expert opinion than high-quality evidence. Indeed, most of the published literature in this field reports single series studies. Very few are large randomised comparative studies. Given this absence of truly strong objective evidence, the patient's own views are all the more important. It is also worth remembering that this is a 'benign' problem. Although it will affect quality of life significantly, it is not life-threatening. Many of the surgical interventions described later carry the risk of complications, of varying degrees of severity. The risk of these must be balanced against the patient's individual condition. A proposed treatment algorithm is shown in Fig. 13.7.

✔ Management of FI is multi-disciplinary, often involving several specialists working to provide holistic care to help the patient cope with the broad range of needs, including consideration of the psychological impact of this potentially stigmatising handicap. With a few exceptions, conservative measures should be used first before more invasive treatments.

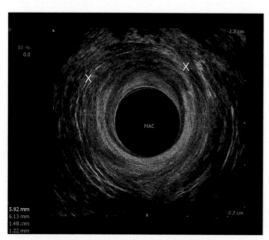

Figure 13.6 Endoanal ultrasonography.

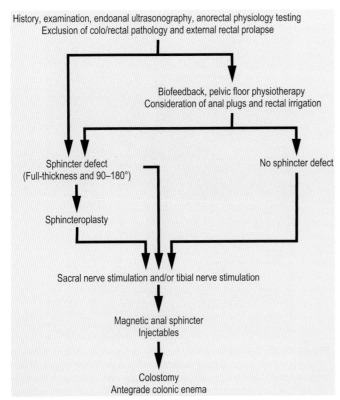

History, examination, endoanal ultrasonography, anorectal physiology testing
Exclusion of colo/rectal pathology and external rectal prolapse

Biofeedback, pelvic floor physiotherapy
Consideration of anal plugs and rectal irrigation

Sphincter defect
(Full-thickness and 90–180°)

No sphincter defect

Sphincteroplasty

Sacral nerve stimulation and/or tibial nerve stimulation

Magnetic anal sphincter
Injectables

Colostomy
Antegrade colonic enema

Figure 13.7 Proposed treatment algorithm for faecal incontinence.

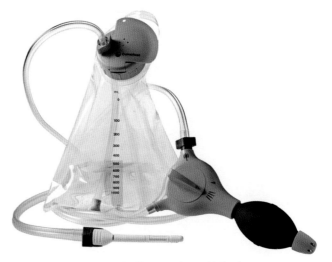

Figure 13.8 Transanal rectal irrigation.

CONSERVATIVE MEASURES

First-line treatment of FI is conservative. These measures can also be used as adjuncts to subsequent surgical procedures.

DIETARY MODIFICATION AND MEDICATIONS

Liquid stools exacerbate FI. An increase in dietary fibre may improve stool consistency. Stool bulking agents (e.g., psyllium) also improve stool consistency and decrease symptoms of incontinence. The recommended dose is 25–30 g/day. A gradual increase in fibre intake will minimise the associated abdominal bloating and discomfort. Dairy products should be avoided in patients with lactose intolerance. Anti-diarrhoeal agents are also useful, and the first drug of choice should be loperamide (0.5–16 mg/day as required). This should be started with low doses (less than 2 mg) to avoid constipation, and loperamide hydrochloride syrup should be considered if fractions of a conventional dose are required. People unable to tolerate loperamide hydrochloride should be offered codeine phosphate or co-phenotrope. Cholestyramine chelates bile salts, the latter being occasionally responsible for diarrhoea, and may be worth a try (in patients having had cholecystectomy or right hemicolectomy).

Small retrograde enemas and suppositories can promote more complete bowel emptying and as a consequence reduce soiling. In more intractable cases, such as spinal cord-injured patients with overflow incontinence from severe faecal impaction, a regular enema programme using specially designed apparatus has proved to be highly effective[31] (Fig. 13.8). Rectal irrigation may also be helpful in those with non-neurogenic incontinence.[32] It may also be useful in situations where the patient has cognitive impairment or in the elderly or infirm, to prevent skin excoriation and infections from frequent soiling.

BIOFEEDBACK AND PELVIC FLOOR MUSCLE RETRAINING

BFB – also known as '*behavioural therapy*' – uses visual, auditory or verbal feedback techniques, with three main goals: strength training, sensory training and coordination training. The treatment protocol should be customised for each patient based upon the supposed underlying pathophysiological mechanism. A set of 10–15 sessions (two per week) is recommended to assess the efficacy of the BFB, with regular 'recall' sessions every 6 months for surveillance of progress. Most importantly, the patient has to exercise at home regularly as he/she knows the type of movements to reproduce. Supportive counselling and practical advice regarding diet and skin care play an important role in the success of BFB. More recently, some units offer group sessions rather than individual consultations. Anecdotal reports suggest that this may be an efficient and effective approach. This may, in part, be due to the reassurance that patients gain from seeing others in the same predicament.

The benefit of BFB varies, with a wide range of improvement reported (64–89%).[8] Exact assessment of its effect is difficult due to the different definitions of success, differing therapeutic regimens, varied selection criteria, fluctuating individual motivations and therapist enthusiasm. Improved rectal sensation after BFB is one of the most consistent predictors for improved continence.

The most recent Cochrane review concluded that the poor quality of published evidence does not allow a definitive assessment of the role of pelvic floor exercises and BFB in the management of FI. Nevertheless, the authors suggested that BFB with limited electrical stimulation is likely to be more beneficial than exercises or electrical stimulation alone. In general, some elements of BFB and sphincter exercises are likely to be beneficial.[33] The current consensus is that BFB as a treatment for FI is possibly effective and is recommended because it is painless and risk-free, after other behavioural and medical management has been tried and inadequate symptom relief has been obtained. Pelvic floor muscle exercises are recommended as an early intervention based upon low cost, no morbidity and some weak evidence suggesting efficacy.

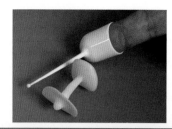

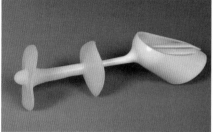

Figure 13.9 The Renew anal insert (with and without applicator).

ANAL INSERT DEVICES

The Peristeen anal inserts (Coloplast Ltd, UK) are disposable devices that expand when soaked with rectal mucus and control continence by blocking the passage of stool. Unfortunately, they can become uncomfortable and are poorly tolerated by many.[34] A newer anal insert, called *the Renew device* (Renew Medical Inc. Ca, USA) (Fig. 13.9) has had encouraging reports. Lukacz and colleagues[35] reported the outcome of a single group study. Eighty percent persisted with this device, with 77% of those who completed the course of treatment reporting a greater than 50% reduction in incontinent episodes. A series from St Mark's reported its use in 30 patients with passive FI who had failed to improve with BFB. At a median of 11 (8–14) weeks, there was an improvement in the St Mark's FI score from 15 (7–18) to 10 (2–18) $P < 0.0001$ and overall satisfaction scores of 80%.[36] The same group reported its use in 15 patients with ileo-anal pouches – all had passive FI. The important finding from this work was a significant improvement in the night time seepage domain of the ICIQ-B assessment tool.[37] The Renew device was compared to tibial nerve stimulation (see later in chapter), in a pilot randomised controlled trial (RCT). Fifty patients with FI were randomised to either percutaneous nerve stimulation (PTNS) or the Renew insert. At 12 weeks, a greater than 50% improvement in symptoms was reported in 78% ($n = 19$) of the Renew group and 48% ($n = 12$) of the PTNS group. This suggested at least equivalence, or even superiority of the Renew insert compared to PTNS.[38] More work is needed to further confirm the benefits of this device.

✅ A patient is referred for surgical consideration after conservative treatment has failed. The surgeon should ensure that these measures of conservative management have been correctly and adequately administered before embarking on surgery.

SURGERY

Surgical treatment for FI is reserved for patients in whom conservative therapy has failed. The available techniques range from direct repair of damaged sphincters (e.g., sphincteroplasty) to techniques that augment the function

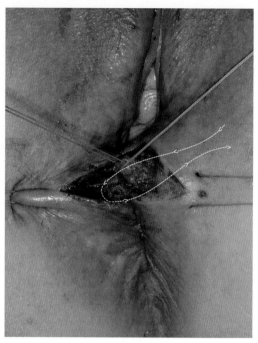

Figure 13.10 Sphincteroplasty for anterior sphincter defect following obstetric injury. Overlapping anal sphincter repair: two edges of detached sphincter muscles dissected free and mobilised with the scar tissue; The U-shaped suturing (*arrows*) uses either non-absorbable or absorbable sutures to bring both muscle ends together.

of (e.g., injectables, sacral nerve modulation and tibial nerve stimulation) or replace the native anal sphincter complex (e.g., artificial bowel sphincter, dynamic graciloplasty or magnetic anal sphincter – these are procedures, which are now rarely used). The relatively lower morbidity of the neuromodulatory treatments such as nerve modulation/stimulation, means that these are often considered first before more invasive treatments. At the end of the spectrum, a stoma should not be perceived as a failure of management and when appropriately chosen can provide a better quality of life for affected patients.

SPHINCTEROPLASTY

'Anal sphincteroplasty' describes a secondary (delayed) repair of the anal sphincter muscles. It is distinct from an 'anal sphincter repair', a term used to describe primary (immediate) repair of the anal sphincters following direct trauma, in the UK often being performed by the attending obstetrician.

Anterior sphincteroplasty following an obstetrical injury is the most common type of reconstruction performed. Overlapping sphincteroplasty is the standard of care (Fig. 13.10). Normally, both the external and internal sphincters are included together in the repair; separation and individual repair of these is not thought to confer any benefit. It is performed under general anaesthesia with the patient either in the prone jack-knife or lithotomy position.[39] An incision is made transversely between the anus and the vaginal introitus. The scar tissue and muscle ends are dissected from the anal canal posteriorly and the vagina anteriorly without separate identification and repair of the internal anal sphincter. Adequate mobilisation is necessary to ensure a tension-free wrap. The scar tissue is then divided, and the two ends are overlapped over the midline and stitched with 2/0 mattress sutures. A levatorplasty can be added, taking great care not to narrow the vagina excessively, which can cause dyspareunia. A 'T'-closure of the skin with interrupted absorbable sutures is often feasible. A small opening can be left in the centre of the wound, or a Penrose drain inserted. A small study of 10 patients suggested that reinforcement of the repair with a small collagen porcine mesh may be beneficial.[40] However, this has not been investigated in larger studies.

✓ Pre-operative counselling should highlight post-operative wound infection and delayed healing as the most common complications.[39]

Sphincteroplasty confers substantial benefits in patients with localised (from 90–180 degrees of circumference) full-thickness sphincter defects. There are no established factors that predict outcome, but it is thought that those with poor function of the residual sphincter muscle pre-operatively are probably unlikely to have a good result. The young patient who attends with a cloaca type defect should be considered for a sphincteroplasty and perineal reconstruction, irrespective of residual function. There may or may not result in a gain in function, but the restoration of anatomy will be of significant benefit to this particular patient group.

The presence of a persistent sphincter defect after repair may be associated with early failure.[41] These may be amenable to a repeat repair.

Short-term outcomes of sphincteroplasty suggest good-to-excellent results in a majority of patients. There is, however, evidence that continence deteriorates over 5–10 years.[42] A systematic review analysed the outcome of over 900 reported repairs. Marked heterogeneity of symptom reporting was found. However, there appeared to be good results initially, which tailed off. There was poor correlation between symptoms and quality of life, and all articles reported high satisfaction scores despite decline in continence.[43] Adjuvant BFB therapy after surgery may improve quality of life and help sustain symptomatic improvement with time. Previous sphincter repair does not seem to affect the clinical outcome of a subsequent repair. In a comparative study, the outcome was similar between patients with or without a previous sphincter repair, with good results obtained in 50% and 58% of patients, respectively.[44] Indeed, the long-term benefit of a repeat sphincter repair was similar to an initial repair.[45] The role of sphincteroplasty when compared to sacral neuromodulation is currently debated.[46]

PELVIC FLOOR REPAIR (POST-ANAL, PRE-ANAL OR TOTAL)

Different types of pelvic floor repair have been described in the past.[47] These are rarely practised today, and are of historical interest only. The aim of the post-anal repair[48] was to increase the length of the anal canal, restore the anorectal angle and recreate the flap valve mechanism, which at the time was thought essential for maintaining faecal continence. Despite initial improvement, the long-term results of post-anal repair or total pelvic floor repair for neurogenic FI have been disappointing. Post-anal repair or total pelvic floor repair now have no place in the treatment of neuropathic FI, as better, less disruptive, options are available.

SPHINCTER RECONSTRUCTION – MUSCLE TRANSPOSITION

Non-stimulated[49] and stimulated muscle transpositions[50] have been devised to replace the anal sphincter (neosphincter) when local repair is not possible or has failed. Transposition of one or both gluteal muscles from the buttock (gluteoplasty) has been used, as well as transposition of the gracilis muscle from the leg, which is wrapped around the anus to form a new sphincter (graciloplasty). Improved results were noted when an implantable electrical stimulator was applied to the transposed gracilis muscle.[50] However, this was not maintained in the medium to longer term. Considerable post-operative morbidity was noted in many of these patients. For these reasons, muscle transposition procedures are rarely performed these days and stimulation devices are no longer available.

ARTIFICIAL SPHINCTERS

Artificial sphincters can be defined as any kind of implanted device intended to replace or reinforce the native sphincter mechanism. They aimed to be a substitute for normal sphincters but because of commercial decisions and probably an inadequate rate of success, they are currently off the market.[51]

Artificial bowel sphincter

Artificial sphincters initially used in humans were silicone, pressure-regulated devices restoring continence through an inflatable cuff placed around the lower rectum or upper anal canal. The majority of the published literature concerns the Acticon Neopshincter™ (American Medical Systems [AMS], Minnetonka, MN, USA) artificial bowel sphincter (ABS). It comprises a fluid-filled cuff that encircles and compresses the anal canal. A pressure-regulating balloon is implanted in the retropubic space of Retzius. A pump placed in the labia majora or scrotum, which is accessible to the patient, controls the system. To initiate defecation, squeezing the pump empties the cuff by transferring fluid into the balloon, permitting passage of stool. The cuff then refills automatically from pressure built up in the balloon.

Few of these, if any, are implanted currently since the device is no longer commercially available. Concerns about the high complication rate, late mechanical failure due to perforation of the cuff, and the availability of less invasive treatments, are likely to be responsible for this. Much of the recent data have described long-term outcome of these devices in expert centres that have mastered the technique; they report satisfactory results.[52] The ABS in its present state has no role in severe FI as it has been superseded by less invasive treatments.

Magnetic anal sphincter

Studied in small trials, the magnetic anal sphincter (MAS; FENIX®, Torax Medical Inc., Shoreview, MN, USA) was a novel device designed to augment the native anal sphincter. It consisted of a series of titanium beads with magnetic cores hermetically sealed inside. The beads are interlinked with independent titanium wires to form a flexible ring that rests around the external anal sphincter in a circular fashion. Early trials suggested promise. However, it is no longer manufactured, and this treatment is not available.

SACRAL NERVE MODULATION

Sacral nerve modulation (SNM) was first described for use in urological disorders and was adapted for use in FI in

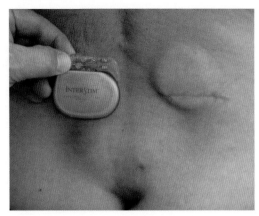

Figure 13.11 Sacral nerve modulation: Interstim™ pulse generator (left) and the implanted generator in a thin patient (right).

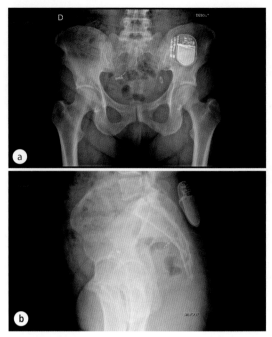

Figure 13.12 Sacral nerve stimulator on plain X-ray: **(a)** anteroposterior and **(b)** lateral views.

1995.[53] The mechanism of action of SNM is unclear. There are no consistent gross anal or pelvic floor motor responses evident in the literature.[54] However, more recent work suggests that it may modulate fine motor activity of the anal sphincter complex, in a way not seen by the usual anorectal physiology assessments. It is believed to work by alteration, or modulation, of ascending spinal sensory pathways. This may have an effect on local colonic and rectal reflexes and also on the sensory cortex.[55] Its effect appears to be genuine. A crossover study in 34 patients comparing active with de-activated devices demonstrated a significant improvement in incontinence symptoms during the active stage.[56]

SNM consists of a *screening phase* of peripheral nerve evaluation (PNE), followed by a second *therapeutic phase* of permanent neurostimulator implantation (Figs. 13.11 and 13.12). In the initial diagnostic phase of PNE, which can be performed under local or general anaesthesia with the patient in the prone position, the S3 foramen is preferentially cannulated under fluoroscopic guidance with an electrode through which stimulation is performed, looking for an appropriate 'bellows response' of the pelvic floor and plantar flexion of the ipsilateral great toe. This is sometimes repeated on the contralateral side to select the best response, with some surgeons routinely screening the S4 position as well. Once a location is decided upon, the electrode is secured in place and connected to a portable external stimulator.[57] The patient then undergoes a 2- or 3-week trial of stimulation while filling out a bowel-habit diary. Only patients with significant clinical improvement, demonstrated by a reduction in frequency of episodes or days of FI of at least 50%, are then selected for the *therapeutic phase*, of permanent stimulator implantation. The permanent stimulator is placed subcutaneously in the gluteal area under local anaesthesia. The pulse generator is activated, and stimulation parameters are set by telemetry. The patient can de-activate it with a small, hand-held device, the 'patient programmer'.

✔ SNM is a minimally invasive technique with low morbidity. The decision to implant a permanent neurostimulator is made on the basis of clinical improvement during test stimulation.

SNM is an attractive treatment option for several reasons. It is minimally invasive, a trial phase allows one to decide on the suitability for permanent implantation, and it has minimal morbidity. Studies have shown that SNM is feasible, with sustainable long-term results. In a series of 228 patients, long-term improvement was seen in 71% at a median follow-up of 84 (70–113) months. The frequency of incontinent episodes per week fell from 7–0.5, and the St Mark's incontinence score improved from a median of 19–6 (both $P <0.001$). Fifty percent of the patients achieved complete continence. However, when the number who underwent test stimulation is taken into account, on an intention-to-treat basis, then full continence was achieved in just over 33% of patients.[58] Another study looked at the outcome of 101 patients at 5 years. Sixty of these patients reported a favourable outcome, and 41 reported an unfavourable outcome. Of these, 24 had their implant de-activated or removed. The authors found that age was a negative predictive factor for success. They found that both an improvement in urgency during the test stage and a good outcome at 6 months were predictive of success. This last finding may highlights the problems associated with patient-reported outcome as a way of judging success of test stimulation.[59] More recent work has suggested that there is a sustained benefit in the even longer term. Recent work from the UK and France has shown the benefits of SNM may be maintained for over 10 years.[60,61]

However, this technique is not free of complications, with reported morbidity including implant site pain (28%), paraesthesia (15%), change in sensation of stimulation (12%) and infection (10%), with less than 5% requiring device explantation. A meta-analysis of 34 studies reported an overall complication rate of 15% in permanently implanted patients, with 3% requiring explantation.[62] The latter results were similarly echoed in a separate study, which reported that at a median follow-up of 33 months, 17.6% of patients required explantation of the device or discontinued treatment entirely.[63]

As encouraging as SNM outcomes may be, this modality is expensive and not all patients respond favourably to PNE. A realistic success rate of PNE is thought to be between 65% and 85%. It is unclear what patient factors are likely to preclude a successful outcome. Therefore patient selection is based on a pragmatic 'trial-and-error' approach, using the PNE test. Test stimulation is indicated not by an underlying physiological condition, but by the existence of an anal sphincter with reduced or absent voluntary squeeze function and intact reflex activity, and nerve–muscle connection.

Contraindications to SNM include pathological conditions of the sacrum preventing adequate electrode placement, skin disease at the area of implantation, severe anal sphincter damage, pregnancy, bleeding risk, psychological instability, low mental capacity and the presence of a cardiac pacemaker or implantable defibrillator.

SNM may be used in those with an anal sphincter defect. A systematic review of the available literature, a total of 119 patients, reported a test stage success rate of 89%. The average number of incontinent episodes per week improved from 12.1–2.3 and the Cleveland Clinic incontinence score (CCIS) improved from 16–3.8.[64]

Recent reports have suggested that SNM may be a useful treatment for low anterior resection syndrome (LARS). A meta-analysis of 10 studies in 2019[65] described an overall median improvement in Cleveland Clinic incontinence score and LARS score of 67% (35–88%). Further work in this area is needed. More recently, rechargeable and MRI compatible SNM systems have become available.[66] Patient selection for the rechargeable devices is still a matter of debate. A standardised approach to lead placement has been decribed.[57] This may have a beneficial effect on outcomes.

✔✔ SNM is an expensive therapy that requires a dedicated team for an optimal outcome. It can yield dramatic improvement in some, and yet provide no benefit in others.[59,62]

PERCUTANEOUS AND TRANSCUTANEOUS TIBIAL NERVE STIMULATION

Another form of neurostimulation, known as *tibial nerve stimulation*, either PTNS or transcutaneous (TTNS), has been investigated (Fig. 13.13). This allows intermittent electrical stimulation of the tibial nerve at the level of the ankle. This has become a popular option for those who have not improved with BFB, and for whom a sphincter repair is not indicated. The percutaneous method requires a needle electrode, whilst the transcutaneous technique uses an electrode pad. The former requires delivery from the hospital outpatient clinic and is the most reported. The latter is cheaper and may be self-administered at home. It is believed that both techniques work by remote stimulation of the sacral plexus via the tibial nerve. This is then thought to mimic the action of sacral nerve modulation.

A large number of single group series have been published. All have reported encouraging results for tibial nerve stimulation in the short term. Hotouras and colleagues[67] reported the outcome of 115 patients who had received 12 sessions of PTNS. At a median follow-up of 26 months, the median CCIS had improved from 12–9.4 (*P* < 0.0001). 'Top-up'

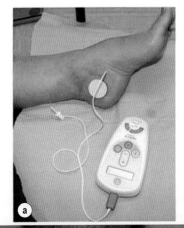
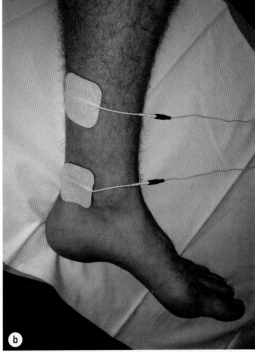

Figure 13.13 **(a)** Percutaneous tibial nerve stimulation; **(b)** transcutaneous tibial nerve stimulation.

treatments were required to maintain efficacy. These were administered at a median of 12 months. The same group[68] reported the outcome of PTNS in those with urge, passive and mixed FI; 25 patients had urge incontinence, the mean CCIS improved significantly from 11–8 (*P* = 0.019), those with mixed incontinence (*n* = 60) also had a significant improvement in outcome (12.8–9.1, *P* < 0.0001). Those with purely passive incontinence (*n* = 15), did not show a significant improvement in CCIS (11.5–9.4, *P* = 0.33).

The effect of TTNS has also been reported. Significant improvements in small group studies were reported by several authors.[69–71] However, a small randomised controlled study attempted to compare PTNS (*n* = 11) with TTNS (*n* = 11) and a sham TTNS (*n* = 8) device.[72] The number of incontinent episodes and urgency improved significantly in the PTNS group when compared to the others (*P* = 0.035). The authors suggested that PTNS is likely to be superior to TTNS.

Unfortunately, doubts have been cast on the effectiveness of tibial nerve stimulation by two large RCTs. Leroi and colleagues[73] compared TTNS with a sham device in a large double-blinded RCT, which investigated 144 patients. No statistically significant difference was seen in the mean number of incontinent episodes. Only 34 (47%) of the active group achieved a reduction of over 30% in a FI severity score against 19 (27%) of the sham group ($P < 0.02$). The CONFIDeNT study[74] reported the outcome of a double-blinded RCT to compare PTNS with a sham device. A total of 227 patients were randomised to either group. Only 39 (38%) of the active group achieved a greater than 50% reduction in incontinent episodes compared to 32 (31%) of the sham group ($P = 0.396$). They concluded that PTNS did not confer any benefit over sham treatment.

However, further subgroup ad-hoc analysis of the CONFIDeNT results suggested that the presence of concurrent obstructed defecation, may adversely affect the outcome of PTNS. When such patients are excluded, there is a definite benefit of PTNS over sham (48.9% vs. 18.2% positive response; $P = 0.002$).[75] In addition to this, a small randomised pilot study compared SNM ($n = 23$) with PTNS ($n = 17$). The authors suggested that both treatment modalities provided some clinical benefit. Eleven of 18 of those who had received SNM and seven of 15 who had received PTNS achieved a greater than 50% improvement in incontinence episodes.[76] More work is needed to establish the place of tibial nerve stimulation in the treatment pathway of FI.

INJECTION THERAPY

Injectable bulking agents were first described for use in FI in 1993. The technique relies on the bulking effect of the injected materials with subsequent fibrosis/collagen deposition helping to enhance continence. These materials are usually injected into either the submucosa or the inter-sphincteric space. It is not clear if clinical localisation or ultrasound guidance is necessary for optimal placement. A variety of materials have been used, including autologous fat, glutaraldehyde cross-linked collagen (Contigen™), pyrolytic carbon beads (Durasphere™) and silicone biomaterial or PTQ™. A Cochrane review looked at the published literature to support their use.[77] Five randomised trials were assessed with the outcome in 382 patients reported; no long-term data were available. Four of the five studies were at an uncertain or high risk of bias. The authors reported some

benefit from the use of dextranomer in stabilised hyaluronic acid compared to placebo, but this was offset by a greater number of adverse events. Despite the relative simplicity of the procedure, the available data suggest that the effects of bulking agents appear to be short-lived and of limited efficacy.

Polyacrylonitrile (Gatekeeper™) is a shape-memory hydrophilic material that enlarges to seven times its initial diameter of 1.2 mm once in contact with human tissue. It can be manufactured into thin rods, which are injected into the inter-sphincteric space. An initial single-centre report showed a sustained improvement in incontinence and quality-of-life scores over a mean follow-up of 33 months.[78] A larger multicentre observational study reported the outcome of this device. At 12 months follow-up, 30/54 (56%) patients achieved a greater than 75% improvement in incontinence symptoms, and seven (13%) achieved continence. The implant extruded in three patients.[79] This technique was developed further into the SphinKeeper (Fig. 13.14). Instead of using four rods, 10 are placed in inter-sphincteric space using a delivery device. A combined series from St Mark's and the Royal London Hospitals in 2020 reported on 27 patients. All had passive FI. In 30%, the delivery device jammed and not all of the implants were delivered. Post-operative EAUS showed that a median of seven implants (0–10) were seen in each patient, with a median of five (0–10) positioned in the optimal inter-sphincteric position. Despite this, the St Mark's FI score improved by a median of 6 points and 14 patients (52%) achieved a greater than 50% improvement in symptoms. This success rate did not appear to be related to implant position.[80]

REGENERATIVE MEDICINE

The use of stem cells and other aspects of regenerative medical therapies in humans have been reported in a small number of papers. These are either cell or cytokine based. Much of this is still currently experimental.

In 2010 Frudinger and colleagues reported the outcome of autologous myoblast cell injection into the anal sphincters of 10 women with FI secondary to obstetrical injury. At 1-year follow-up, improvements in quality-of-life scores and a 13.7 point (confidence interval, 16.3–11.2) improvement in the Wexner FI score were reported.[81] This improvement was

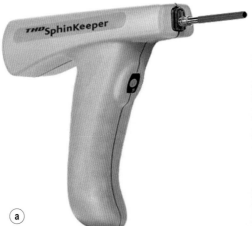
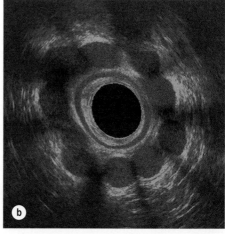

Figure 13.14 (a, b) Sphinkeeper delivery device with loaded implantable rod.

maintained at 5-year follow-up.[82] Further promising work was reported by Boyer and colleagues in 2018. Twenty-four patients were randomised to receiving either placebo or autologous derived skeletal myoblast anal sphincter injections. At 12 months, an initial placebo effect in the placebo group had receded to demonstrate significant improvements in Wexner FI score in the treatment arm (6.5 vs. 15; $P = 0.006$) compared to baseline and not in the placebo arm (14 vs. 15; $P = 0.35$).[83]

The cytokine CXCL12, or stromal derived growth factor 1, has received much attention. Its role in vivo is to attract stem cells and progenitor cells to the site of injury and stimulate tissue regeneration. Work from the Cleveland Clinic, Ohio USA suggested that in a rodent model, application of this, on its own, without additional cell-based therapy may be all that is needed for anal sphincter regeneration.[84]

STOMA FORMATION

ANTEGRADE CONTINENCE ENEMA

This procedure was first described in 1990 for children.[85] The concept of irrigation is to ensure emptying of the colon and/or rectum to prevent seepage of stool. Various procedures have been described to provide access to the right colon. Initially, the appendix was used to create a continent stoma, an 'appendicostomy', by invaginating the tip of the appendix into the caecum to create a one-way valve. The base of the appendix is then brought out to the abdominal wall and the patient can then introduce antegrade enemas. Other options now include a caecal or ileal tube.[86] This procedure can also be performed percutaneously guided by a colonoscope during which a specially designed catheter (CHAIT Trapdoor™) is introduced into the caecum using the following method: (1) fixation of the caecum to the abdominal wall using anchors, (2) dilatation of the caecostomy site and (3) placement of a CHAIT trapdoor catheter.[87] This minimally invasive approach has been shown to be safe and useful for both paediatric patients and adults.

In a recent long-term review of 75 adult patients, with a median follow-up of 4 years, up to 91% of patients were still performing antegrade enemas, while maintaining a significant reduction in incontinence scores compared to preoperative values.[88] However, some morbidity has been reported with this procedure, the most common being wound infection and leakage from the ministoma.

END STOMA

A stoma is appropriate for patients with severe end-stage FI in which all other available treatments have failed, are inappropriate because of comorbidities, or when preferred by the patient. While a stoma may be associated with significant psychosocial issues and stoma-related complications, it can allow the patient to resume normal activities and improves quality of life. In a survey of patients who had a colostomy created to manage their FI, 83% reported a significant improvement in lifestyle and 84% would choose to have the stoma again.[89] An end sigmoid colostomy without proctectomy is usually recommended as a procedure of choice for patients who elect to have a colostomy. A colostomy, however, can result in its own problems in some patients, such as diversion proctitis and mucus leakage, which may necessitate

a secondary proctectomy. The use of laparoscopic surgery has reduced the morbidity associated with this procedure. The use of a prophylactic mesh may reduce the, once near certain, chance of a parastomal hernia developing.[90]

✔ A colostomy can be a good option for patients who suffer from severe FI, offering symptom relief with improved quality of life.

CONCLUSION

Despite all the currently available treatment procedures presented and discussed earlier, each patient requires an individualised management approach, taking into account their own needs and preferences. Evidence is unfortunately not robust for most assessment and treatment methods described. Thus, decision-making often relies on expert opinion and personal experience, which should in turn be in the context of a multi/trans-disciplinary team of specialists. This is essential for optimising patient outcomes, with the colorectal surgeon being only a part of the support process.

There is active research in this field and new treatments will soon be available. In the future, these may involve the use of stem-cell therapy and newer sphincter augmentation technologies. Improvement in our understanding of how neuromodulation works will allow more refined electrical stimulation/modulation treatments to be developed. A better evidence base is also needed. Large randomised comparative studies although difficult to set, are needed to evaluate the new treatments when they emerge.

Key points

- Faecal incontinence (FI) is defined as the involuntary loss of solid or liquid stool.
- The frequency and severity of incontinence episodes and urgency, best assessed with stool diaries (and eventually electronically), guide the treatment choice.
- FI is multifactorial: the identification of mechanism and cause of FI is key for subsequent management.
- Conservative management including dietary counselling, medication and pelvic floor retraining is first line. Psychosocial support plays an important role in management of FI.
- Overlapping sphincteroplasty can be offered to patients with significant FI and a documented sphincter injury, frequently due to obstetrical trauma. Most patients improve after sphincteroplasty, but outcomes deteriorate over time.
- Sacral nerve modulation is an effective therapy for patients with significant FI in whom conservative management fails. The technique has the advantage of allowing a therapeutic trial before permanent stimulator implantation.
- Colostomy provides restoration of a more normal lifestyle and improves quality of life. An end sigmoidostomy alone is recommended. Antegrade colonic enemas can also be an option in refractory FI.
- In time, new technologies such as regenerative medicine and the SphinKeeper device may offer effective treatment options.

 References available at http://ebooks.health.elsevier.com/

▶ RECOMMENDED VIDEOS

- SNM placement – https://www.youtube.com/watch?v=EnF5NJaQ-3k.
- Anal sphincteroplasty – https://www.youtube.com/watch?v=oiiZ0HoeVPc.

KEY REFERENCES

[23] Carrington EV, et al. The International Anorectal Physiology Working Group (IAPWG) recommendations: standardized testing protocol and the London classification for disorders of anorectal function. Neuro Gastroenterol Motil 2020;32(1):e13679.

[43] Glasgow S, Lowry A. Long-term outcomes of anal sphincter repair for fecal incontinence: a systematic review. Dis Colon Rectum 2012;55(4):482–90.

[61] Desprez C, et al. Ten-year evaluation of a large retrospective cohort treated by sacral nerve modulation for fecal incontinence: results of a French Multicenter Study. Ann Surg 2022;275(4):735–42.

[74] Knowles CH, et al. Percutaneous tibial nerve stimulation versus sham electrical stimulation for the treatment of faecal incontinence in adults (CONFIDeNT): a double-blind, multicentre, pragmatic, parallel-group, randomised controlled trial. Lancet 2015;386(10004):1640–8.

Pelvic floor surgery for the colorectal surgeon

14

Alison J. Hainsworth | Andrew B. Williams

INTRODUCTION

Pelvic floor pathology is multifactorial and often multi-compartmental. Pelvic floor dysfunction includes pathology of the anterior, middle and posterior pelvic floor compartments. Posterior pelvic floor pathology includes defaecatory dysfunction with obstructed defaecation (evacuatory difficulties with or without concomitant faecal incontinence) and rectal prolapse.

Pelvic floor defaecatory dysfunction may be caused by anatomical pathologies (rectocele, intussusception, enterocoele, sigmoidocele, rectal prolapse, perineal descent), functional abnormalities (dyssynergy, poor coordination, poor propulsion) or both.[1] Pelvic pain, bowel motility disorders and psychological contributors are also implicated. Patients primarily presenting with bowel related complaints may also have concurrent vaginal and urinary symptoms.

All aspects must be addressed and treatment of urogynaecological pathology in isolation is likely to have an adverse impact on defaecatory function, and vice versa.[2] Careful assessment and treatment planning in a multi-disciplinary team meeting and dedicated pelvic floor clinic are essential.[3] Ideal care involves specialist urologists, gynaecologists and colorectal surgeons, together with allied specialities including radiology, physiotherapy, specialist nursing expertise, physiology, gastroenterology, psychiatry and chronic pain clinics.

✔ Pelvic floor pathology is multifactorial and multi-compartmental. All aspects must be addressed, and treatment planned by the multi-disciplinary team. A multi-disciplinary team meeting and dedicated pelvic floor clinic are essential.

ASSESSMENT

Patients can be assessed by subjective measures (symptom assessment) and objective measures (assessment of the structure and function of the bowel and anorectum) (Table 14.1).

SYMPTOM ASSESSMENT

Symptom assessment can be carried out by clinical history, bowel diaries, visual analogue scores and questionnaires. A careful urogynaecological and obstetrical history and assessment of the impact upon the patient's quality of life must be included.

The Rome IV diagnostic criteria should be fulfilled for a diagnosis of functional defaecation disorder.[4] The Pelvic Floor Consortium, supported by the International Consultation on Incontinence, recommend assessment with both the Patient Assessment of Quality of Life Symptoms (PAC-SYM) questionnaire and Constipation Severity Instrument, as well as an assessment of quality of life, for patients with bowel evacuatory difficulties and constipation.[5] The International Consultation on Incontinence Modular Questionnaire Bowel Score assesses bowel symptoms, the bother they inflict and health-related quality of life (www.iciq.net).[6] In addition, the Obstructed Defaecation Syndrome (ODS) score can assess evacuatory difficulties and monitor symptoms post-operatively.[7]

✔ The Pelvic Floor Consortium is a panel of international experts who have reviewed all symptom scores available. They recommend assessment with both the PAC-SYM questionnaire and Constipation Severity Instrument, as well as an assessment of quality of life, for patients with bowel evacuatory difficulties and constipation. The overall battery of validated instruments for the assessment of all pelvic floor disorder symptoms have been combined to produce an Initial Measurement of Patient-Reported Pelvic Floor Complaints Tool.[5]

EXAMINATION

Careful examination with general, abdominal and anorectal examination should be performed. Rectal examination is useful to rule out any rectal mass as well as the assessment of scarring from previous obstetrical trauma or surgery, concurrent sepsis or fistula, perineal descent and anal tone at rest and voluntary squeeze.[8]

Rigid sigmoidoscopy and proctoscopy examine for masses and a solitary rectal ulcer and may detect intussusception whilst asking the patient to bear down.

PRELIMINARY INVESTIGATION

Any change in bowel habit or defaecatory difficulties should be investigated by a colonoscopy or computed tomography (CT) colonoscopy to rule out underlying pathology, such as malignancy.[8] Where there is rectal prolapse, a flexible sigmoidoscopy should be performed to exclude any proximal structural abnormality or mass.

Table 14.1   The investigations used for patients with pelvic floor defaecatory dysfunction

Investigation	Role	Advantages	Disadvantages
Colonic Transit Studies	To distinguish between slow transit constipation and evacuatory difficulties	Easily accessible, simple investigation	Crude investigation which may not appreciate patients with mixed pathology
Anorectal Physiology			
Anorectal Manometry	To assess the function of the anal sphincters	Highlights concurrent anal sphincter weakness which should be addressed prior to surgical interventions	Requires specialist equipment and training Results may not correlate with symptoms
Rectal Balloon studies	To assess dyssynergy and rectal compliance and sensitivity	Highlights concurrent rectal hyposensitivity	Results may not influence treatments
Imaging			
Endoanal Ultrasound	Assess the structure of the anal sphincter	Assess the integrity of the anal sphincter and examine for concurrent obstetric anal sphincter injury, sepsis and fistula	Requires specialist equipment and training
Integrated Total Pelvic Floor Ultrasound	Dynamic visualisation of entire pelvic floor as an alternative to defaecatory imaging	Dynamic visualisation of anatomical changes and changes to the anorectal angle Simple to perform, cheap, safe, portable, well tolerated by patients compared to proctography. Can be performed in a one stop clinic with simultaneous endoanal assessment of anal sphincter integrity	Does not observe defaecatory dynamics. User dependent
Defaecation Proctography	Dynamic assessment of anatomical and functional aspects	Dynamic visualisation of anatomical changes and rectal emptying. Performed in the upright physiological position	Multicompartmental visualisation is invasive. May overestimate pathology There is debate regarding normal parameters. Radiation exposure
MRI	Defaecation MRI - dynamic assessment of anatomical and functional aspects Dynamic MRI – Dynamic assessment of anatomical aspects	Multicompartmental assessment No radiation	Posterior pathology underestimated without rectal evacuation Anterior pathology underestimated in the supine position Limited access to open configuration systems

COLONIC TRANSIT STUDIES

Colonic transit studies aim to differentiate between slow transit constipation and evacuatory disorders. Colonic transit time is assessed by the ingestion of radio-opaque markers and sequential abdominal X-rays. There are differing protocols but usually patients who expel 80% of markers on day 5 are labelled with normal colonic transit. Retained markers may be scattered throughout the colon (suggesting slow transit constipation) or accumulated in the rectum or rectosigmoid (suggesting functional outlet obstruction).[8]

ANORECTAL PHYSIOLOGY

Anorectal physiology includes anorectal manometry and the measurement of rectal sensation and compliance.

Anorectal manometry is the use of a catheter in the anorectum to measure pressure along the anal canal. A variety of systems exist to do this with the two most commonly used

ones being water perfused systems or solid-state devices, which are described in the previous chapter. Both systems are used to measure the strength of the anal sphincters both at rest (resting tone; predominantly generated by the internal anal sphincter) and on maximal voluntary squeeze (squeeze pressure; generated by the striated components of the anal canal and pelvic floor).[8] Patients with obstructive defaecation may possess concomitant anal sphincter damage and reduced resting and squeeze pressures.

The measurement of rectal and anal pressures during balloon expulsion can be used to evaluate dyssynergy. Dyssynergy is divided into four subtypes; type I – adequate increased rectal pressure with a paradoxical rise in anal pressure, type II – inadequate increase in rectal pressure (poor propulsive forces) with a paradoxical rise in anal pressure, type III – adequate increase in rectal pressure with a failure of reduction in anal pressure and type IV – inadequate increase in rectal pressure (poor propulsive force) with a failure of reduction in anal pressure).[9]

Rectal balloon testing is the most common way of measuring rectal sensation and compliance. Compliance reflects rectal wall distensibility and is the volumetric response of the rectum when

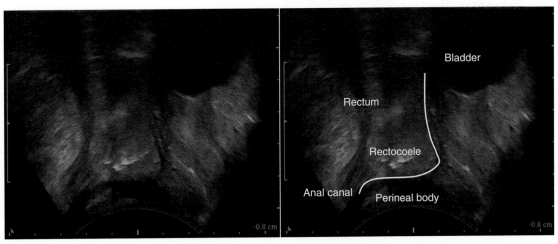

Figure 14.1 Transperineal ultrasound.

subjected to increased intra-luminal pressure.[10] There is conflicting evidence regarding compliance and obstructive defaecation; compliance may be normal or increased with rectocele.

✔ The international anorectal physiology working group have published a standardised testing protocol for the performance and interpretation of anorectal function testing with anorectal manometry and the balloon expulsion test.[11]

ANAL ENDOSONOGRAPHY/ENDORECTAL ULTRASOUND

Routine endoanal ultrasound is performed with a transducer (endoprobe) in the anal canal providing either axial or sagittal images along the anal canal. A volume of data is acquired during an automated withdrawal of the endoprobe with the rotating axial scan or the sagittal array, which sweeps through 360 degrees. This volume of data can be interrogated in any plane for assessment of anal sphincter integrity, obstetrical injury and associated repairs, fistulae or sepsis.[12] It is important to appreciate these pathologies before embarking on treatment of defaecatory dysfunction and prolapse. The internal sphincter may be hypertrophied in patients with straining or rectal prolapse. The interpretation of which must take into account that the thickness of the internal sphincter increases with age: the normal width for a patient aged 55 years or younger is 2.4–2.7 mm; in an older patient the normal range is 2.8–3.4 mm.

INTEGRATED TOTAL PELVIC FLOOR ULTRASOUND

Integrated total pelvic floor ultrasound (TPFUS) is the dynamic assessment of the entire pelvic floor with transperineal, transvaginal and endoanal ultrasound.[13] It is cheap, accessible and can be performed in a one stop clinic alongside anorectal physiology and endoanal ultrasound. TPFUS is routinely used for anterior and middle compartmental dysfunction (e.g., cystocoele). However, it is now also emerging as an alternative to defaecatory imaging for anatomical (rectocele, intussusception, rectal prolapse, enterocoele, sigmoidocele and perineal descent) and functional (changes in the anorectal angle) aspects.[14] The patient is asked to squeeze up and then perform the Valsalva manoeuvre; some specialists

routinely instil and encourage expulsion of rectal gel to improve accuracy of detection of intussusception and rectocele.

TRANSPERINEAL ULTRASOUND (FIG. 14.1)

Transperineal ultrasound allows the global assessment of the entire pelvic floor in real time. It is the most useful element of TPFUS for the assessment of the patient with defaecatory dysfunction. It is non-invasive and potentially more acceptable to patients than defaecatory imaging.[15] It allows visualisation of anterior, middle and posterior pelvic floor compartments in the longitudinal and transverse sections and dynamic assessment of cystocoele, vaginal vault prolapse, enterocoele, rectocele, intussusception, rectal prolapse, dyssynergy and perineal descent without contrast. Comparisons with defaecatory imaging have shown than transperineal ultrasound may be a useful screening tool for defaecatory dysfunction and may avoid further imaging in some patients.[14,15]

TRANSVAGINAL ULTRASOUND

Murad-Regadas et al. report on dynamic three-dimensional endovaginal scanning for the near perfect detection of rectocele, enterocoele and intussusception compared to defaecation proctography.[16] There are concerns however that the vaginal probe may prevent the full prolapse of structures or impede the Valsalva manoeuvre.

PROCTOGRAPHY – DEFECOGRAPHY/ EVACUATION PROCTOGRAPHY

Defaecation proctography (defaecation barium proctography, fluoroscopic evacuatory proctography, defecography) is a dynamic investigation of rectal emptying. A mixture of barium paste and either porridge oats or potato starch to try to simulate the consistency of stool is instilled in the rectum and the subject sits on a commode and evacuates whilst the process is recorded on cineradiography or fluororadiography.[17]

Advantages include the examination of defaecatory dynamics in the upright physiological position. Defaecation proctography, with rectal and oral contrast, allows the visualisation of anatomical abnormalities (namely rectocele, intussusception,

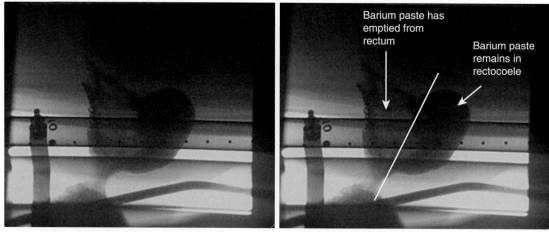

Figure 14.2 Defaecation proctography.

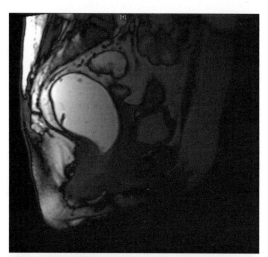

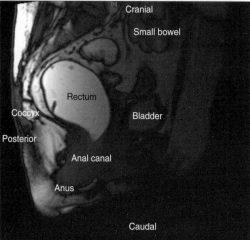

Figure 14.3 Defaecation magnetic resonance imaging (MRI).

rectal prolapse, enterocoele, sigmoidocele and perineal descent) and functional problems (changes in the anorectal angle, the extent and duration of rectal emptying and 'trapping' of stool within a rectocele) (Fig. 14.2). Multi-compartmental visualisation is invasive, though possible by contrast opacification of the vagina (dynamic colpoproctography), bladder (dynamic cystoproctography) or peritoneal cavity.

Defaecation proctography has substantial diagnostic and therapeutic benefit regarding diagnosis and determining management.[18] However, there are concerns that pathology may be over-diagnosed. Patient embarrassment may affect defaecatory dynamics (more complete evacuation of rectocele is observed after evacuation in a private bathroom than during defecography[19]). There is also debate surrounding the association of pathological findings with symptoms and normal proctographic parameters (rectoceles have been found in asymptomatic subjects[20,21]). Findings should be interpreted in context and with caution.

DEFAECATION MAGNETIC RESONANCE IMAGING

Defaecation magnetic resonance imaging (MRI) (the expulsion of aqueous sonographic gel), or dynamic MRI (relaxing, straining) is an alternative to defaecation proctography (Fig. 14.3). MRI allows multi-compartmental assessment in multiple planes, including visualisation of co-existing anterior and middle compartment pathology in high resolution without radiation. Markers, tampons, catheters and contrast opacification of the vagina, bladder and small bowel are possible but usually unnecessary, however, it is usually performed with the patient in the supine position (not physiological for bowel evacuation).

Posterior compartment pathology (e.g., intussusception) is underestimated without contrast evacuation (evacuation may be difficult in a supine closed configuration system).[22] Anterior compartment pathology (e.g., cystocoele) does not require contrast evacuation but may be underestimated with supine imaging.[23] The expense and access to open configuration systems, which allow upright assessment means that MRI has not superseded conventional proctography.

✓ The pelvic floor consortium has published a consensus document for the interpretation of evacuation proctography.[24] Guidelines for the interpretation and use of MRI defecography and integrated total pelvic floor ultrasound are due to be published shortly.

✓ There is not one perfect test for patients with pelvic floor defaecatory dysfunction. The link between findings on imaging and symptoms is not absolute and there may be overlap between findings in symptomatic patients and those in asymptomatic individuals. Findings on imaging must be interpreted with caution and in context.

RECTAL PROLAPSE

Rectal prolapse is the external protrusion of the rectum through the anus. Prolapse is either mucosal, where only the mucosal layer prolapses, or full thickness, with circumferential protrusion through the anus of all linings of the rectal wall. Rectal prolapse is most common in elderly women. Risk factors include connective tissue disorders (e.g., Marfan's and Ehler's–Danlos syndromes), anorexia nervosa, high body mass index and high birthweight during vaginal deliveries.

MUCOSAL PROLAPSE

Mucosal prolapse may occur in isolation but is commonly seen with obstructive defaecation and solitary rectal ulcer syndrome. It may cause perianal discomfort, passage of mucus or blood, constipation and straining at stool. Treatment initially involves bulking agents, increased fibre intake and improving toileting techniques. If surgery is required, outpatient procedures such as suction banding or day case procedures such as surgical excision or plication of the prolapse may be used.[25,26] Patients with mucosal prolapse and obstructive defaecation may be treated with the procedure for prolapse and haemorrhoids (PPH) or stapled transanal rectal resection (STARR).[27]

FULL-THICKNESS RECTAL PROLAPSE

Although conservative treatment with increased fibre intake and the use of bulking laxatives may improve symptoms, the definitive treatment is almost exclusively surgical. The Cochrane Library's review on prolapse surgery failed to identify any trials comparing surgery to non-operative management.[28] Rectal prolapse may be defined as either 'high take off' where the origin of the prolapse is high in the rectum, which progressively intussuscepts until it becomes evident through the anus, or 'low take off', where the edge of the rectum at the anal verge everts and turns back on its self (akin to folding the cuff of a sweater back). In the former condition when the prolapse is out, an examining digit can be inserted into a sulcus between the anal canal and the prolapsing rectum. In low take off prolapse the edge of the prolapse is contiguous with the anal margin and no sulcus exists.

Surgery may be via an abdominal or perineal approach. High take off prolapse usually mandates an abdominal operation as perineal surgery is seldom able to access the apex of the intussusception.

RECTAL PROLAPSE SURGERY

CHOICE OF ABDOMINAL OR PERINEAL SURGICAL APPROACHES

The approach is influenced by the anatomy of the prolapse (see earlier), the preference of the surgeon and patient factors including co-morbidity, age, gender and sexual activity. Most surgeons used to prefer perineal procedures in elderly or frail patients and abdominal approaches in fit patients,[29] although there is increasing evidence that laparoscopic procedures are safe in the elderly. Other considerations include concurrent genital prolapse, constipation, evacuatory difficulties, faecal incontinence and previous pelvic floor injury. Resection rectopexy has traditionally been recommended for patients with both constipation and rectal prolapse, although there is little objective evidence to support this practice. Men may prefer perineal procedures to avoid potential erectile dysfunction following rectal mobilisation during abdominal approaches.

✔✔ A meta-analysis of randomised controlled trials in prolapse surgery was published by the Cochrane Library in 2015 but identified only 15 trials with 1007 patients.[28] The reviewers set out to address abdominal versus perineal approaches, rectopexy methods, open versus laparoscopic approaches, and no resection versus resection. The paucity of data, small sample sizes and methodological problems resulted in few useful conclusions. There was no difference in recurrence rates between abdominal and perineal approaches. Quality of life was poorly reported in all trials. The authors concluded that longer follow-up and larger rigorous trials are needed to improve the evidence base and optimise surgical treatment of full-thickness rectal prolapse.

✔✔ The UK's PROSPER trial recruited 293 patients in a pragmatic trial design where randomisation occurred at either one or two steps within the treatment pathway: 48 patients were randomised to abdominal versus perineal approach, 78 to abdominal resection versus suture rectopexy, and 212 to perineal procedures: Delorme's versus Altemeier's.[30] Recurrence rates overall were high but all procedures were associated with an improvement in quality of life. No approach was found to be superior with respect to recurrence of prolapse, quality of life or impact on faecal incontinence.

PERINEAL APPROACHES

The principal perineal approaches are the Delorme's and Altemeier's procedures. The Delorme's procedure involves resection of the sleeve of redundant rectal mucosa and plication of the prolapsed muscle wall without resection.[31] The Altemeier's procedure (perineal rectosigmoidectomy) involves dissection into the peritoneal cavity via the prolapsed peritoneal lining of the pouch of Douglas, followed by excision of the rectum and sigmoid colon and a coloanal anastomosis[32] (Fig. 14.4). Simultaneous pelvic floor repair or levatorplasty may be performed to treat incontinence.

Delorme's procedure has remained in favour; it is well tolerated in the elderly, has low morbidity and mortality, and minimal impact on continence and bowel function. Recurrence rates are high (5–26.5%), although the procedure may be repeated.[33]

✔✔ A randomised trial of Delorme's procedure versus Delorme's procedure with levatorplasty in 82 patients found a significant improvement in post-operative symptoms of faecal incontinence, and a trend to lower recurrence rates at 12 months, with levatorplasty.[33]

Altemeier's procedure carries the potential complication of pelvic sepsis from anastomotic dehiscence, but appears well tolerated, even in the elderly. Complication rates are 12–14%, mortality rates are low, and continence is improved in half of patients. Recurrence rates are high (10–16%).[34]

✔✔ A randomised trial of 20 participants compared Altemeier's procedure with abdominal resection rectopexy, both with pelvic floor repair.[35] One patient in the Altemeier's arm had recurrent full-thickness prolapse although two patients in each arm developed mucosal prolapse. Both groups experienced significant post-operative morbidity, but incontinence significantly improved only in the abdominal resection rectopexy group.

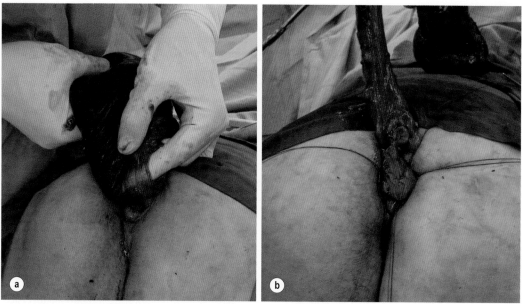

Figure 14.4   **(a)** Division of peritoneal reflection during Altemeier's procedure. **(b)** Division of peritoneal reflection during Altemeier's procedure. (Reproduced by permission of Dr Tracy Hull, Cleveland Clinic, Cleveland, Ohio.)

ABDOMINAL APPROACHES

Abdominal surgery may be performed either open or laparoscopically. Abdominal rectopexy entails rectal mobilisation and fixation to the sacrum with either sutures or mesh.

> ✓✓ A randomised trial of 252 patients confirmed the traditional view that fixation of the rectum to the sacrum (rectopexy) is an integral part of the success of prolapse repair by the transabdominal route.[36]

Rectopexy may be performed either posteriorly with Ivalon sponge (Wells' procedure), fascia lata (Orr Loygue operation) or non-absorbable mesh, or anteriorly with an anterior mesh sling around the rectum to the sacrum (Ripstein's procedure) or ventral mesh rectopexy (VMR). Working on the premise that rectal prolapse is always initiated by anterior rectal wall intussusception, ventral rectosacropexy with no other rectal mobilisation was introduced. Full mobilisation of the posterior rectum during rectopexy is often associated with deterioration or de novo constipation and so many would combine this with a sigmoid resection to offset this change (Frykman Goldberg procedure), which inevitably increases the risk of complications related to the handsewn or stapled anastomosis at the sacral promontory.

> ✓ A multicentre pooled analysis of 643 patients who underwent abdominal procedures for rectal prolapse over a 22-year period found age, gender, surgical technique, means of approach (open or laparoscopic) and method of rectopexy had no impact on recurrence rates.[37] Nevertheless, this study was retrospective and underpowered.

Defaecatory disorders are common after abdominal rectopexy and may present either as novel or worsening constipation, evacuatory difficulties or faecal incontinence. Although many studies include analysis of these

problems, the extent of the problem is difficult to quantify. The latest Cochrane review suggests that lateral ligament division (with potential rectal denervation and worsening constipation) is associated with lower recurrence rates.[28]

Numerous studies examine different methods of rectal fixation during rectopexy. The principal concern with mesh is infection and extrusion. Although the incidence of infection is low,[38] the consequences are serious when it occurs. Complete peritoneal closure over non-absorbable meshes may also reduce the incidence of post-operative small-bowel obstruction.

Resection is usually performed in combination with suture rectopexy in view of the theoretical excess risk of infection if non-absorbable mesh is used for the rectopexy. Comparison of resection rectopexy with suture rectopexy has shown a lower incidence of post-operative constipation with resection rectopexy but no difference in quality of life between the two procedures.[28]

LAPAROSCOPIC APPROACHES

Laparoscopic procedures are associated with fewer complications and shorter length of stay.[28] A meta-analysis comparing open to laparoscopic rectopexy analysed 688 patients from 12 studies (only one was prospective and randomised).[39] The rectopexy techniques included resection, suture and mesh. The meta-analysis concluded that laparoscopic rectopexy was safe, took longer and had comparable recurrent prolapse rates compared to open surgery. Surgeon preference for the laparoscopic abdominal approach has become well-established in the UK.[40]

Improved quality of life is an essential outcome after prolapse surgery but, to date, has only been reported in one trial.[30]

Only one trial has compared the laparoscopic procedures of posterior sutured rectopexy and VMR: 75 patients with full-thickness prolapse were randomised. The primary outcome selected was change between pre- and post-operative obstructive defaecation syndrome scores. There was no difference in functional outcomes, complication rates or recurrence rates at 12 months. Colonic transit time increased in both groups, but to a significantly lesser extent in the ventral rectopexy arm. These approaches are discussed in more detail later.

A feasibility study has examined the technique of robot-assisted laparoscopic rectopexy and concluded that robotic rectopexy can be safely undertaken with similar functional outcomes but higher recurrence rates than open rectopexy.[41] A small trial of laparoscopic MVR (LMVR) versus robotic (RMVR) in 30 patients, of whom only six had full-thickness prolapse, found that the robotic approach was safe and produced good anatomical correction, but without assessing functional outcomes.[42] The additional cost of robotic surgery still needs justification with health economic modelling.

MULTI-COMPARTMENTAL PROLAPSE

The surgical management of combined rectal and urogenital prolapse is probably best carried out from an abdominal approach and laparoscopic repairs are particularly suitable for repairing abnormalities of the rectum, vagina, bladder and pelvic floor. The advantages of laparoscopic approaches in these patients include nerve-sparing surgery and minimally invasive surgery. A combined approach may also serve to lessen the impact of prolapse repair in one compartment on symptoms in another. If mesh is used, ideally procedures that open the vagina should be avoided to reduce the chances of mesh erosion. Vaginal hysterectomy in the setting of combined rectal and urogynaecological prolapse surgery may be associated with higher morbidity.

RECURRENT RECTAL PROLAPSE

Recurrence rates following rectal prolapse surgery vary widely. As all of the approaches carry a risk of recurrent rectal prolapse, a number of patients will come to a second procedure. There is, however, little in the reported literature on management of recurrent rectal prolapse. Abdominal approaches are used more commonly than perineal approaches for recurrent full-thickness prolapse by some groups, while others point out that perineal procedures can be safely repeated. Recurrent prolapse in more than one compartment may be best treated by an abdominal approach. Irrespective of approach, surgery for recurrent prolapse carries a significant risk of post-operative bowel dysfunction, either with obstructive or incontinent symptoms. Ultimately, patients with end-stage recurrent rectal prolapse may gain significant improvement in quality of life with an anal Tiersche suture to close the anus and prevent prolapse together with a de-functioning colostomy, often formed laparoscopically.

OBSTRUCTED DEFAECATION

The cardinal symptoms of obstructive defaecation are straining at stool, incomplete evacuation and the need for rectal, vaginal or perineal digitation to achieve evacuation. According to the Rome IV committee, a diagnosis of functional defaecatory disorder can be made after the following

are fulfilled for 3 months (symptom onset at least 6 months prior);

1. Two or more of the following for at least 25% of defaecations: a. straining, b. lumpy or hard stools, c. sensation of incomplete evacuation, d. sensation of anorectal obstruction/blockage, e. manual manoeuvres to facilitate defaecations (e.g., digital evacuation, support of the pelvic floor) or f. fewer than three defecations per week.
2. Loose stools are rarely present without the use of laxatives.
3. Insufficient criteria for irritable bowel syndrome (abdominal pain and bloating may be present but are not predominant).[4]

Obstructed defaecation may be caused by anatomical abnormalities (namely an anterior rectocele, intussusception, enterocoele, perineal descent and pelvic organ or rectal prolapse), functional abnormalities (pelvic floor dyssynergia, poor propulsion) or a combination of both.[8]

Paradoxical contraction of the puborectalis muscle during straining at stool is better termed *pelvic floor dyssynergia*. It is now apparent that poor propulsive factors also contribute (with or without increased resistance to expulsion). The Rome IV criteria recognise that symptoms may be attributed to either 'dyssynergic defaecation' or 'inadequate defaecatory propulsion'. Pelvic floor dyssynergy is more commonly associated with urogynaecological, gastrointestinal and psychological problems than with slow-transit constipation. Many 'constipated' patients will have improvement in their symptoms with treatment of obstructive defaecation.

Symptoms of obstructive defaecation may mask a number of occult disorders including anxiety and depression, gynaecological prolapse, rectal hyposensitivity and slow-transit constipation. There is a significant association between constipation, ODS and a history of previous eating disorder or abuse, be that physical, sexual or psychological. Many problems associated with obstructive defaecation may not be immediately apparent. Recognition and anticipation of occult pathology allows treatment to be tailored to the individual patient.

RECTOCELE

A rectocele is a hernia of the anterior rectal wall bulging into the rectovaginal septum. It arises from muscular and nerve damage sustained during vaginal delivery, as a result of hormonal changes following the menopause, or due to paradoxical contraction of puborectalis. Rectoceles occur due to a pressure gradient between the rectum and vagina during coughing and straining and weakness in the puborectalis and bulbocavernosus muscles.[43] Suspensory surgery on the anterior vaginal wall (e.g., anterior colporrhaphy) may predispose to the development of a rectocele. Posterior rectoceles are rare, and usually result from traumatic injury or surgical interventions breaching the anococcygeal ligament.

Symptoms associated with rectocele include difficulty in evacuation, constipation, the need for perineal or vaginal digitation/support during defaecation and rectal discomfort. Concomitant faecal incontinence may be due to the involuntary expulsion of the material trapped in the rectocele after defaecation (defaecatory soiling)[44] or an associated intussusception preventing anal closure.[45] Rectoceles vary in size, both in the extent of protrusion into the vagina and in the length of involvement of the rectovaginal septum, but size does not correlate with symptom severity.

An anterior rectocele is common in patients with obstructive defaecation, but may also occur in asymptomatic patients.[20,21] The link between Barium trapping in a rectocele (incomplete evacuation of a rectocele on defaecation proctography despite rectal emptying) and symptoms is sadly lacking, with a pocket of up to 2 cm considered within normal limits.

RECTAL INTUSSUSCEPTION

Rectal intussusception refers to invagination of the rectal wall during the act of defaecation. The bowel wall will descend to a varying degree, which is classified according to the leading edge of the intussusception. The intussusception may remain entirely within the rectum (recto-rectal intussusception), protrude into the anal canal (recto-anal intussusception) or protrude through the anus (full-thickness high take-off rectal prolapse). Intussusception may be classified on defaecation proctography according to the Oxford Radiological Grading System where severity is determined by the extent of the infolding rectal wall in relation to the anal canal; grade I–II is recto-rectal intussusception, grade III–IV is recto-anal intussusception and grade V is high take-off external rectal prolapse.[46] Recto-rectal intussusception is a normal variant.[20]

Rectal intussusception may be associated with symptoms of obstructive defaecation. This may be caused by occlusion of the rectal lumen[45] or the high incidence of concurrent rectocele.[45] However, there is little correlation between the degree of intussusception on evacuation defaecography and symptom severity, and rectal intussusception is also seen in asymptomatic individuals.[20,21]

Half of patients with intussusception suffer with incontinence.[45] The reasons behind this are not clear but it may be due to the infolding rectal folds leading to rectal distention, the associated chronic straining causing pudendal neuropathy, inflammation from a solitary rectal ulcer causing urgency or prolapsing rectal mucosa opening the anal canal.[45]

ENTEROCOELE

The peritoneum of the pouch of Douglas may herniate and contain small bowel (an enterocoele). This is a marker of global pelvic floor weakness and co-exists with other pelvic floor disorders.[47] It is caused by previous pelvic surgery, traction from a prolapsing pelvic organ, intussusception or straining.

Symptoms attributed to enterocoele are vague and non-specific and include incomplete evacuation, post-evacuatory discomfort, pelvic pain and heaviness. The bowel can also descend onto the rectum and contribute to rectal prolapse. The relevance of an enterocoele is controversial as an enterocoele, which descends onto the rectum during defaecation proctography does not necessarily impede evacuation.[48]

SOLITARY RECTAL ULCER SYNDROME

Solitary rectal ulcer syndrome (SRUS) may be caused by paradoxical contraction of the anal sphincter muscle during defaecation, is frequently associated with anal digitation and results in anterior mucosal trauma and ulceration. It is characterised by classical symptoms, endoscopic findings and histopathological changes.[49] Treatment involves dietary changes, bulking agents and biofeedback to reverse the underlying defaecatory disorder. Surgical intervention is only rarely indicated and should only be used for patients with concomitant demonstrable prolapse or intractable symptoms refractory to conservative management. A number of surgical options have been described in SRUS management, including transanal excision of the ulcer, stapled mucosal resection, modified anterior Delorme's procedure, abdominal rectopexy and colostomy formation. Simple resection of the ulcer without biofeedback does not resolve the symptoms. Laparoscopic mesh rectopexy may offer some hope for these patients with improvement in symptoms in around three-quarters of patients.[50]

CONSERVATIVE TREATMENT

The mainstay of treatment is conservative with medical treatment with dietary manipulation, the use of laxatives, suppositories, adjuncts such as rectal irrigation and biofeedback training. The majority of patients with symptoms of obstructive defaecation and an associated rectocele will respond to dietary manipulation and biofeedback.[51] Surgery should be reserved for patients with a correctable anatomical abnormality in whom conservative measures fail.

SURGICAL APPROACHES

Evacuatory difficulties secondary to anatomical abnormalities (i.e., rectocele or intussusception) may be treated by the restoration of normal anatomy.[52] The National Institute for Health and Care Research (NIHR) CapaCITY working Group and Pelvic Floor Society produced a series of systematic reviews, which aimed to assess outcomes for constipation treated with hitching procedures for the rectum (rectal suspension),[52] rectal wall excisional procedures (rectal excision),[53] rectovaginal reinforcement procedures[54] and sacral nerve stimulation.[55] Surgery for obstructed defaecation has been categorised according to these approaches later.

HITCHING PROCEDURES FOR THE RECTUM (RECTAL SUSPENSION)

Resuspension of the rectum aims to hitch up the prolapsing or redundant rectal wall to straighten the intussusception or efface the rectocele.[52] This can be achieved by VMR (LVMR] or RVMR) or resection rectopexy (laparoscopic or open).

Laparoscopic ventral rectopexy involves peritoneal mobilisation over the pouch of Douglas to gain access via the rectovaginal septum to the pelvic floor, mesh fixation to the septum distally and with either sutures or a ProTack™ stapling device proximally to the sacrum, and extra-peritonealisation of the mesh by full peritoneal closure. A simultaneous colporrhaphy to treat an enterocele or vaginal prolapse may be performed by anchoring the posterior vagina to the mesh with sutures.

This approach remains controversial because the link between anatomical abnormalities and symptoms is not absolute and rectal suspension for rectal prolapse is linked with new constipation. This may be caused by either fibrosis of the rectal wall secondary to foreign material (i.e., mesh) or disruption of the lateral suspensory ligaments of the rectum, which contain nerves.[52] The use of sutures rather than mesh and resection of colon rather than simple rectopexy aim to reduce these factors. A laparoscopic or robotic approach has been favoured rather than open surgery because of more rapid recovery and better visibility of the pelvis.

Proponents of ventral rectopexy for full-thickness rectal prolapse propose that avoidance of posterior mobilisation reduces rectal denervation and may lessen post-operative symptoms of constipation.[56] Improvement of constipation symptoms after rectopexy in patients with external prolapse has led to the introduction of ventral rectopexy as a treatment for other disorders associated with obstructed defaecation, including internal rectal intussusception and rectocele.[56]

RVMR has been carried out with equivalent functional outcomes and though more expensive than LVMR, it may be cost effective in the long term.[57] A systematic review comparing LVMR to RVMR showed that the robotic approach takes longer but with no significant added benefit over laparoscopy.[58]

The NIHR CapaCITY working group conducted a systematic review of hitching procedures in 2017, which included 18 articles from 1995–2015 with outcomes from 1238 patients.[52] Selection criteria for patients were variable and data on harms were inconsistently reported. However, length of surgery was 1.5–3.5 hours, length of stay 4–5 days and morbidity 5–15%. Data on efficacy were inconsistently reported but there was good or satisfactory global patient satisfaction outcomes in 83% of patients. After LVMR, 86% of patients reported improvements in constipation. Healing of a solitary rectal ulcer associated with intussusception (reported on 75 patients from two studies) was achieved in 80%. After LVMR or RVMR, high-grade rectal intussusception was corrected in 80–100% of cases. Anatomical recurrence occurred in 2–7% of patients. Patient selection was inconsistently documented although perceived to be vital in predicting outcomes. There were no high-quality studies identified; the majority of studies were observational with uncertain methodology and poor definitions, which made comparison of outcomes difficult. The team concluded that future work is required with high-quality studies to identify those clinical and radiological features, which can predict optimal outcomes.

Consequently Knowles et al. designed a multicenter, stepped-wedge randomised trial of LVMR for patients with intussusception and constipation.[59] Outcomes are awaited and will include pre-operative determinants of outcome and health economics.

VMR may be performed using synthetic or biological mesh. Since the systematic review by the CapaCITY working group, there has been increased interest in mesh-related complications following pelvic surgery. This is discussed and outlined later.

✔ The systemic review of hitching procedures (i.e., LVMR or RVMR or resection rectopexy) for obstructed defaecation by the NIHR CapaCITY working group included 18 articles from 1995–2015 with outcomes from 1238 patients. Recurrence rates appeared reasonable at 0–15.6%. Morbidity rates ranged from 5–15% with mesh complications in 0.5% of patients. However, data on harms were inconsistently reported and there was a paucity of good quality studies.[52]

RECTAL WALL EXCISIONAL PROCEDURES (RECTAL EXCISION)

Surgical excision of the redundant rectal wall that either balloons out (i.e., rectocele) or prolapses in (i.e., intussusception) aims to restore 'normal anatomy'.[53] This can be achieved by the STARR procedure, the use of a modified stapler called the *Contour Transtar* and the intra-anal Delorme's procedure.

STARR was first used in obstructive defaecation following the introduction of the PPH technique. The latter uses a circular stapling device called *Proximate PPH-01*™ made by Ethicon Endo Surgery®.[60]

STARR is normally carried out in the Lloyd–Davies position, although some surgeons prefer the prone jack-knife or Kraske position. STARR consists of a full-thickness circumferential resection of the lower rectum using stapling devices, either with a PPH technique with protection of the rectovaginal septum, or a circumferential technique involving four or five firings of a curved linear stapler (Contour Transtar™, Ethicon Endo-Surgery®). With either method, the end result should be a circumferential row of staples.[1] Any bleeding points are oversewn manually with an absorbable suture.

One of the major concerns about the STARR technique is that it is performed blind and so poses a potential threat to structures lying anterior to the rectal wall in the pouch of Douglas. As an enterocele is a fairly common finding in patients with pelvic floor disorders, it is important to establish the presence of an enterocele with defaecography or MRI before performing a STARR procedure. A German group has advocated the use of laparoscopic surveillance during the STARR procedure in patients known to have an enterocele pre-operatively.[61] Early concern about the STARR procedure arose from a report of 29 patients of whom half had severe post-operative complications or recurrent symptoms.[62] The authors discussed potential errors in technique, including the possibility of stapling too close to the dentate line, undetected co-pathology including pelvic floor dyssynergia, or poor patient selection, and suggested that parity, pelvic floor dyssynergia and anxiety states were risk factors predisposing to failure of STARR. Small rectal diameter, marked pelvic floor descent and low sphincter pressures are also poor prognostic indicators for STARR, whereas rectocele, enterocele and intussusception are positive predictors for a favourable outcome

Early concerns regarding a lack of evidence base for the use of STARR led in 2009 to the European STARR registry, which reported the combined UK, Italian and German 1-year follow-up results of 2224 patients who had undergone surgery.[63] The mean age was 54.7 years and 83.3% of patients were female. While significant improvements were seen in obstructive defaecation and symptom severity scores and in quality-of-life assessment, the complication rate was high at 36%. Complications included urgency (20%), persistent pain (7.1%), urinary retention (6.9%), post-operative bleeding (5%), sepsis (4.4%), staple-line complications (3.5%) and incontinence (1.8%). Single cases each of rectal necrosis and rectovaginal fistula were reported although there was no peri-operative mortality. The conclusions urged better methods of patient selection and optimisation of technique to reduce post-operative defaecatory urgency and pain. Outcomes after Transtar suggests a lower complication rate of 11%.[64]

The systematic review of rectal excision procedures by the NIHR CapaCITY working group included 47 studies with outcomes provided on 8340 patients.[17] The quality of evidence was better than other studies related to surgery for constipation though still relatively poor for a systematic review. Morbidity rate was 16.9% (0–61%), with lower rates after Transtar (8.9%) (although this needs to be confirmed with better research). A reduction in the obstructed defaecation syndrome score was seen in 68–70% of patients. The group proposed that complication rates may have been exaggerated in previous reports; the most common complication was faecal urgency at 10%, long-term pain was seen in less than 2% and rectovaginal fistula was rare (one in 1600 patients). The conclusions drawn were that rectal excisional surgery is appropriate in the presence of a rectocele, with or without intussusception, in patients who have failed conservative measures. It was not possible to advise which method was superior in terms of efficacy and harms, and further studies are required. The group also advised that reliance on unvalidated scoring systems is not satisfactory and that future studies should use disease-specific and generic quality-of-life scoring instruments.

The National Institute for Health and Care Excellence guidelines recommend that there is sufficient evidence to support the safety and efficacy of STARR for obstructed defaecation syndrome and that it can be used within the normal arrangements for clinical governance and consent.[53,65]

✔✔ The systematic review of rectal excision procedures by the CapaCITY working group examined 47 studies on 8340 patients and concluded that complication rates may have been exaggerated previously. Morbidity rate was 16.9% with a rate of faecal urgency of 10%. Rectal excisional surgery was recommended in patients with a rectocele, with or without concurrent intussusception, who have failed conservative measures. It was not possible to advise which excisional surgery is superior.[53]

RECTOVAGINAL REINFORCEMENT PROCEDURES

The correction of a rectocele by reinforcing the barrier between the rectum and the vagina (i.e., the rectovaginal

septum) can be achieved by approaches via the posterior vaginal (posterior repair) (Fig. 14.5), the perineum (transperineal repair) or the anus (transanal repair).[54]

Vaginal repairs involve an incision along the posterior vaginal wall, the plication of the redundant tissue outside the bowel wall and the reconstruction of the vaginal wall. The levator ani and pelvic side walls can also be reinforced although this may be associated with dyspareunia.[54] Transperineal repair, with a curved incision over the perineal body, allows simultaneous sphincteroplasty. A transanal repair can be performed via the Sarles procedure (an elliptical transanal mucocutaneous flap, plication of the anterior rectal muscle with non-absorbable sutures, resection of redundant mucosa and re-application of the flap to the anal verge with absorbable sutures [like an anterior Delorme's operation]) or the Block procedure (full-thickness suture plication of the rectocele with absorbable sutures). Transanal approaches may compromise the integrity of the sphincter complex with consequent faecal incontinence.

A retrospective multicentre study examined the results of rectocele repair in 317 patients by transanal approaches (n = 141), perineal levatorplasty (n = 126) or combined transanal repair and perineal levatorplasty (n = 50).[66] None of the procedures was functionally superior, but bleeding complications were more common in transanal procedures, and dyspareunia and delayed perineal wound healing were more frequent after perineal levatorplasty. About half of the patients studied who had pre-operative faecal incontinence and who underwent perineal levatorplasty had improved continence scores post-operatively.

Two small randomised trials have compared transanal rectocele repair with posterior colporrhaphy in 57 and 30 patients, respectively, with both trials favouring the vaginal approach. Limited evidence reported in a recently updated Cochrane review suggested that vaginal approaches to rectocele repair may offer better anatomical restoration than transanal repair but the functional outcomes remain uncertain.[67] Use of mesh is associated with less awareness of prolapse but there is a significant mesh erosion rate.[67]

A trial did not find in favour of using biological mesh to augment rectocele repair.[68] A randomised trial in

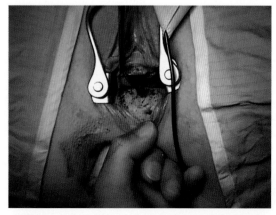

Figure 14.5   Posterior vaginal (posterior repair).

multiparous women with obstructed defaecation randomised patients to three different types of rectocele repair: transperineal repair with or without levatorplasty and transanal repair. All three methods improved the anatomical appearances of rectocele on defecography but transperineal repair with levatorplasty was associated with the best functional outcome.[69]

The CapaCITY working group conducted a systematic review on rectovaginal reinforcement procedures and examined 43 articles on 3346 patients.[54] The majority of studies were observational and comparative. Average length of procedures were 20–169 minutes and length of stay 1–15 days. Complications occurred in 7–17% of patients (bleeding in 0–4%, haematoma or sepsis in 0–2%, fistulation was extremely rare and mesh erosion was common but only reported on in two studies). Long-term outcomes were poorly reported and dyspareunia was reported too inconsistently to make any meaningful conclusions although it may be central in the decision making process for the patient. There were two procedure related deaths in 3209 patients. Data on efficacy was inconsistently measured but 78% reported a satisfactory or good outcome and 30–50% reported reduced symptoms of straining, incomplete evacuation and vaginal digitation. Seventeen percent developed anatomical recurrence. Patient selection was inconsistently documented and there was no evidence to support better outcomes based on selection of patients with a particular sized rectocele. There was insufficient evidence to prefer one type of procedure over another. The team concluded that larger trials are needed to inform future clinical decision making and to define the functional and radiological parameters, which impact treatment outcomes.

✓✓ The systematic review of rectovaginal reinforcement procedures conducted by the CapaCITY working group examined 43 patients in 3346 patients. There was only one high-quality study; the rest were observational studies and comparisons. There was insufficient evidence to prefer one study over another and no evidence to base patient selection on a particular size of rectocele. It was concluded that large trials are required in the future.

SACRAL NERVE STIMULATION

✓✓ The CapaCITY working group conducted a systematic review on the use of sacral nerve stimulation in constipation and identified seven articles with outcomes in 375 patients.[55] The studies were poor quality with morbidity of between 13 and 34% and a removal rate of 8–23%. This systematic review could not identify any particular phenotypes, which would respond favourably to sacral nerve stimulation. Further robust trials since this review have urged even greater caution.

MESH AND PELVIC FLOOR SURGERY

Previously, the use of mesh formed a key component of many pelvic floor surgeries. In terms of posterior compartment pathology, VMR has been the most performed mesh procedure. It has become more evident that pelvic mesh may be associated with morbidities such as mesh erosion, pelvic sepsis and chronic pelvic pain. This has resulted in intense global scrutiny and the publication of the 'Cumberlege review' – 'First Do No Harm'. This report was conducted over 2 years and included the exploration of the use of pelvic mesh, which was found to have caused crippling, life changing complications. The report made nine key recommendations centring on the culture of informed consent and patient safety.[70]

Whilst evidence suggests that mesh morbidity associated with VMR is lower than those seen with transvaginal mesh (the main subject of concern) and abdomino-pelvic procedures for urogenital prolapse (e.g., sacrocolpopexy), there are published national recommendations for VMR from the Pelvic Floor Society in the UK.[71] A multi-disciplinary team approach, enhanced consent, comprehensive patient information leaflets, adequately trained pelvic floor surgeons, careful choice of suture material, a preference for biological mesh and careful recording of outcomes on a national registry are all recommended to optimise outcomes and minimise harm. These recent developments also mean that alternatives to mesh surgery are being explored. Part of the aforementioned recommendations include the development and mandatory use of an NHS hosted pelvic mesh registry and database, which is presently under construction.

FUTURE DEVELOPMENTS

The mainstay of treatment for obstructed defaecation will continue to be conservative. The systematic reviews of surgery for obstructed defaecation performed by the CapaCITY working group highlighted the need for future good quality studies to aid clinical decision making and surgical planning for patients who exhaust conservative treatment options. The Cumberlege report and controversy surrounding the use of pelvic mesh means that alternatives to mesh should also be explored. A national pelvic mesh registry and enhanced consent are requirements for the use of mesh going forwards.

In the UK, the largest drive from the Pelvic Floor Society is equal access and uniformity to pelvic floor services across the country. The Covid pandemic has further heightened the disparity between different services and the geographical variations, which exist.

The primary goal should continue to be a holistic, multi-disciplinary approach with minimal morbidity, patient-centred care and enhanced consent.

Key points

- Patients being considered for surgical management of functional disorders of defaecation are best managed within the setting of a multi-disciplinary clinic or team.
- Subjective assessment includes symptom assessment with patient questionnaires.
- The management of full-thickness prolapse is almost exclusively surgical.
- Correcting full-thickness rectal prolapse results in improved quality of life.
- There is no current evidence to support the superiority of abdominal or perineal approaches to rectal prolapse repair.
- Laparoscopic approaches to abdominal rectopexy are as effective as open approaches and may have benefits in terms of recovery times and lower morbidity.
- Further evidence is needed to determine whether laparoscopic ventral rectopexy is superior to posterior rectopexy in terms of functional outcomes.
- Conservative measures are the mainstay of treatment for obstructed defaecation. Surgery may offer symptomatic relief in carefully selected patients with obstructive defaecation syndrome.
- Surgery for obstructed defaecation can be categorised as rectal suspension, rectal wall excisional procedures and rectovaginal reinforcement procedures. Systematic reviews for each of these have shown a paucity of high-quality studies.
- A multi-disciplinary approach, enhanced consent, patient information leaflets, adequately trained surgeons, careful choice of suture material, a preference for biological mesh and the recording of outcomes on a national registry are recommended for VMR.

 References available at http://ebooks.health.elsevier.com/

ACKNOWLEDEGMENTS

We would like to thank Nicola S. Fearnhead and Alexis M. P. Schizas for their previous versions of the book chapters entitled 'Functional Problems and their Surgical Management' and 'Anorectal Investigation'.

▶ RECOMMENDED VIDEO

- Ventral mesh rectopexy https://youtu.be/VZxf8VCoaCk

KEY REFERENCES

[5] Bordeianou LG, Anger J, Boutros M, Birnbaum E, Carmichael JC, Connell K, et al. Measuring pelvic floor disorder symptoms using patient-reported instruments: proceedings of the consensus meeting of the pelvic floor consortium of the American Society of Colon and Rectal Surgeons, the International Continence Society, the American Urogynecologic Society, and the Society of Urodynamics, Female Pelvic Medicine And Urogenital Reconstruction. Tech Coloproctol 2020;24(1):5–22.

The Pelvic Floor Consortium is a panel of international experts who have reviewed all symptom scores available and made recommendations regarding the questionnaire assessment of patients with pelvic floor dysfunction.

[28] Tou S, Brown SR, Nelson RL. Surgery for complete (full-thickness) rectal prolapse in adults. Cochrane Database Syst Rev 2015;11:CD001758.

Cochrane meta-analysis of randomised controlled trials in prolapse surgery identified 15 trials with 1007 patients. There was no difference in recurrence rates between abdominal and perineal approaches.

[30] Senapati A, Gray RG, Middleton LJ, Harding J, Hills RK, Armitage NCM, et al. PROSPER: a randomised comparison of surgical treatments for rectal prolapse. Colorectal Dis 2013;15(7):858–68.

The largest reported randomised study in rectal prolapse surgery did not favour any specific procedure or approach but did demonstrate an improvement in quality of life after prolapse repair. Recurrence rates overall were higher than anticipated.

[33] Youssef M, Thabet W, El Nakeeb A, Magdy A, Alla EA, El Nabeey MA, et al. Comparative study between Delorme operation with or without postanal repair and levateroplasty in treatment of complete rectal prolapse. Int J Surg 2013;11(1):52–8.

Showed significant improvement in faecal incontinence with levatorplasty.

[35] Deen KI, Grant E, Billingham C, Keighley MR. Abdominal resection rectopexy with pelvic floor repair versus perineal rectosigmoidectomy and pelvic floor repair for full-thickness rectal prolapse. Br J Surg 1994;81(2):302–4.

A randomised controlled trial of Altemeier's procedure with pelvic floor repair compared to abdominal resection rectopexy with pelvic floor repair. Similar recurrent prolapse rates and significant post-operative morbidity were observed in both groups. Incontinence significantly improved in the resection rectopexy group only.

[52] Grossi U, Knowles CH, Mason J, Lacy-Colson J, Brown SR, NIHR CapaCiTY working group, et al. Surgery for constipation: systematic review and practice recommendations: results II: hitching procedures for the rectum (rectal suspension). Colorectal Dis 2017;19(Suppl. 3):37–48.

A systematic review for rectal suspension surgery for obstructed defaecation. There were 18 articles identified of 1238 patients. Morbidity rates ranged from 5–15% with mesh complications in 0.5% of patients. The studies included were poor quality and methodologically robust trials are required to aid future clinical decision making.

[53] Mercer-Jones M, Grossi U, Pares D, Vollebregt PF, Mason J, Knowles CH, et al. Surgery for constipation: systematic review and practice recommendations: results III: rectal wall excisional procedures (Rectal Excision). Colorectal Dis 2017;19(Suppl. 3):49–72.

A systematic review for rectal wall excisional procedures for obstructed defaecation. Forty-seven studies were identified, providing outcomes in 8340 patients. The review concluded that rectal wall excisional procedures are safe with little major morbidity.

[54] Grossi U, Horrocks EJ, Mason J, Knowles CH, Williams AB, NIHR CapaCiTY working group, et al. Surgery for constipation: systematic review and practice recommendations: results IV: rectovaginal reinforcement procedures. Colorectal Dis 2017;19(Suppl. 3):73–91.

A systematic review for rectovaginal reinforcement procedures for obstructed defaecation, conducted by the CapaCITY working group. The review examined 43 articles on 3346 patients. The majority of studies were observational and comparative. Seventy-eight percent reported a satisfactory or good outcome and 17% developed anatomical recurrence. Larger trials are needed to inform future clinical decision making.

[55] Pilkington SA, Emmett C, Knowles CH, Mason J, Yiannakou Y, NIHR CapaCiTY working group, et al. Surgery for constipation: systematic review and practice recommendations: results V: sacral nerve stimulation. Colorectal Dis 2017;19(Suppl. 3):92–100.

A systematic review on sacral nerve stimulation for constipation performed by the CapaCITY working group. Seven articles were included with outcomes in 375 patients. This review could not identify any particular phenotypes, which would respond favourably to sacral nerve stimulation. Further robust trials since this review urge even greater caution.

[70] First Do No Harm: The report of the Independent Medicines and Medical Devices Safety Review [Internet]. Available from: www.immdsreview.org.uk/downloads/IMMDSReview_Web.pdf.

A report was conducted over 2 years, which included the exploration of the use of pelvic mesh. Pelvic mesh was found to have caused crippling, life changing complications and nine key recommendations were made centring on the culture of informed consent and patient safety.

[71] Mercer-Jones MA, Brown SR, Knowles CH, Williams AB. Position statement by the pelvic floor society on behalf of the association of coloproctology of great Britain and Ireland on the use of mesh in ventral mesh rectopexy. Colorectal Dis 2020;22(10):1429–35.

A position statement from the Pelvic Floor Society in the UK published recommendations for the use of mesh in ventral mesh rectopexy. These included a multi-disciplinary team approach, enhanced consent, comprehensive patient information leaflets, adequately trained pelvic floor surgeons, careful choice of suture material, a preference for biological mesh and careful recording of outcomes on a national registry.

Functional problems and their medical management

15

Anton V. Emmanuel

INTRODUCTION

Symptoms related to functional gastrointestinal disorders (FGIDs) are highly prevalent. In community-based studies, up to 22% of 'normal' UK subjects can be diagnosed as having irritable bowel syndrome (IBS) and up to 28% have functional constipation.[1] These disorders are constellations of symptoms – they are not diseases. As such, the emphasis of management of these patients is based on simple principles: the exclusion of organic disease, making a confident diagnosis, explaining why symptoms occur, alteration of lifestyle where appropriate and avoidance of surgery. Education about healthy lifestyle behaviours, reassurance that the symptoms are not due to a life-threatening disease such as cancer and establishment of a therapeutic relationship are essential, and patients have a greater expectation of benefit from lifestyle modification than drugs. This chapter will deal primarily with IBS and functional constipation, leaving the treatment of faecal incontinence to Chapter 13. Similarly, rectal prolapse, which is a frequent co-morbidity of chronic constipation, is dealt with in Chapter 14.

The prevalence of functional disorders depends on the exact diagnostic criteria used; the current standards are the Rome IV criteria.[2] These have updated the previous core diagnostic criteria for IBS: namely the presence of abdominal pain, altered bowel function (in terms of altered stool form or frequency) and a temporal relationship between pain and function. The new criteria require 'pain' rather than just 'discomfort' and that the pain is present at least once a week. The definition of functional constipation requires the presence of at least two of the following: less than three bowel actions a week, need to strain or manually assist evacuation on >25% of occasions, passage of hard stools on >25% of occasions or a sensation of abnormal evacuation on >25% of occasions. These symptoms need to be chronic, and organic disease needs to have been excluded. Although these criteria can be criticised for being over-inclusive, what is clear is that FGIDs represent a major burden on secondary and tertiary outpatient clinics and IBS is the commonest diagnosis in gastrointestinal clinics.[3] An important confounding factor to be borne in mind when reviewing the literature on FGIDs is that the overwhelming majority of studies originate from tertiary centres. Patients attending such institutions are known to have disproportionately high scores on scales of depression, health-related anxiety and somatisation,[4] representing a potentially biased, self-selected group. One further exacerbating variable in assessing studies of FGIDs is that there is a notoriously high placebo response, ranging from 30–80%.[5]

IRRITABLE BOWEL SYNDROME

The key to successful management of IBS is empathic reassurance. This will need to be individually directed according to the patient's symptoms, beliefs and anxieties.[6] Early and positive diagnosis is essential. Helpful factors in establishing a diagnosis are: (i) presence of symptoms for more than 6 months; (ii) frequent consultations for non-gastrointestinal symptoms; (iii) self-report that stress aggravates symptoms.

A key component of the reassurance is provision of a simple explanation of the benign nature and prognosis of the condition. Patients should be advised that no more than 2% of patients need their diagnosis of IBS to be revised at 30 years of follow-up.[1] Equally, it is important to remember that 88% of patients had recurring episodes of gastrointestinal symptoms, and so reassurance should be allied to advice about the need for long-term symptom control.[1]

INVESTIGATION

The presence of alarm features such as symptom onset after age 50 years, rectal bleeding, significant weight loss or abdominal mass mandates serological and luminal investigation to exclude organic disease. Investigations in these frequently young patients (the majority of patients at presentation are aged less than 35 years[1]) should otherwise be avoided since they may both exacerbate patients' anxieties and undermine their confidence in the clinician. The search for a simple diagnostic test of IBS remains, and faecal calprotectin has emerged as a possible candidate to differentiate IBS from an organic cause of diarrhoea.[7] The three hallmark features of IBS are:[8]

- Abdominal pain (not just discomfort)
- Altered bowel pattern (constipation or diarrhoea or both)
- Temporal relationship between pain and altered bowel function

✓ An important diagnosis to consider, especially in the presence of low-grade anaemia, is coeliac disease.[9]

✓ Microscopic colitis should be a differential diagnosis in an older patient with diarrhoea (especially if nocturnal), weight loss and a history of autoimmune disease and recent commencement of a non-steroidal or proton-pump inhibitor.[10]

Approximately 5% of patients fulfilling IBS diagnostic criteria will have histological evidence of coeliac disease

169

compared to 0.5% of controls without IBS symptoms,[9] 13% have reduced faecal elastase, suggestive of pancreatic exocrine insufficiency,[11] and 28% have bile acid malabsorption.[12]

TREATMENT

A stepwise approach to care is advocated, recognising that many patients with mild symptoms, and even some with more severe ones, will respond to such an approach.[13]

LIFESTYLE MODIFICATION

The low FODMAPs diet has emerged in a series of randomised clinical trials as an effective treatment for patients with IBS, especially for the symptoms of bloating, flatulence and abdominal discomfort.[14] Careful dietary adherence supported by specialised dietitians appears to be vital for the success of the diet. Long-term data with the low FODMAPs diet are not available and strict FODMAP restriction is associated with inadequate nutrient intake (e.g., calcium) and potential alteration of gut microbiota.[14] Another helpful dietary intervention worth considering in diarrhoea-predominant IBS patients (d-IBS) is reduction of excess caffeine and sorbitol (found in chewing gum and sweeteners).[15]

Studies have been carried out on the effect of dietary fibre augmentation in some constipation-predominant IBS (c-IBS) patients.[16,17] Early placebo-controlled cross-over studies showed some acceleration of transit but no significant effect on symptoms.[16] Later studies have corroborated the absence of beneficial effect on symptoms and suggested that there is an increase in abdominal bloating, discomfort and flatulence during dietary fibre supplementation.[17] In summary, the effect of dietary fibre in IBS is not significantly beneficial, and the diet is frequently difficult to adhere to in the long term.[18] Current guidelines generally recommend avoiding fibre supplementation in IBS patients (www.nice.org/uk/CG061).

PHARMACOLOGICAL TREATMENTS

Most patients with FGIDs do not need regular drug therapy. The strongest evidence for a single agent in IBS patients is in d-IBS, where loperamide is a well-tolerated and effective treatment of diarrhoea and urgency.[19]

The popular aetiological theory that IBS symptoms relate to gut spasm has led to a huge number of uniformly low-quality studies of anti-spasmodics in IBS patients. These have been subject to meta-analysis.[20] In essence, what can be concluded is that, even allowing for publication bias in favour of positive studies, the evidence is of only modest benefit for anti-cholinergic (such as dicycloverine, hyoscine) or anti-spasmodic drugs (mebeverine, peppermint) over placebo in treating the symptoms of IBS.

In contrast, the data for the efficacy of tricyclic anti-depressants show unequivocal benefit in favour of low-dose usage of these agents.[21] Doses of amitriptyline or nortriptyline of 10–50 mg act at both the central (anxiety and depression) and peripheral (neuromodulatory) mechanisms of IBS.

The putative mechanisms of action of tricyclic agents are through an effect on gut serotonin receptors and visceral sensitivity.

Many drugs that agonise or antagonise serotonin receptors have been developed, and the effect of all these drugs amounts to about 20% advantage over placebo.[22]

There is good evidence supporting the use of ondansetron for d-IBS.[23] Serotonin agents are amongst a number of emerging agents targeting enteric neurotransmitter receptors, some of which may have a role in relieving the sensory symptoms of IBS.[22] In contrast to studies of low-dose tricyclics, standard doses of newer anti-depressants (selective serotonin re-uptake inhibitors) lead to a less impressive improvement in IBS, and at greater cost.[21,24] Linaclotide is licensed for use in patients with constipation-predominant IBS.[13] Finally, early evidence suggests the possibility that some probiotic strains of bacteria may have a beneficial influence in patients with IBS, though this is very much emerging information.[25]

PSYCHOLOGICAL TREATMENTS

Cognitive behavioural therapy directed towards bowel symptoms, and gut-focused hypnotherapy are effective in treating women with IBS, with a 'number needed to treat' of 3.[21,26]

The essence of such treatment is that it is gut focused, since general cognitive behavioural and relaxation therapies are no more effective than standard care. A study by Creed also showed that such treatment is cost-effective and beneficial in the long term.[26]

A number of studies in the literature show the value of hypnotherapy in IBS with benefit in the long-term setting, at up to 6 years following the cessation of therapy.[27]

In brief, three-quarters of patients report symptom alleviation after hypnotherapy, and over 80% of these responders remain well at a median follow-up of 5 years.[21,27]

SURGERY

Patients with IBS are disproportionately more likely to undergo abdominal and pelvic surgery than age- and sex-matched controls.[28,29] IBS patients have a prevalence of cholecystectomy of 4.6% compared with 2.4% in controls, and a prevalence of hysterectomy of 18% versus 12% in controls. There is also evidence that IBS patients are more likely to undergo appendicectomy (35% prevalence compared to 8% in control patients with ulcerative colitis [which is lower than the normal prevalence of appendicectomy]).[29] Furthermore, these procedures are more likely to yield normal findings macroscopically and histologically in IBS patients.[6]

Recent years have seen the re-emergence of the Se-HCAT test to assess for bile acid malabsorption as a cause of symptoms in some patients with IBS, especially when there are symptoms of nocturnal diarrhoea and faecal incontinence in a patient with previous biliary disease.[30]

Abdominal or pelvic surgery may predispose to the development of functional symptoms through mechanical, neural or hormonal impairments. Heaton et al. reported that 44% of subjects develop new symptoms of urgency after cholecystectomy and 27% report constipation symptoms beginning after hysterectomy.[31] In contrast, women undergoing gynaecological surgery for non-pain indications did not develop IBS more often than non-operated controls.[32] What these studies do highlight is the key importance of trying to minimise surgery in patients with FGIDs. In those patients who do undergo an operation, it is implicit that there is complete explanation of the possibility of developing new symptoms post-operatively. The corollary of this is that patients in whom there is a high suspicion of FGID (based on symptoms and normal investigations) should be dissuaded from undergoing diagnostic laparoscopy, which is not usually revealing, and which may result in new complaints.

FUNCTIONAL CONSTIPATION

Estimates from the USA suggest that 1.2% of the population consult a physician every year with the complaint of constipation.[33] Healthcare costs are high (>$7500 per year at 2007 levels) since 85% of these consultations result in the prescription of a laxative.[34] This figure does not include the cost of over-the-counter laxatives nor the costs of specialist investigation and work absenteeism. What these figures reflect is the importance of the role of the hospital specialist in identifying appropriate patients to put through further investigation and specific treatments.

In terms of pathophysiology, functional constipation is considered to be due to either slow whole-gut transit ('colonic inertia'), rectal evacuatory dysfunction or a combination of both of these abnormalities. The commonest cause of slow transit in general practice is as a side-effect of drug therapy for other reasons. The commonest culprit drugs are opiates, anti-cholinergics, anti-hypertensives, iron supplements, antacids and non-steroidal anti-inflammatory drugs.[35]

INVESTIGATION

As in the case of patients with IBS, luminal investigation is reserved for patients with a short history or alarm symptoms, in whom there is the need to exclude colorectal cancer. In addition to the drug causes listed earlier, which can be identified from careful history-taking, the other common associations are with neurological disease (multiple sclerosis, Parkinson's disease and diabetic autonomic neuropathy). Causes of constipation that can be identified from simple serological testing include hypothyroidism, hypercalcaemia and hypokalaemia.

Whereas the diagnosis of IBS is one of exclusion, there are investigations available both to define the pathophysiological abnormality and confirm the presence of constipation. Colonic transit can be simply measured by use of radio-opaque markers followed by a plain abdominal x-ray. One well-described assessment comprises ingestion of three sets of radiologically distinct markers at 24-hour intervals and an abdominal x-ray taken 120 hours after the first ingestion; retention of more than the normal range for any one of the three sets of markers reflects slow transit. The test is cheap, sensitive and reproducible, and provides clinically

helpful information in the management of patients with constipation.[36]

Defaecating proctography (using barium or magnetic resonance contrast gel) and the balloon expulsion test are means of quantifying the anatomical and physiological disturbances of rectal evacuation in patients with functional constipation. Abnormalities such as paradoxical anal sphincter contraction, impaired pelvic floor relaxation, anal intussusception and rectal prolapse can be demonstrated by these techniques.[36] No firm evidence exists as to the value of these abnormalities in the management of patients with constipation.[36] To date, there is no evidence to support the advantage of high resolution anal manometry as a diagnostic modality to aid characterisation or therapy.[37] The place of anorectal manometry in patients with chronic constipation is primarily in the exclusion of Hirschsprung's disease, by confirming the presence of an intact recto-anal inhibitory reflex.[36]

TREATMENT

DIETARY FIBRE SUPPLEMENTATION

This is the traditional first line of therapy for chronic constipation, and by the time of specialist referral, most patients would have already undertaken trials of such therapy. Fibre supplementation increases gut transit and stool bulk by a fraction of the starting value, and as such is only effective in patients with mild constipation.[38] In those small numbers of patients seen in hospital who have not tried fibre supplementation, advice needs to be offered about a gradual stepwise increase in fibre intake. Patients need to be counselled that the effect is not apparent until therapy has been established for several weeks.

✔ Patients need to continue with the diet in the long term,[39] and there is evidence that this can be difficult for a significant proportion. Increasing liquid intake and attempting to maintain regular meal-time patterns seem also to have a place in improving symptoms, although the evidence is strongest in the elderly.[38]

LAXATIVES, SUPPOSITORIES, ENEMAS AND NOVEL PROKINETICS

There are widely held misconceptions of the danger of 'self-poisoning' without a daily bowel action. Given the limited evidence base for the use of laxatives, the first step in the management of constipation is to discourage laxative overuse.[35] The effect of laxatives in chronic constipation is modest at best. Only a very small number of trials have compared a laxative regimen with placebo, and meta-analysis would not be statistically or clinically meaningful.[35] Compared to the dearth of placebo-controlled studies, there are a number of open and blinded comparisons between different laxatives. These have been reviewed,[35] and as might be predicted the opinion of the reviewers is that methodological flaws and inconsistencies prevent meaningful conclusions being drawn. The conclusions that can be drawn are listed later. Overall, there is an increase in stool frequency with bulking agents of 1.4 bowel movements per week, and with other laxative classes of 1.5 bowel movements per week.

Bulk laxatives have a limited role in chronic constipation. They should be reserved for patients who are unable to consume adequate dietary fibre. They have no role in either patients with severe constipation or those who need rapid relief of symptoms.

✓ **Osmotic agents** comprise either poorly absorbed ionic salts or non-absorbed sugars and alcohols. Dose titration is possible with osmotic laxatives, which have a particular place in the management of megacolon and megarectum once the patient has been disimpacted.

✓ **Stimulant laxatives** (anthranoid compounds such as senna, or polyphenolic compounds such as bisacodyl) usually have an effect on stool output within 24 hours of ingestion, and are most suitable for occasional, rather than regular, use.

The effect of these drugs is unpredictable and dose escalation is often required. Nevertheless, they appear to be harmless and are frequently used in chronic severe constipation. What is clear is that the previous fears that chronic use of anthranoid laxatives may result in enteric nerve damage is highly unlikely.[40] **Stool softeners** and **compound mixtures** of the aforementioned classes of laxative are also commonly used, although their efficacy has not been rigorously demonstrated.

Some **suppositories** induce a chemically induced reflex rectal contraction. **Enemas** act either by stimulating rectal contraction or by softening hard stool.[41]

✓ Suppositories and enemas can be effective in alleviating the symptoms of evacuation difficulty if dietary modification and behavioural therapy have been unsuccessful. Used on an as-required basis, enemas have a particular place in managing rectal impaction.

Prucalopride is an effective **prokinetic** for patients with chronic constipation refractory to laxative therapy.[42] Chloride channel agents such as linaclotide (and lubiprostone, which is no longer available in many countries) have also been shown in large-scale randomised trials to have efficacy in similar populations.[43] All these drugs improve transit and pain/bloating symptoms, although the optimal duration of treatment remains uncertain. There seems to be efficacy both in patients with transit delay and those with pelvic floor dyssynergia.[43] Peripherally acting mu-opioid receptor antagonists have also been developed with a beneficial effect on patients with opioid induced constipation.[43]

✓✓ In laxative refractory patients, novel prokinetic and secretagogue drugs offer a therapeutic alternative to behavioural therapy or surgery.[42,43]

BEHAVIOURAL THERAPY (BIOFEEDBACK)

Gut-directed behavioural therapy, biofeedback, is now an established therapy for functional constipation, and in a number of specialist centres is first-line therapy for new referrals.[44,45] Biofeedback is a learning strategy based on operant conditioning. The main focus is on abdominal and pelvic coordination, and it is undoubtedly beneficial in patients with dyssynergic evacuation,[44] but it also seems beneficial in patients with slow transit.[45]

✓✓ Short- and long-term benefit is evident in over 60% of unselected patients in specialist centres.[10,45,46]

The effect of treatment is seen not only in symptoms (improved bowel frequency, reduced need to strain), but also in terms of reduced laxative use and improved quality-of-life scores.[10]

Biofeedback seems to have its effect through alteration of a variety of pathophysiological disturbances. There is evidence that successful outcome with biofeedback is associated with specifically improved autonomic innervation to the colon, and improved transit time for patients with slow and normal transit.[10]

✓ In addition, treatment may improve pelvic floor coordination,[45] thereby allowing antegrade peristalsis and preventing retrograde movement of colonic content. What is important is that biofeedback is successful not just in patients with mild symptoms, but also in those with intractable symptoms who are being considered for surgery.[46]

✓ Transanal irrigation has emerged as a therapy for patients with both functional constipation and constipation secondary to neurological disease such as multiple sclerosis and spinal cord injury (neurogenic bowel dysfunction).

SURGICAL TREATMENT FOR CONSTIPATION

Surgery for rectal evacuation symptoms in the context of structural anorectal disturbance is described in Chapter 14. In those patients with proven slow transit who have failed to respond to dietary modification, biofeedback, long-term trials of laxatives and prokinetics, the traditional algorithm dictates consideration of a surgical approach. The standard surgical procedure has been total colectomy (performed to the level of the sacral promontory) and ileorectal anastomosis.[47] Ileorectostomy is reported as being more successful than ileosigmoidostomy in terms of successful relief of constipation and, providing greater than 7–10 cm of rectum is left intact, then bowel frequency and urgency are not unacceptably frequent.[47]

Almost every major colorectal institution and a huge number of other centres have published on their experience of subtotal colectomy for slow transit constipation. Results vary widely, with satisfaction rates varying from 39–100%.[45] Whilst median scores of bowel frequency tend to show statistically significant improvements, what these composite figures mask are the facts that, firstly, approximately one in three patients do not improve at all and, secondly that some patients develop diarrhoea.

The strongest argument against colectomy for slow transit constipation is that the disorder is a pan-enteric one, and so mere removal of the colon is unlikely to yield sustained benefit.[48,49]

There are two unequivocal conclusions that come out of the welter of small studies in the literature. Firstly, adverse effects occur in over half of all patients. Most common is episodic subacute small-bowel obstruction (occurring in up to two-thirds in some series), need for further abdominal surgery (in up to one-third of patients), persisting constipation (in up to one-quarter), diarrhoea (in up to one-quarter) and faecal incontinence (in up to 10%).

The second conclusion, related to the incidence of adverse events, is the importance of careful patient selection.

Thus, of the many patients complaining of constipation in the community, only a tiny proportion (approximately 1%) are referred to tertiary care, of whom only a small fraction (less than 5%) might benefit from surgical treatment.[50] Patient selection must initially be on clinical grounds (including careful consideration of potential psychiatric disorders) and the physiological demonstration of slow transit. Some authors have recommended extensive anorectal sensory and motor physiological testing, defaecating proctography and upper gut motility studies to aid identification of subgroups in whom surgery may be more successful.[51] In contrast, Rantis et al.[52] identified only 23% of patients in whom such extensive testing altered clinical management; additionally, the cost of this testing was great (US $140 000 in 1997).

In view of the controversy about subtotal colectomy, a vogue for alternative surgical therapies arose. Two particular surgical approaches have received sustained study: stoma formation and segmental colonic resection. However, the data on efficacy and morbidity of these techniques are little different and no less controversial than those for subtotal colectomy.[53] There is unequivocally no place for division of the puborectalis in an attempt to treat rectal evacuatory dysfunction.[54]

A less invasive surgical approach to functional constipation has been the antegrade continence enema (the Malone procedure). Initially used in patients with constipation secondary to neurological disease, the technique has been widely reported in functional constipation.[55] Patients intubate their stoma (appendix or plastic conduit) and irrigate with either water or a stimulant or osmotic laxative. Although there are stomal complications in over 50% of patients (stenosis, mucus leak, pain), three-quarters of patients report 'high' or 'very high' satisfaction with the procedure.[55]

Current trials of medical therapy for FGIDs require quality-of-life data to complement conventional efficacy data. The surgical literature to date shows that although stool frequency may improve, gut-specific quality of life does not.[56]

PUTATIVE TREATMENTS FOR CONSTIPATION

Recent surgical developments have looked at modifications of subtotal colectomy. Small, short-term studies have shown that ileosigmoid or anti-peristaltic caecorectal anastomoses may improve bowel frequency and quality of life.[57]

In some patients with constipation, the presence of intussusception on proctography may provoke the decision to undertake laparoscopic ventral mesh rectopexy. Long-term data are not available, and it is evident that there are mesh-related complications,[58] so at this time, caution is advocated.

Sacral nerve stimulation for constipation has been studied, but disappointing long-term data have meant that the treatment is no longer supported for this indication.[59]

IDIOPATHIC MEGARECTUM AND MEGACOLON

Megarectum and megacolon are uncommon clinical conditions of unknown aetiology that present typically, but not exclusively, with intractable constipation in the first two decades of life.[60] Other conditions presenting with constipation in the context of gut dilatation (e.g., Hirschsprung's disease, chronic intestinal pseudo-obstruction) are not included since the aetiology of these disorders is known. Patients with idiopathic megarectum tend to present with faecal incontinence in the context of recurrent faecal impaction frequently requiring surgical disimpaction. In contrast, patients with idiopathic megacolon more frequently present with abdominal pain and distension in the context of chronic constipation.[60]

The majority of patients with idiopathic megarectum and megacolon can be successfully managed by disimpaction followed by the use of osmotic laxatives. The osmotic agent needs titration in order that the patient obtains a semiformed ('porridgey') stool that is passed three times a day. Occasionally, rectal evacuation techniques (such as suppository use or biofeedback therapy) are required actually to empty the rectum of the semiformed stool.[61]

When medical therapy fails (due to compliance failure or lack of success in avoiding recurrent impaction), surgical therapy is warranted. A number of surgical procedures have been performed, with variable reports of success. As with reports of surgery for idiopathic constipation, the longer the duration of follow-up, the worse the documented outcome. Anorectal physiology, whole-gut transit studies and evacuation proctography do not help identify patients who may benefit or help with choice of surgical procedure.[62] Anorectal physiology testing does have a role in identifying the presence of a recto-anal inhibitory reflex, which excludes the differential diagnosis of Hirschsprung's disease.

With regard to resectional surgery, colectomy offers good results in the majority of patients (80%), with ileorectal anastomosis yielding the greatest levels of patient satisfaction.[62]

Outcomes with the Duhamel procedure, anal myomectomy and restorative proctocolectomy are also favourable in the majority of cases, approaching 70% in the majority of series. Restorative proctocolectomy is suitable in patients with dilatation of both the colon and rectum, whilst the recent procedure of vertical reduction rectoplasty has been proposed for those with dilatation confined to the rectum.[62]

In situations where initial surgery has failed, formation of a stoma (colostomy or ileostomy) is associated with excellent results.[63]

Stoma formation as a primary procedure is also successful in the vast majority of cases.[63] The ultimate choice of surgical procedure will depend on available expertise, patient physical and psychological factors, and the patient's choice.

Key points

- Since dietary manipulation will usually have been undertaken unsuccessfully by the time patients are referred to hospital care, it is seldom beneficial to pursue this form of therapy again.
- There is an expanding differential before making a diagnosis of IBS – coeliac disease, bile acid malabsorption and microscopic colitis.
- Drug therapy is rarely needed in treating patients with IBS.
- Loperamide is unequivocally beneficial in patients with loose stools and urgency.
- Low-dose tricyclic anti-depressants are effective in relieving functional abdominal pain.
- A comprehensive approach to therapy of functional disorders requires close liaison with psychological services.
- Tailored laxatives are preferable to empiric treatment with particular agents.
- Novel prokinetic and secretagogue drugs offer an alternative therapy in laxative refractory cases.
- Biofeedback is effective in almost two-thirds of patients with constipation, whether caused by slow transit or evacuatory dysfunction.
- Subtotal colectomy and ileorectal anastomosis are beneficial in a small number of highly selected patients with idiopathic constipation, although surgical morbidity is frequently high.
- The majority of patients with idiopathic megarectum and megacolon can be managed by disimpaction and initiation of osmotic laxatives.

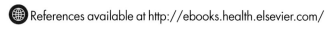 References available at http://ebooks.health.elsevier.com/

KEY REFERENCES

[14] Nanayakkara WS, Skidmore PM, O'Brien L, et al. Efficacy of the low FODMAP diet for treating irritable bowel syndrome: the evidence to date. Clin Exp Gastroenterol 2016;9:131–42.

The low FODMAPs diet restricts the amount of osmotically-active and rapidly fermentable substrate, and hence can improve symptoms of loose stool and gaseousness in some IBS patients.

[17] Snook J, Shepherd HA. Bran supplementation in the treatment of irritable bowel syndrome. Aliment Pharm Ther 1994;8:511–4.

Whilst some patients can expect improvement in stool output with bran, the majority of patients experience an increase in abdominal distension and discomfort.

[19] Cann PA, Read NW, Holdsworth CD, et al. Role of loperamide and placebo in management of irritable bowel syndrome. Dig Dis Sci 1984;29:239–47.

Loperamide is effective in slowing gut transit, reducing stool frequency and urgency in patients with IBS.

[21] Ford AC, Quigley EM, Lacy BE, et al. Effect of antidepressants and psychological therapies, including hypnotherapy, in irritable bowel syndrome: systematic review and meta-analysis. Am J Gastroenterol 2014;109:1350–65.

Meta-analysis of studies using a variety of tricyclic antidepressants in varying doses in patients with FGIDs showing clear benefit for low-dose tricyclics over placebo.

[22] Spiller R, Aziz Q, Creed F, et al. Guidelines on the irritable bowel syndrome: mechanisms and practical management. Gut 2007;56:1770–98.

Practical review of management options available for IBS, encompassing minimum investigation, pharmacological, dietary and lifestyle treatment.

[43] Emmanuel AV, Tack J, Quigley EM, et al. Pharmacological management of constipation. Neurogastroenterol Motil 2009;21 (Suppl. 2):41–54.

A pragmatic approach to using laxatives, based on a combination of what is known about mechanism of action and the available literature on evidence.

[45] Chiotakakou-Faliakou E, Kamm MA, Roy AJ, et al. Biofeedback provides long term benefit for patients with intractable slow and normal transit constipation. Gut 1998;42:517–21.

Demonstration of long-term efficacy of biofeedback in patients who have an initially good response to treatment.

[48] Knowles CH, Scott M, Lunniss PJ. Outcome of colectomy for slow transit constipation. Ann Surg 1999;230:627–38.

Systematic review of most of the small reports of subtotal colectomy showing that efficacy is inversely related to duration of follow-up. A rationale for patient selection is presented.

[59] Zerbib F, Siproudhis L, Lehur PA, et al. Randomised clinical trial of sacral nerve stimulation for refractory constipation. Br J Surg 2017;104(3):205–13.

Definitive evidence of the lack of long-term response to sympathetic nervous system in patients with constipation, despite initial transient benefit.

[60] Gattuso JM, Kamm MA. Clinical features of idiopathic megarectum and idiopathic megacolon. Gut 1997;41:93–9.

The only true prospective comparison of symptoms, pathophysiology and management between patients with idiopathic megarectum and megacolon.

[62] Gladman MA, Scott SM, Lunniss PJ, et al. Systematic review of surgical options for idiopathic megarectum and megacolon. Ann Surg 2005;241:562–74.

A definitive systematic review of the published data on surgical procedures for idiopathic megacolon and megarectum in adults.

Anal fistula 16

Phil Tozer

INTRODUCTION

Anorectal sepsis is common, presenting as either an acute abscess or a chronic anal fistula. Treatment in most involves only a small risk of minor complications, but a minority can present a major challenge to both sufferer and surgeon.

Although fistula-in-ano may be found in association with a variety of specific conditions, the majority in the UK are idiopathic or cryptoglandular, their exact aetiology having not been fully proven, although the diseased anal gland in the inter-sphincteric space is considered central. Research interest in factors encouraging fistula formation, and perhaps more importantly persistence, is growing. Fistulas may either be seen in association or confused with Crohn's disease, tuberculosis, pilonidal disease, hidradenitis suppurativa, lymphogranuloma venereum, pre-sacral dermoid or rectal duplication, actinomycosis, trauma and foreign bodies.[1] An important association is malignancy, which may manifest as a discharging opening on the perineum from a pelvic source, but which may (very rarely) also arise in long-standing fistulas, of whatever aetiology.

Incidence is not known, as most data come from tertiary referral centres. Perhaps the most accurate information comes from Scandinavia, where incidences of between 8.6 and 10 per 10 000 have been reported. There is a male predominance, most series reporting a male to female ratio between 2:1 and 4:1. No sex differences in histology or distribution of anal glands has been found, and there seem to be no differences in circulating sex hormone concentrations between sufferers of either sex or healthy controls. Anal fistulas most commonly afflict people in their third, fourth or fifth decades.[2–4]

The overall morbidity from fistula is difficult to assess in either individual or economic terms. For most patients with simple fistulas, the time spent off work with the initial abscess and subsequent fistula management may be relatively short. However, it is not uncommon for a patient with a complex fistula to have had multiple hospital admissions and operations over several years, with a substantial impact on their professional and personal lives. For these patients, tertiary referral centres with the necessary expertise are essential, with such expertise lying in the hands not only of the surgeons, but also the nurses, radiologists, physiologists and psychologists.

AETIOLOGY

The current hypothesis centres on the anal gland. These have been shown to secrete mucin, but with a different composition from that secreted by rectal mucosa. Current thinking blames anal glands situated in the inter-sphincteric space; these may constitute one-third to two-thirds of the total number of glands found in an anal canal.[3] Eisenhammer[5] considered all non-specific abscesses and fistulas to be the result of extension of sepsis from an intra-muscular or inter-sphincteric anal gland, the sepsis being unable to drain spontaneously into the anal lumen because of infective obstruction of its connecting duct across the internal sphincter.

✔ Parks[6] proposed that, should the initial abscess in relation to the inter-sphincteric anal gland subside, the diseased gland might become the seat of chronic infection with subsequent fistula formation. The fistula is thus a granulation tissue-lined tract kept open by the infective source, which is the abscess around a diseased anal gland in the inter-sphincteric space. Parks[6] studied 30 consecutive cases of anal fistula and found cystic dilatation of anal glands in eight, which he attributed to acquired duct dilatation or more probably a congenital abnormality, a precursor to infection within a mucin-filled cavity.

The importance of bacterial infection in fistula aetiology or persistence remains unclear. Although infection and its effective drainage are the primary problems in the acute stage and failure to treat secondary extensions and abscesses will inevitably lead to recurrence, the possibility that the anal gland becomes the seat of chronic infection in the established fistula has little support in the only two studies directed at this aspect of the hypothesis.[7,8] Subsequent assessments of the fistula tract microbiota using molecular techniques have also failed to demonstrate live bacteria, but have found evidence of inflammation derived from the fistula lumen, and of antibodies to and macrophages containing bacterial cell wall products.[9,10] Another reason why idiopathic fistulas might persist is that they become (at least partly) epithelialised, a factor responsible for failure of healing of fistulas at other sites in the body. A histological study of the inter-sphincteric component of 18 consecutive idiopathic anal fistulas showed that although an association between anal gland and fistula may be demonstrated in a minority of cases, epithelialisation from either or both ends of the fistula tract is a more common finding.[11]

A multifactorial pathogenesis is likely, with inflammation (probably initiated by bacterial components), a failure of wound repair, and structural features such as epithelialisation driving *persistence*, which may be more relevant than the initial infective process itself.[12] This question remains the subject of focused research in fistula units.

Spread of sepsis from an acutely infected anal gland may occur in any of the three planes: vertical, horizontal or circumferential. Caudal spread is the simplest and most usual way by which infection is thought to disseminate to present acutely as a perianal abscess (labelled [A] in Fig. 16.1). Cephalad extension in the same space will result in a high inter-muscular abscess (labelled [B] in Fig. 16.1) or a supra-levator pararectal (or pelvirectal) abscess (labelled [C] in Fig. 16.1), depending on the relation of the sepsis to the longitudinal muscle layer. Lateral spread across the external sphincter will reach the ischioanal fossa (labelled [D] in Fig. 16.1), where further caudal spread will result in the abscess pointing at the skin as an ischioanal abscess; upward spread may penetrate the levators to reach the supra-levator pararectal space. Circumferential spread (Fig. 16.2) may occur in any of the three planes: inter-muscular (synonymous with intra-muscular and equivalent to inter-sphincteric but with no restriction to a level beneath the anorectal ring), ischioanal or supra-levator. All those conditions that Eisenhammer[13] considered not to be of cryptoglandular origin, he placed into the miscellaneous group of acute anorectal non-cryptoglandular non-fistulous abscesses (Fig. 16.3). These included the submucous abscess (arising from an infected haemorrhoid, sclerotherapy or trauma), the mucocutaneous or marginal abscess (infected haematoma), the perianal abscess (follicular skin infection), some ischiorectal abscesses (primary infection or foreign body) and the pelvirectal supra-levator abscess originating from pelvic disease. Another source of inter-sphincteric fistula is the anal fissure. When examining a fissure, the surgeon should 'pinch' it between thumb and forefinger to identify whether a 'pea' is felt and look for an external opening just outside the anal verge. If an abscess cavity or fistula is found to arise from the fissure, it may be laid open, healing both pathologies.

One further source worthy of mention is the pre-sacral cystic lesion (dermoid cyst, duplication cyst, tailgut cyst and others) usually recognisable on sagittal fat saturated T2 magnetic resonance imaging (MRI) images. These are rare and sometimes small enough to elude diagnosis. Such lesions do not normally need biopsy, as MRI appearances can usually differentiate benign disease from (rare) malignant transformation. Their management is beyond the scope of this chapter but when associated with a fistula (because of secondary infection or biopsy), they may require excision as part of the fistula treatment.

MANAGEMENT OF ACUTE SEPSIS

Although the majority of chronic anal fistulas are preceded by an episode of acute anorectal sepsis, acute sepsis does not inevitably lead to fistula formation.[14] Once thought to be one in three, the reported rate of recurrent abscess or fistula development following simple incision and drainage of primary abscess derived from Hospital Episode Statistics (HES) data is 17%. The optimal management of acute sepsis should reside in an understanding of aetiology. Pilonidal infection, hidradenitis and perianal Crohn's disease are usually fairly easy to recognise by history and examination, although it is worth noting that 10% of perianal disease in Crohn's presents before luminal symptoms. Further, Crohn's was diagnosed (after a 14-month delay) in 3% of patients presenting with a primary anorectal abscess in the same HES data.[15]

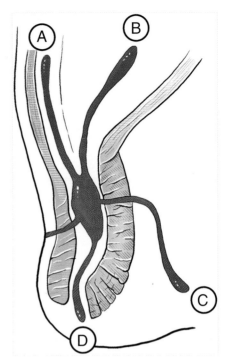

Figure 16.1 The possible courses of spread of sepsis from the diseased anal gland in the inter-sphincteric space. See text for explanation.

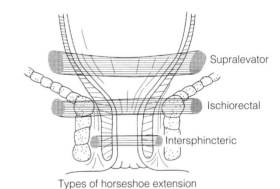

Types of horseshoe extension

Figure 16.2 The three planes in which sepsis may spread circumferentially. (Reproduced from Parks AG, Gordon PH, Hardcastle JD. A classification of fistula-in-ano. Br J Surg. 1976;63:1-12. © British Journal of Surgery Society Ltd. Permission is granted by John Wiley & Sons Ltd on behalf of the BJSS Ltd.)

Patients with acute anorectal sepsis usually present to the emergency department rather than the outpatient clinic, with more pain than constitutional upset likely in perianal abscess, and the opposite with ischioanal fossa abscess. Examination may reveal tender induration over the abscess rather than an exquisitely tender, well-defined lump. Sepsis higher up in the sphincter complex may present with rectal pain, and possibly disturbance of micturition, and there may be no external signs of pathology.

The previous practice of microbiological assessment is now rarely undertaken at the time of incision and drainage as the findings of such assessment would not change management and the evidence base underpinning assertions regarding the risk of fistula persistence is limited.

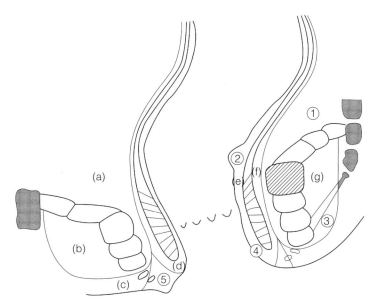

Figure 16.3 The acute anorectal non-cryptoglandular non-fistulous abscesses of Eisenhammer: *(a)* pelvirectal supra-levator space; *(b)* ischiorectal space; *(c)* perianal or superficial ischiorectal space; *(d)* marginal or mucocutaneous space; *(e)* submucous space; *(f)* inter-muscular (syn. Inter-sphincteric) space; *(g)* deep post-anal space. *1*, Pelvirectal supra-levator abscess; *2*, submucous abscess; *3*, ischiorectal abscess; *4*, mucocutaneous or marginal abscess; *5*, perianal or subcutaneous abscess.

Drainage should be wide and should not disrupt the sphincter complex, so that a circumanal incision is often most appropriate. Internal drainage may be more suitable where the abscess is high inter-sphincteric or supra-sphincteric, but if the cavity is in the ischioanal fossa or is close to the skin, external drainage is warranted.

There is much debate over whether an internal opening should be sought at the time of abscess drainage. Two systematic reviews have been dedicated to this question. Those who advocate a more aggressive approach to acute sepsis do so on the basis that incision and drainage can only be effective if the abscess is not cryptoglandular (since a cryptoglandular abscess is really the acute presentation of a fistula),[13] that definitive treatment in the initial stage obviates further surgery, and that such a policy reduces the incidence of complex fistulas arising due to incompletely drained sepsis. The reported recurrence/fistula rate following primary fistulotomy (0–7%) supports this. There are drawbacks, however: internal openings are evident in only about one-third of cases; the acute situation facilitates creation of false tracts and internal openings; and the unknown proportion of patients with cryptoglandular sepsis who might be cured by incision and drainage alone would not be well served by a procedure associated with a greater risk of flatus incontinence and soiling.

The randomised controlled trials of immediate fistula treatment (reviewed in references[17,18]) had a control arm of abscess drainage alone in which only 9–29% of patients presented post-operatively with a persistent fistula, whereas 83–100% of patients in the immediate fistula treatment arms were found to have a tract that was treated at the initial procedure. Iatrogenic injury may account for the higher rate of fistula detection in the immediate fistulotomy arm but, more likely, is an appreciation of the difference between aetiology and persistence. The 17% fistula persistence rate sits neatly in the centre of the range described earlier (9–29%) and it seems likely that the acute fistula will simply heal in all others. Fistulotomy or seton insertion ensures that these patients will be unnecessarily exposed to the risks of fistula surgery such as continence impairment. The minimal benefit to those who would develop a persistent fistula and could then be treated with the same operation at a later date does not seem to justify this.

✓✓ Meta-analysis of these trials[16,17] concluded that fistulotomy resulted in reduction in risk of recurrence at final follow-up without a higher risk of flatus incontinence and soiling (relative risk [RR], 2.46; 95% confidence interval [CI], 0.75–8.06; $P = 0.14$) but (1) some of the studies did find a significant difference in continence between the two groups, (2) continence is notoriously poorly recorded in studies of fistula treatment and (3) the wider literature clearly demonstrates a risk of minor continence impairment of one in three after fistulotomy. It seems, therefore that these reviews conflate two groups of patients: those who will go on to suffer with a chronic fistula and those that would never suffer again after abscess drainage, and that the latter group is put at an unnecessary risk.

Some advocate a policy (in experienced hands) of simple incision when a fistula is not evident, and primary fistulotomy when a fistula is evident and low (or placement of a draining loose seton if there is any doubt about the level, or concern about continence), as long as the patient has been adequately counselled. However, it is probably more sensible to avoid fistula treatment in any form unless a chronic tract in the context of recurrent abscess formation is found. In the latter circumstance, spontaneous regression seems unlikely and fistula treatment (after adequate counselling) will not be disadvantageous.

Since 3% of patients with acute primary abscesses are diagnosed with Crohn's disease a year or so later, this presentation represents an opportunity for early diagnosis. Signs and symptoms, or a family history of Crohn's disease should prompt investigation. Faecal calprotectin and abscess/fistula biopsy are simple first steps, but ongoing suspicion should be investigated with ileocolonoscopy.

CLASSIFICATION OF ANAL FISTULA

Successful surgical management of anal fistula depends upon accurate knowledge of anal sphincter anatomy and the fistula's course through it.

✓ The most comprehensive, practical and widely used classification is that devised by Sir Alan Parks at St Mark's Hospital, based on a study of 400 fistulas treated there.[18]

The cryptoglandular hypothesis and the presence of inter-sphincteric sepsis is central to this classification. Four main groups exist: inter-sphincteric, trans-sphincteric, supra-sphincteric and extra-sphincteric. These can be further subdivided according to the presence and course of secondary extensions.

Inter-sphincteric fistulas (Fig. 16.4; 45% of the original St Mark's series) are usually simple; others have a high blind tract, a high opening into the rectum or no perineal opening, or even have pelvic extension, or arise from pelvic disease. Trans-sphincteric fistulas (Fig. 16.5; 29%) have a primary tract that passes through the external sphincter at varying levels into the ischioanal fossa. Such fistulas may be uncomplicated, consisting only of the primary tract, or can have a high blind tract that may terminate below or above the levator ani muscles. Supra-sphincteric fistulas (Fig. 16.6; 20%) run up to a level above puborectalis and then curl down through the levators and ischioanal fossa to reach the skin. Extra-sphincteric fistulas (Fig. 16.7; 5%) run without relation to the sphincters and are classified according to their pathogenesis. In addition to horizontal and vertical spread, sepsis may spread circumferentially in the inter-sphincteric, ischioanal or pararectal spaces.

The St Mark's classification does have drawbacks, but these are of little clinical significance. Superficial fistulas and those associated with bridged fissures are not acknowledged by a classification whose emphasis is the inter-sphincteric space, but both may be laid open. There can be clinical difficulty in differentiating between a simple inter-sphincteric fistula and a very low trans-sphincteric fistula that crosses the lowermost fibres of the external sphincter. Some question whether supra-sphincteric tracts can be part of a classification based on cryptoglandular pathology (arguing that many are iatrogenic). The extreme rarity of supra-sphincteric fistulas and the difficulty of distinguishing them from high trans-sphincteric tracts raise doubts about their very existence. However, clinical differentiation from high trans-sphincteric fistulas is immaterial since the same methods of treatment are used.

Additional anatomical features have become more relevant as the surgical options have increased; cephalad obliquity, inter-sphincteric complexity, the size of the internal opening and diameter of the tract are all relevant in some

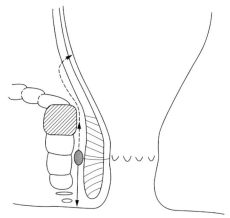

Figure 16.4 The possible courses of an inter-sphincteric fistula. (Reproduced from Marks CG, Ritchie JR. Anal fistulas at St Mark's Hospital. Br J Surg. 1977; 64:84-91. © British Journal of Surgery Society Ltd. Permission is granted by John Wiley & Sons Ltd on behalf on the BJSS Ltd.)

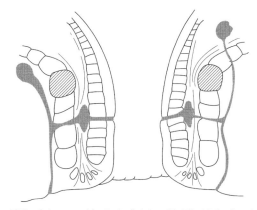

Figure 16.5 A trans-sphincteric fistula with blind infra-levator ischiorectal extension (*left*) and supra-levator pararectal extension (*right*). (Reproduced from Parks AG, Gordon PH, Hardcastle JD. A classification of fistula-in-ano. Br J Surg. 1976; 63:1-12. © British Journal of Surgery Society Ltd. Permission is granted by John Wiley & Sons Ltd on behalf on the BJSS Ltd.)

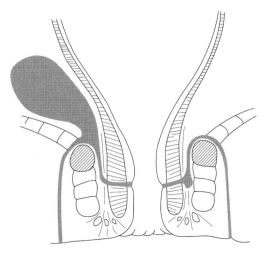

Figure 16.6 Simple supra-sphincteric fistula (*right*) and more complex form with associated secondary pelvic abscess (*left*). (Reproduced from Parks AG, Gordon PH, Hardcastle JD. A classification of fistula-in-ano. Br J Surg. 1976;63:1-12. © British Journal of Surgery Society Ltd. Permission is granted by John Wiley & Sons Ltd on behalf on the BJSS Ltd.)

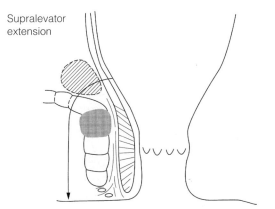

Supralevator
extension

Figure 16.7 Extra-sphincteric fistula running without relation to the sphincter complex. (Reproduced from Marks CG, Ritchie JK. Anal fistulas at St Mark's Hospital. Br J Surg. 1977;64:84-91. © British Journal of Surgery Society Ltd. Permission is granted by John Wiley & Sons Ltd on behalf on the BJSS Ltd.)

surgical situations. Inclusion of all such factors would create a new classification system too complex to be of widespread value.

ASSESSMENT

CLINICAL

A full history and examination, including proctosigmoidoscopy, are essential to exclude any associated conditions. The normal bowel habit and any risk of deterioration in the future (such as the presence of irritable bowel syndrome, inflammatory bowel disease or simply a tendency towards a loose stool) should be identified. A patient who passes a hard stool twice a week will tolerate a greater degree of sphincter disturbance than another who opens their bowel three times a day to loose stool. Clinical assessment of the fistula involves five essential points, enumerated by Goodsall and Miles:

1. location of the internal opening (IO);
2. location of the external opening (EO);
3. course of the primary tract;
4. presence of secondary extensions;
5. presence of other diseases complicating the fistula.

The relative positions of the external and internal openings indicate the likely course of the primary tract, and the presence of any palpable induration, especially supra-levator, should alert the surgeon to a secondary tract. The distance of the external opening from the anal verge may assist in differentiating an inter-sphincteric from a trans-sphincteric fistula; the greater the distance, the greater the likelihood of a complex cephalad extension.[3] Goodsall's rule generally applies in that the likely site of the internal opening can be predicted by the position around the anal circumference of the external opening. Exceptions to this rule include anteriorly located openings more than 3 cm from the anal verge (which may be anterior extensions of posterior horseshoe fistulas) and fistulas associated with other diseases, especially Crohn's and malignancy.

The first is to identify the position of the external opening(s). Next, the perianal area should be carefully palpated with a well-lubricated finger to feel for the presence and direction of induration, which will indicate the course of the primary tract (Fig. 16.8). If the tract is not palpable, it is likely the fistula is not inter-sphincteric or low trans-sphincteric. Digital examination within the anorectal lumen is then performed to locate indentation/induration marking the site of the internal opening. Asking the patient to contract the anal sphincters allows assessment of the position of the primary tract in relation to the puborectalis sling (posteriorly) or upper border of the external anal sphincter (anteriorly), although it must be remembered that in trans-sphincteric fistulas the level of the internal opening may not be the same as that at which the primary tract crosses the external sphincter (which may be higher, especially if the internal opening is above the dentate line). The finger is then advanced into the rectum and supra-levator induration sought (it feels like bone and is more noticeable when it is unilateral as there is asymmetry; Fig. 16.9). Digital assessment of the primary tract by an experienced coloproctologist has been shown to be 85% accurate.[19]

Examination under anaesthesia complements examination in the awake patient. The internal opening may be easily seen at proctoscopy, aided if necessary, by gentle downward retraction of the dentate line, which may expose openings concealed by prominent valves or papillae. Lateral traction of an opened Eisenhammer proctoscope may reveal dimpling at the internal opening due to its underlying fibrous inelasticity. Massage of the tract may reveal the site of the internal opening as a bead of pus. If the tract is simple, a probe may traverse its entire length, but if the probe comes to lie above or remote from the dentate line, a direct association between the tract and the adjacent anoderm cannot be assumed.[20] Instillation of dilute hydrogen peroxide is the easiest way of locating the internal opening, as staining (e.g., with methylene blue) is avoided.[20,21]

Careful probing can delineate primary and secondary tracts. If the internal and external openings are easily detected but the probe cannot traverse the tract, it is possible that there is a high extension, and a probe passed from each opening may then delineate the primary tract. Failure to negotiate probes around a horseshoe posterior trans-sphincteric fistula suggests at least one acute bend in the tract, within the inter-sphincteric space and crossing the external sphincter, or in the roof of the ischioanal fossa, in which case, anatomy will only be defined once surgery is under way (Fig. 16.10) and may be assisted by fistuloscopy. Persistence of granulation tissue after curettage during the operation is an indication of a secondary extension, as it indicates that the granulation comes from the extension and therefore cannot be removed by curettage within the primary tract.[21]

If the tract in a primary fistula can be palpated from external to internal opening without any other induration being present, it is likely that the tract is simple and low, whether inter-sphincteric or trans-sphincteric. Anything else represents potential complexity and should prompt imaging, as should recurrence or a plan to undertake a sphincter preserving procedure.

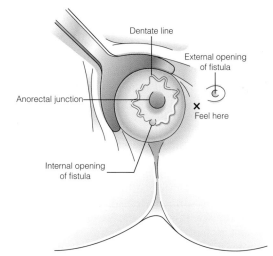

Figure 16.8 Palpating for the direction and depth of the primary tract. (Reproduced from Phillips RKS. Operative management of low cryptoglandular fistula-in-ano. Operat Tech Gen Surg. 2001;3(3):134-41. With permission from Elsevier.)

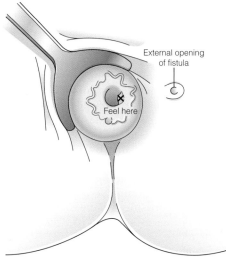

Figure 16.9 Palpating for the presence of induration, indicating either a high primary tract or secondary extension in the roof of the ischiorectal fossa or supra-levator space. (Reproduced from Phillips RKS. Operative management of low cryptoglandular fistula-in-ano. Operat Tech Gen Surg. 2001;3(3):134-41. With permission from Elsevier.)

IMAGING

Previous surgery leads to scarring and deformity, as well as the creation of unusual tracts, which can make clinical assessment extremely difficult. Also, sphincter preserving techniques such as 'ligation of the inter-sphincteric fistula tract' (LIFT) or laser fistula treatment (of which FiLaC is one example), rely on a simple, single tract and confirmation of the anatomy is sensible to reduce the risk of failure due to occult extensions. The advent of endoanal ultrasound (EAUS) and MRI, however, has resulted in a plethora of reports assessing and comparing imaging modalities, which have been comprehensively reviewed.[22]

These modalities have rendered fistulography almost obsolete. Computed tomography (CT) is indicated only

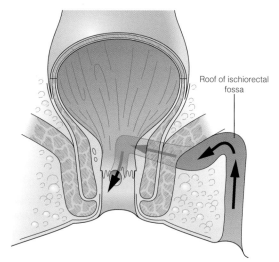

Figure 16.10 Trans-sphincteric horseshoe fistulas may have several sharp bends along their course, preventing exact delineation unless the ischiorectal fossa is opened widely (to reach the acute bend in the roof of the ischiorectal fossa), and often necessitating dislocation of the posterior sphincter from its ligamentous attachments (to ascertain the site at which the tract crosses the external sphincter). (Reproduced from Phillips RKS. Operative management of low cryptoglandular fistula-in-ano. Operat Tech Gen Surg. 2001;3(3):134-41. With permission from Elsevier.)

when the fistula arises from an intra-abdominal or pelvic source.

EAUS is relatively cheap and easy to perform, but operator-dependent with limited focal range, making evaluation of pathology beyond the sphincters (laterally or above) difficult. These are the same areas from which difficulty in clinical assessment often arises. Also, sepsis and scarring from prior surgery can confuse fistula assessment. EAUS is superior to MRI in assessing sphincter integrity. Three-dimensional (3D) EAUS is practiced successfully by some surgeons in the clinic and the operating room, but the repeatability and accessibility of MRI make it the most useful modality. Three-D MRI, volume and activity assessment are under investigation and may enhance the value of MRI further in education, surgical planning and medical treatment monitoring.

Short tau inversion recovery (STIR) sequencing (a fat-suppression technique) to highlight the presence of pus and granulation tissue without the need for any contrast media[23] was used in a prospective study involving 35 patients that favourably compared MRI interpretations with the independently documented operative findings.[24] Schwartz et al. compared the accuracy of MRI, EAUS and examination under anaesthetic in a prospective cohort and found that a combination of any two yielded accuracy of 100%.[25]

Further prospective studies have confirmed that the technique certainly challenges operative assessment by an experienced coloproctologist as the gold standard. A prospective study has demonstrated a therapeutic impact of MRI in the management of patients treated for primary anal fistulas,[26] although the therapeutic impact is much greater when used to assess recurrent fistulas.[27]

The value of imaging prior to sphincter preserving procedures to identify specific anatomical features, which preclude or favour a given operation has been suggested,[28] and work on a minimum dataset for MRI reporting (and requesting) may help standardise the information offered to the fistula surgeon.[29] A collaborative approach with surgeon and radiologist reviewing images together and planning surgery accordingly seems sensible.

The accuracy of MRI also means that we are now able to refute or confirm the presence of sepsis in those patients with symptoms, but in whom clinical examination is unrewarding, and in the prospective assessment of newer methods of attempted fistula eradication.

PHYSIOLOGICAL

The correlation between subjective assessment of an individual's continence and physiological measurements recorded in a laboratory remains limited, and the influence of these measurements on outcome when a given operation is undertaken is unknown. Some argue for physiological assessment (anal canal length, pressures along it, anorectal sensitivity, sphincter integrity and pudendal nerve conduction studies) in the clinical context of a patient with a complex fistula (or at risk of functional compromise); others (including the author) find little or no value in it, since it is not clear what a given set of anorectal physiology results indicate regarding options for surgery, other than that a weak sphincter would be weakened further by fistulotomy, which is usually clinically apparent.

✔️ Milligan and Morgan[30] stressed the importance of the anorectal ring in fistula surgery: 'If this ring be cut, loss of control surely results, yet as long as the narrowest complete ring of muscle remains, control is preserved. All the anal sphincter muscles below this ring may be divided in any manner without harmful loss of control.' Whether their patients and an in-depth assessment of quality of life centring on continence would support this statement is less clear, and certainly many patients now fear even a modest loss of control.

Complete division of the puborectalis sling in suprasphincteric and extra-sphincteric fistulas results in total incontinence. It is often said that the higher the level at which the primary tract crosses the sphincter complex, the greater the possibility of impaired function after fistulotomy, and the weaker the sphincters before surgical intervention, the greater the likelihood of such morbidity. A similar line of thinking argues that the amount of muscle divided at fistulotomy is an important determinant of resultant function. In fact, as with liver resection, it is the amount left behind, which is crucial and really quite high fistulas may be laid open with good results in appropriately assessed, counselled and willing patients.

Traditionally, greater importance has been apportioned to the external than the internal anal sphincter in the context of muscle preservation in fistula surgery. Indeed, the importance of eradication of the presumed aetiological source, the diseased anal gland in the inter-sphincteric space, led Parks[6] to advocate internal sphincterectomy (excision of that segment of internal sphincter overlying the diseased gland) as an essential part of surgical management. Nowadays, most surgeons divide rather than excise the circular muscle, but the concept of getting rid of the inter-sphincteric source remains widely held.

To determine the physiological and functional effects of fistula surgery, a prospective study[31] of 37 patients successfully treated for either inter-sphincteric (15 patients) or trans-sphincteric fistulas was performed. All patients underwent division of the internal anal sphincter and anoderm below the level of the primary tract; 15 of the 22 patients with trans-sphincteric fistulas also underwent division of the external sphincter, at least to the level of the dentate line, whereas the remaining seven patients with trans-sphincteric fistulas were successfully treated without external sphincter division. As might be predicted, distal anal canal and maximum resting pressures were reduced to a similar extent in all patients, whether the internal alone or both sphincters were divided. The addition of external sphincter division in the 15 patients who underwent fistulotomy of trans-sphincteric tracts did, however, result in significant reductions in distal anal canal and maximum squeeze pressures.

Functional outcome was not related to division of the external sphincter, with an equal incidence of minor disturbances of continence reported by those in whom it had been preserved (53% vs. 50%, respectively). Furthermore, the severity of post-operative symptoms was no different between the two groups, being related to reduced post-operative resting pressures, reduced maximum resting pressure and higher thresholds of anal electrosensitivity in the sector of surgery, rather than to post-operative squeeze pressures.

We have demonstrated similar findings in subsequent studies of fistulotomy[32,33] in which a one in three or one in four risk of flatus incontinence and mucus leakage or 'skid marks' in the underwear occurs with division of any amount of internal or external sphincter as long as a minimum length of external sphincter is left behind (2 cm as a rule but less in some cases), and in the presence of a normal bowel habit. This forms the basis of informed consent for fistulotomy.

Total sphincter conservation would be optimal in terms of functional outcome, but the drawback is that no sphincter-preserving method heals the underlying fistula as surely as lay-open. This is important, because although the studies discussed earlier revealed a relatively high incidence of (minor) functional disturbance, the vast majority of patients were satisfied with their management and tolerated a reduction in function as a reasonable price to pay to be rid of chronic anal sepsis. When asked prospectively, patients are frightened by the term 'incontinence' and generally seek to avoid it.[34] It is important, instead, to outline the anticipated functional result and to be descriptive (e.g., wind might escape inadvertently and there might be 'skid marks' in the underwear), avoiding using emotive words such as 'incontinence' and also to acknowledge that patients at different stages of their 'journey' will have different goals and differing willingness to accept a risk of functional impairment to obtain cure.

PRINCIPLES OF FISTULA SURGERY

Acute sepsis is an indication for urgent surgical drainage, usually followed by early fistula treatment. However, in cases where a more complex procedure than lay-open is contemplated, acute sepsis should be eradicated, leaving well-established chronic tracts. A loose seton may be required to achieve adequate drainage of the primary tract. Secondary tracts should be either laid open, curetted or drained, according to their position in relation to the levators. Often, authors recommend parenteral antibiotics peri-operatively and post-operatively for any of the more complex reconstructive procedures.

In the UK, fistula surgery is usually performed under general anaesthesia, but in North America, local or regional anaesthesia is widely used. There is some advantage of light general anaesthesia in that it is still possible to gauge muscle tone and determine how much muscle might remain were the fistula to be laid open. Similarly, in the UK most anal fistula surgery is performed with the patient in the lithotomy position, although the prone jack-knife position is favoured by some. The operative findings and treatment should be recorded; the St Mark's Hospital fistula operation sheet (Fig. 16.11) based on the Parks classification provides an excellent standardised format for documentation.

SURGICAL TREATMENT – GENERAL PRINCIPLES AND INTERPRETING THE EVIDENCE

Lay-open remains the surest way of eliminating an anal fistula. However, the risk of functional impairment, whether to stool (which is rare and can generally be avoided) or to flatus with marking of the underwear (which occurs at a rate of one in three when muscle is divided) may cause some to hesitate. Others prefer this risk to that of recurrence, particularly when the fistula is already recurrent or longstanding.[35] The multiplicity of techniques designed to preserve sphincter function and at the same time eradicate fistula pathology (the so-called *sphincter-preserving procedures* or *SPPs*), reflects their relative lack of success. A degree of caution and scepticism may be appropriately apportioned when assessing reported results of the various approaches, since:

1. patient populations may be markedly different;
2. fistula classification may be variable;

ST. MARK'S HOSPITAL
FISTULA OPERATION NOTES

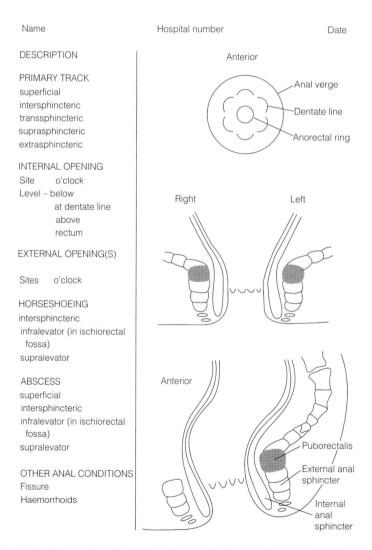

Figure 16.11   The St Mark's Hospital fistula operation sheet. (Reproduced with thanks to Mr James P.S. Thomson, Emeritus Consultant Surgeon, St Mark's.)

3. reports of successes may not be tempered by honest reporting of failures;
4. reports of success in terms of fistula cure have historically not always been accompanied by reports of changes in continence;
5. despite the increasing drive for evidence-based medicine, the use of adequately powered prospective randomised trials is perhaps rarely achievable, because of individual fistula (and sphincter) variability and individual surgeon preference and skill;
6. follow-up may be inadequate and MRI confirmation of healing, which can substitute for longer follow-up, may also be lacking;
7. assessment of continence is often hampered by a lack of clarity regarding pre-operative continence and therefore a post-operative change, confusion regarding discharge and pad use due to the fistula being mistaken for incontinence in scoring systems, and the use of average scores pre- and post-operatively across the whole study cohort, which may dilute and obscure a significant continence impairment in a small minority.

The 'sphincter preserving' procedures do not succeed in permanently eradicating the fistula as often as fistulotomy, but some are also unable to demonstrate that they are truly protective of the patient's continence. This may be due to a degree of injury to the sphincter complex but may also relate to other aspects of the continence mechanism. It is possible to consider these procedures according to the element of fistula pathology to which they are directed. For example, the advancement flap and LIFT procedure disconnect the tract from the gut tube (potentially causing a degree of sphincter damage in the process). The glues and plugs fill the space. Stem cells are thought to exert an anti-inflammatory effect but also to facilitate the wound repair process. Video-assisted anal fistula treatment (VAAFT) and laser fistula closure obliterate the luminal aspect of the tract to encourage healthy tissue to heal. Another way to classify fistula operations is according to their intent (cure or palliation) and their impact on the sphincter (whether truly sphincter preserving or not). For example, fistulotomy with or without reconstruction and tight/cutting setons are non-SPPs, whereas plug, VAAFT and laser are SPPs. LIFT carries a very small risk to continence and advancement flaps a slightly greater one, but still broadly represent SPPs. Loose setons are not placed with curative intent.

To improve outcomes, many reparative techniques include elements thought (but rarely proven) to enhance healing or avoid complications, or to address an additional aspect of pathology. The use of antibiotics, mechanical bowel preparation and 'tract preparation' are examples.

TRACT PREPARATION AND RATIONALISATION

Tract preparation is an increasingly explicit concept in surgical fistula trials. If one assumes that epithelialisation will prevent healing or that a secondary extension or undrained collection will induce early recurrence, a period of seton drainage followed by thorough debridement of the luminal aspect of the tract should improve the chance of success. This question has been considered in a number of studies of seton drainage before transanal

advancement flap repair, with some identifying a benefit and others not.[36] A study randomising patients to a full programme of tract preparation with evidence of success (which might be measured by resolution of secondary extensions or abscesses, or reduction in inflammatory activity) before definitive surgery is required to answer this question.

Some techniques (such as the plug, LIFT or FiLaC) probably require a particular tract anatomy (such as a single, straight, trans-sphincteric tract) to be successful. In these cases, tract preparation involves complete healing of secondary extensions (usually by laying open with seton drainage of the primary tract) before the definitive operation can be attempted.

This process of 'rationalisation' is traditionally performed by wide drainage or laying open. In the ischioanal fossa, this is straight forward and carries no risk of continence impairment, although the wounds may be large and take time to heal, and 'medialisation' of the external opening towards the anus often leads to bifurcation outside the sphincter complex with new and old openings persisting. These can be laid open again, or a long seton placed in the first instance instead.

Pararectal extensions, which arise entirely above the sphincter complex can be laid open into the rectum with relative impunity. Bleeding can be a problem and jaw diathermy or ultrasonic devices may be useful. Inter-sphincteric complexity is also usually laid open internally but doing so will bring about the same concerns regarding minor continence impairment (flatus incontinence, minor mucus leakage) as fistulotomy of an inter-sphincteric fistula. Patients may accept this risk in return for a 95% chance of cure (as with fistulotomy) but may be less willing when the residual primary tract is too high to lay open, and an SPP is needed to attempt closure. In that case, they may ultimately be left with a continence impairment and a persistent fistula; the worst of both worlds. The first stage procedure in which the internal lay open is performed is the moment when the patient takes on the risk without yet obtaining a high chance of a benefit, and therefore is the key point of no return. There is value in identifying and highlighting this moment to the patient, who may instead choose to leave the inter-sphincteric extension and stick with a permanent loose seton as the lesser of two evils. Some effort is underway to assess the value of rationalisation by minimally invasive techniques such as VAAFT. The extensions can be identified and treated with cautery, widely drained and sometimes treated in this way on multiple occasions, to try to reduce the complexity and eradicate extensions. Whilst this is an attractive prospect, no reports have yet described this technique, and personal experience is underwhelming.

CHOICES, CONSENT AND GOALS

When offering options to patients, a surgeon will consider the fistula, the patient's bowel habit and their underlying disease factors as described earlier. Ultimately, there will be three principal routes of treatment to offer, of which one or more may be unsuitable. These are fistulotomy, permanent loose seton drainage or a sphincter preserving procedure. As these are discussed with the patient, it is crucial that their goals are explored. Does the patient simply wish to be rid of pain and abscess episodes? Would she/he rather undergo a single operation to draw a line under things and accept the functional impairment, which may result? Is the primary goal to avoid any impairment to continence?

A frank conversation in which these broad options are honestly discussed is a key element of the management of a fistula patient. For the surgeon to understand clearly the options that can be offered is only half the story – the patient controls the rest, and the joint decision making, which follows informs and empowers both parties.

THE LOOSE SETON

Setons may be loose, tight or chemical. Only the former protects continence. Setons are useful:

* as a holding measure to prevent abscess formation and drain acute sepsis;
* to help identify the tract in an awake patient when the muscle involved can be more accurately assessed;
* to guide the VAAFT scope through a complex tract;
* to prepare a tract before an attempt at definitive fistula repair;
* as part of a strategy of symptom control in the management of Crohn's anal fistula;
* as a long-term solution for patients who cannot or do not wish to undergo further attempts at repair

Historical procedures in which the internal sphincter was divided and a seton left through the external anal sphincter, the latter being removed at 2–3 months if healing was progressing well, were based on the principle that the pathology in the inter-sphincteric space having been dealt with, the rest of the tract would settle. They are of little interest now and were not successful in the long term.

With a loose seton in place, there are several options available: (i) the patient may be happy living with a 'controlled' fistula with a long-term draining seton. Our preference is for a permanent loose seton made of No.1 Ethibond with just one surgeon's knot and the 'whiskers' secured with 2/0 silk, to avoid bulkiness and to give comfort (nylon setons tend to be sharp, Silastic setons have bulky knots); (ii) a sphincter-sparing procedure might be considered; (iii) a fistulotomy may be performed (if appropriate); or (iv) fistulotomy may be combined with the raising of a defunctioning colostomy, time allowed for full healing, before sphincter repair and then restoration of intestinal continuity at a final stage. The decision made must be between the individual patient and the surgeon.

SPHINCTER DIVIDING OPERATIONS

FISTULOTOMY

Fistulotomy means laying open and allowing to heal by secondary intention and it is very likely to heal any fistula, but this success rate is tempered by sphincter division and the associated risks of continence disturbance. If fistulotomy is being considered, it is important to be aware of pre-existing bowel habit to help judge how much muscle should be preserved at surgery. In principle, high trans-sphincteric (especially anterior tracts in women) and supra-sphincteric tracts should generally not be considered for fistulotomy. Inter-sphincteric and low trans-sphincteric tracts are probably best treated by this method.

The surgeon should assess the fistula with a probe or a seton right through the fistula to determine whether it can be safely laid open based on the amount of muscle that would remain and a knowledge of the patient's bowel habit and wishes. Hydrogen peroxide, the passage of a second probe through the other opening and the use of lachrymal probes may make it easier to traverse the difficult tract. The internal opening is often lower than one assumes; the tract may turn caudad in the inter-sphincteric space, and some tracts narrow at this point like an hourglass and will not allow a Lockhart–Mummery probe to pass but will accept a lachrymal probe. If the tract is not traversed easily despite these measures, it is better to try another day than to create a false passage, a new opening and potentially an incurable fistula.

Marsupialisation, that is, suturing the divided wound edge to the edges of the curetted fibrous tract, results in a smaller wound and faster healing.[37,38]

Secondary extensions from the primary tract can be dealt with in 2 ways. The traditional method in the UK is to lay these open widely to allow maximal drainage, which is followed by healing by secondary intention. As long as the external sphincter is intact, the residual scarring after healing is remarkably little. In the United States, the use of incisions, counter-incisions and the placement of encircling drains is sometimes preferred; these drains are left in for 2–4 weeks, with more rapid healing and less deformity claimed.

In rare cases, a patient with a substantial history and ongoing, severe symptoms, may opt for fistulotomy despite a more significant risk to their continence, perhaps necessitating stoma formation. This is a difficult decision in benign disease and most patients would eschew the offer, but in experienced hands, it has a place and brings long awaited relief to a tiny minority in whom nothing else works.

FISTULOTOMY AND IMMEDIATE RECONSTITUTION

Parkash et al.[39] reported a series of 120 patients treated by fistulotomy, immediate reconstruction of the divided musculature and primary wound closure. The results were impressive: 88% of wounds had healed by 2 weeks, there was a 4% recurrence rate and all patients were satisfied with the functional outcome. However, 118 of the 120 fistulas were classified as low inter-sphincteric or simple trans-sphincteric, and the authors acknowledged that similar success would not be expected with more complex fistulas. The technique has been applied to a small cohort of patients with recurrent complex fistulas, not amenable to fistulotomy, with good results in terms of healing, manometric and functional outcomes, and with no report of dehiscence of the reconstituted sphincter.[40] More recently, Roig et al. published parallel case series of rectal advancement flap and fistulectomy with immediate sphincter repair for complex cryptoglandular fistula. In the fistulectomy and sphincter repair group, the new minor incontinence (soiling and flatus incontinence) rate following surgery was around 20% despite similar resting tone pre- and post-surgery.[41]

These and other studies have been reviewed and similarly strong success rates and continence preservation have been shown, but higher tracts are both more likely to recur and carry a greater risk of continence disturbance. It remains a concern that the true continence impairment rate in high fistulae, the only ones in which patients benefit from reconstruction, is higher than usually reported, due to poor reporting of fistula height and of post-operative continence change in many studies.[42] However, this technique may be particularly useful in those with a pre-existing sphincter injury and continence deficit, in whom continence may improve.[43]

FISTULECTOMY

The technique of fistulectomy, which excises rather than incises the fistula tract, has been criticised on the basis that the greater tissue loss leads to delayed healing.[44]

However, Lewis[45] advocates core-out fistulectomy rather than excision of the tract.

Although rarely for primary repair, this technique is useful when the primary tract is difficult to follow, and as part of other procedures such as LIFT or in direct repair of a rectovaginal fistula, for example, with a Martius or omental flap.

THE TIGHT SETON

The rationale of the tight or cutting seton is similar to that of the staged fistulotomy technique, in that the divided muscle is not allowed to spring apart but there is supposed to be gradual severance through the sphincter followed by fibrosis. Its value lies in two principles: first that it preserves continence, and second that it reduces perineal deformity. Whilst the second may carry some merit, the former is highly questionable.

Goldberg and Garcia-Aquilar[46] recommended the use of a tight seton whenever the fistula encircles more than 30% of the sphincter complex and when local sepsis or fibrosis precludes the raising of an advancement flap. The portion of the tract outside the sphincters is laid open, although others in the United States have recommended Penrose drainage of horseshoe extensions. The anoderm and perianal skin overlying that portion of the sphincter encircled by the seton are incised and the inter-sphincteric space drained by internal sphincterotomy, extended cephalad if necessary to drain any high inter-sphincteric (inter-muscular) extension. Tightening of the seton does not commence until any suppuration has resolved, usually at 3-weeks post-operatively. Tightening is repeated every 2 weeks using a silk tie or Barron band until the seton has cut through.

Goldberg described the use of the cutting seton in 13 patients with trans-sphincteric fistulas between 1988 and 1992 and found that the average time for the seton to cut through was 16 weeks (range 8–36 weeks) with no recurrences at a median follow-up of 24 months (range 4–60 months). This was tempered by a relatively high incidence of functional morbidity: one patient suffered major incontinence, and a further seven patients (54%) complained of minor persistent loss of control to flatus or episodic loss of liquid stool.

The critical aspects of management by the cutting seton must be firstly the elimination of acute sepsis and secondary extensions before sphincter division, and secondly the speed with which the seton cuts through the sphincter. In a series of 24 patients with high trans-sphincteric fistulas,

Christensen et al.[47] tightened the seton every second day; 62% of patients reported some degree of incontinence postoperatively, including 29% who wore a pad constantly. The 'snug' Silastic (elastic) seton method, in which the muscle is cut through much more slowly but without the need for tightening, in the treatment of inter- and trans-sphincteric fistulas, was associated with healing in all cases, but with a 25% incidence of continence disturbance in the 16 patients followed up at a median 42 months after the seton had cut through.[48] The rates of sphincter disturbance described are similar to those seen with simple fistulotomy and therefore any benefit over single-stage fistulotomy is unclear. Another consideration is the time taken to heal and, in the case of the tight seton, the discomfort of tightening. As a result, it is difficult to define a clear role for this technique. We consider that the tight seton should not be used with high fistulas. Essentially, the decision to be made is whether a fistula can be laid open. If it can, then probably there is no advantage to laying it open slowly. If it cannot, then a tight seton will lead to significant faecal incontinence. National and international guidelines in general do not support this technique.

THE CHEMICAL SETON

This method, enjoying a resurgence in India where it is known as *Ksharasootra*, involves weekly re-insertion of a thread along the fistula tract. The thread is prepared in a multistage process involving layers of agents derived from plants. Apart from its anti-bacterial and anti-inflammatory properties, the alkalinity of the thread (about pH 9.5) appears to be the means by which the thread slowly cuts through the tissues at about 1 cm of tract every 6 days.

In a randomised trial involving 502 patients,[49] apart from a longer healing time (8 weeks vs. 4 weeks), the results of this outpatient treatment were comparable with fistulotomy (incontinence rate 5% vs. 9%; recurrence rate at 1 year 4% vs. 11%).

Recurrences usually occur for the same reasons as after conventional surgery, such as a missed secondary tract or another internal opening, but the economic advantages of such a method in a developing country are obvious. For low fistulas, however, a randomised study from Singapore concluded that the method has no advantage over conventional fistulotomy.[50]

SPHINCTER PRESERVING PROCEDURES

The sphincter preserving procedures offer a chance to heal a fistula without (substantial) muscle damage. Some preserve muscle more completely than others and each has different risks, fistulae for which it is suitable and technical requirements. There are many sphincter preserving procedures since none is reliably effective in high enough proportions across different institutions. Each has been introduced with great excitement and high success rates, which have rarely been maintained when the technique is generalised. Some have failed completely (such as fibrin glue) and others continue because of minimal negative effects, despite a modest success rate.

In practice, the 'newer techniques' offer fewer risks but with a less robust evidence base, so that even though the estimated success rate is no greater than 50%, we feel less confident in that number than for the 'more established techniques' (LIFT and flaps), which carry slightly greater risks (Table 16.1). In general, a new technique should offer no less a chance of success than the existing SPPs, and must offer no greater risk, to be of value.

ADVANCEMENT FLAPS

Elting[51] described advancement flaps in anal fistula in 1912, supported by two principles: severing the communication with the bowel, and adequate closure of that communication with eradication of all diseased tissue in the anorectal wall. To these, modern surgeons have added adequate flap vascularity and anastomosis of the flap to a site well distal to the site of the (previously excised) internal opening. Modifications have included the use of full-thickness rectal flaps, partial-thickness flaps, curved incisions and rhomboid flaps, with or without closure of the defect in and outside the external sphincter,[52] and distally based flaps (anocutaneous flaps transposed upwards). Some authors argue that the flap should include part if not all of the underlying internal sphincter to maintain vascularity, but this may have an impact on continence.[41] In general, thicker flaps are more likely to be successful but also to impair continence to a minor degree. Apart from the presence of acute sepsis, a large internal opening is considered a contraindication as the risk of anastomotic breakdown is high,[53] and a heavily scarred, indurated perineum precludes adequate mobilisation.

Physiological assessment has revealed that the technique may be associated with reduced resting[54] and squeeze[55]

pressures, and success rates in terms of fistula healing decrease with time.[56]

Smoking has been shown to increase recurrence[57] and Mizrahi et al. found that Crohn's disease was also associated with failure.[58]

Advancement flap surgery is facilitated when there is a degree of perineal descent or internal intussusception, both of which can be identified in the outpatient setting. In their absence, we would not usually recommend this technique.

In a large series reported in 2010, Mitalas et al. describe successful healing in around two-thirds of 278 consecutive patients with high trans-sphincteric fistulas operated on in two tertiary referral units in the Netherlands.[36] This probably represents a realistic, high-quality series.

✅ A more recent meta-analysis of almost 800 patients demonstrated success in around three quarters of patients with idiopathic fistula, and around six in 10 with Crohn's disease, and newly developed continence impairment in around 8% across both groups.[59] The issues discussed earlier, which limit the quality of evidence with regard to 'healing' and incontinence apply here, despite the best efforts of the authors.

INTER-SPHINCTERIC APPROACHES

In 1993 an inter-sphincteric approach was published from St Mark's Hospital with reasonable results. The LIFT operation is similar and combines disconnection of the

Table 16.1 Sphincter preserving procedures

Technique	Evidence base	Ideal fistula / Contraindications	Continence impact	Other risks
LIFT	Established technique	Straight TS tract / Past or present IS complexity, very high tract, IAS loss/wide IO	1.6% minor impairment	'Upstaging' of fistula
Advancement flap	Established technique	High, single IO with good rectal wall mobility / Fixed tissues, very low or multiple IOs	1 in 3 risk of minor impairment (less if mucosal only)	Greater risk of failure with thinner flaps, can leave a very large tract if flap retracts
Plug	Less robust evidence base	Straight TS tract / Any side branch or cavity	None	Can leave a larger tract although often helps tract settle somewhat even in failure
Laser	Less robust evidence base	Straight, narrow TS tract / Any side branch or cavity, marked angulation	None	Can leave a large tract although often helps tract settle somewhat even in failure
VAAFT	Less robust evidence base	Straight, wide TS tract, some complexity may be acceptable / Tract too narrow for scope to pass, marked angulation	None	Can leave a large tract although often helps tract settle somewhat even in failure
MSCs	New but stronger evidence base	pCD only at present, suitable for quite complex fistulae / Currently only available in trials in the UK	None	Logistical and cost implications are substantial

IAS, Internal anal sphincter; IO, internal opening; IS, intersphincteric; LIFT, ligation of the inter-sphincteric fistula tract; MSC, mesenchymal stem cell; pCD, perianal Crohn's disease; TS, trans-sphincteric; VAAFT, video-assisted anal fistula treatment.

tract from the gut with destruction of the culprit inter-sphincteric gland. An inter-sphincteric approach is made, with ligation (or transfixion) and division of the tract as it traverses the inter-sphincteric space. The external component is curetted and left open to drain whereas the inter-sphincteric wound is closed. Initial series of low fistulas demonstrated success rates in excess of 90% and then 80% without impairment of continence, but more complex tracts demonstrated a more modest success rate of 57%, also with preserved continence.

✔✔ A recent systematic review including almost 500 patients suggests a success rate for LIFT of 65–70% with a new continence impairment rate of 1.6%.[59] Some heterogeneity in technique and length of follow-up limits these findings but the technique is cheap and safe. The addition of a bioprosthetic implant in the inter-sphincteric space does not seem to confer a benefit.

If the tract is very high, there is a risk of injury to the rectum (or vagina) during blind passage of a right-angle clip cephalad to the fistula. A 'deep wide cup' internal opening represents loss of the internal anal sphincter at the site of the internal opening and therefore a loss of the space in which the LIFT procedure is performed. These features represent contraindications to the operation, as do inter-sphincteric complexity or scarring.

Recurrence/failure takes the form either of breakdown of the inter-sphincteric wound, inter-sphincteric recurrence of the fistula through the inter-sphincteric wound alone ('downstaging'), trans-sphincteric recurrence through the original tract or 'upstaging' of the fistula with a new tract in the inter-sphincteric wound appearing in addition to the main tract. If the fistula is 'downstaged' to an inter-sphincteric tract alone, fistulotomy may become suitable.[60]

INFILL MATERIALS – GLUES AND PLUGS

Enthusiastic initial reports have not always stood the test of time.[61] In fact, the literature describing fibrin glue and the fistula plug are remarkably similar, both suggesting initial success rates in the order of 80%, which have fallen over the years to around 40%. Both approaches are highly attractive, as they require little surgical skill, but their weakness is their uncertain success rate. They may be used as an adjunct to advancement flap surgery. There are many considerations: biocompatibility; rate of decomposition/integration with host tissues; and how to prepare the host environment (drill/core-out/curette the tract or leave it alone, prior identification and drainage/eradication of secondary extensions, and so on).[62]

FIBRIN GLUE

Several reviews have discussed the variable efficacy reported for fibrin glue.[63–65] The 2010 Cochrane review of the surgical management of anal fistula evaluated two randomised trials of fibrin glue (versus fistulotomy and advancement flap repair). Fibrin glue was inferior in both and its place in the surgical armamentarium is questionable – indeed glue has substantially fallen out of favour. The glue theoretically fills the tract, promoting healing through fibroblast migration and activation and the formation of a collagen

meshwork. Curettage to remove granulation tissue and debris is stressed. Difficulty with this and complete occlusion of secondary tracts may account for failure. Early absorption or leakage from the fistula will also lead to recurrence and often occurs.[66] Post-operative MRI, despite clinical healing, has shown much lower true healing rates, in the order of 10–20%.[67]

BIOPROSTHETIC PLUGS

The anal fistula plug also sprang onto the scene with great optimism, with success rates of 80% reported. Subsequent success rates are very variable, and proponents argue that surgical technique may be at fault, issuing consensus statements to try to improve outcome.[68]

The plug has been compared with an advancement flap in two randomised trials. One closed prematurely because of an unacceptable failure rate with the plug,[69] while in the other, recurrence with a plug was also higher.[70]

Plug extrusion inevitably leads to failure and is thought to contribute to high recurrence rates in some studies. This may explain the association between a tract length of over 4 cm and a three-fold increase in success rate.[71] In this study, the 43% success rate was disappointing, particularly given the small number of plug extrusions and the presence of an experienced plug surgeon at every case. However, the 61% success rate in the group with a long tract and the median 2-year follow-up are more encouraging. In other studies, longer-term follow-up and MRI assessment have demonstrated a lower healing rate than was initially clinically apparent.[72,73]

✔✔ The results of the FIAT trial,[74] which included around 300 patients, have not changed the landscape, demonstrating a success rate at 12 months of around 50% for plug, and similar to the surgeon's preference group, which included fistulotomy, cutting seton and LIFT. In fact, fistulotomy seemed to produce more healing and LIFT a little less. Despite the primary outcome (being Faecal Incontinence Quality of Life) favouring the plug over fistulotomy, no difference was seen between the two groups. Complications at 6 weeks were twice as likely in the plug group. The overall cost of the two seems to be fairly similar, particularly perhaps when assuming the ongoing costs of a failed repair in the life of a fistula patient.

NEWER TECHNIQUES

A key consideration with the newer techniques is whether they will suffer the same deterioration in outcome seen in the glue and plug literature as their own evidence base matures. In the interim, their expanded utility and lack of substantial risks make them attractive, but their use should be associated with honest consenting and reporting of results.

VIDEO-ASSISTED ANAL FISTULA TREATMENT

VAAFT was developed by Meinero and first published in 2006.[75] It involves the introduction of a rigid fistuloscope into the tract through the external opening, with saline or glycine irrigation to open the tract, which can then be followed. The scope has a working channel, which can accommodate forceps, brush or diathermy. The surgeon passes the scope into all accessible tracts and can undertake lavage, biopsy and cauterisation. Meinero initially described closure of the internal opening with an advancement flap. The procedure has two phases: diagnostic and therapeutic. In evaluating this technique, it is important to recognise the value of the two phases separately but in general a 'success rate' meaning healing of the fistula is described – in this case the term cVAAFT (curative) is used.

In fact, the main value of this technique may prove to be its wide utility:

1. For passing setons through very tortuous tracts[76]
2. For biopsies in deep cavities and tracts
3. For palliating tracts (pVAAFT), for example, in Crohn's disease[77]
4. For the identification and eradication of otherwise occult secondary extensions (dVAAFT)
5. As a form of advanced tract preparation before another definitive technique is performed

In the Crohn's patient, the goal of treatment may be symptom control rather than fistula healing, and the pVAAFT technique carries value in symptom reduction as part of a multi-disciplinary approach.[77] The dVAAFT technique aims to eradicate extensions, which might otherwise involve wide drainage or sphincter division to achieve. Data are awaited but our own experience is mixed.

In terms of a healing rate after VAAFT, the two largest series report healing in around 75% at short-term follow-up, which seems to have been maintained at 1 year.[77] Complications are minor and the most common is perineal oedema caused by extravasation of irrigation fluid. This raises the question of iatrogenic tract formation, which has not yet been widely reported. The technique also carries great value in training and for the surgeon's understanding of the fistula and indeed fistulae.

LASER FISTULA CLOSURE (INCLUDING FILAC: FISTULA TRACT LASER CLOSURE)

FiLaC was initially described in 2011 by Wilhelm and uses a radial emitting laser to obliterate the luminal aspect of the fistula to a known depth, throughout its length.[78] The technique was initially combined with closure of the internal opening by advancement flap but this was subsequently replaced with simple suture closure with no change to the success rate noted. The procedure is quick and easy. There is some pain postoperatively and the probes and laser are expensive. Success rates initially ranged from around 70–80%, but Wilhelm's 5-year experience showed a primary healing rate of around 65%.[79] Further assessment, particularly in Crohn's patients and in randomised trials, is required and will help establish the place of this technique. The fistula must be narrow and simple for optimal use, according to most proponents. A more recent systematic review suggests that Wilhelm's outcomes are accurate[80] but as with other SPPs, we reserve judgement until the technique is more mature.

OVER-THE-SCOPE CLIP

Over-the-scope clip (OTSC) was first published in 2012 by Prosst and Ehni, who describe placement of a Nitinol clip over a denuded area around the internal opening, closing it and disconnecting the tract from the gut. The largest series to date was published by Prosst in 2016 and described a success rate of 79% in primary fistulas.[81] This fell to 26% in recurrent fistulas, 20% in rectovaginal fistulas and 45% in the presence of inflammatory bowel disease, although all these groups were much smaller. Clip migration and elective removal because of pain, soiling or for unexplained patient choice imply that the clip is not quite so well tolerated as the developers claim. One study[82] had very poor results with significant complications but the surgeons were inexperienced in the technique and included mostly very complex patients. A systematic review found three studies[80] and more recent publications have not substantially improved understanding yet.

STEM CELLS

Adipose-derived mesenchymal stem cells (ASC) have been used in both cryptoglandular and Crohn's anal fistulas. In 2009 Garcia-Olmo reported a randomised phase II trial of fibrin glue with ASCs versus glue alone and subsequently reported long-term follow-up.[83] In the ASC group, 17 of 24 patients' fistulas closed at 8 weeks compared to three of 25 in the glue alone group. Two of the ASC group successes then relapsed at 1 year. In the long-term follow-up study, three were lost to follow-up and five relapsed so that of the original 17 successes, seven remained closed at the end of approximately 40 months' follow-up compared to two of the original three successes in the glue alone group.

✔ In Crohn's disease, the ADMIRE CD group published a multicentre double-blind randomised trial of ASC injection versus placebo.[84] This large study with more than 100 patients in each arm used a combined clinical and radiological outcome measure and found remission in 50% in the treatment arm versus 34% in the control arm. Longer follow-up data suggest these closure rates persist out to 2 years. The ADMIRE II study and INSPIRE registry aim to increase numbers and follow-up length, and include real world data, however, both are industry sponsored.

Whilst evidence of long-term success is limited, these studies suggest the potential of this technique. The anti-inflammatory, pro-wound healing action of stem cells may alter the immune environment surrounding the fistulas, encouraging healing. Whether in isolation or to enhance definitive surgical or medical treatment, stem cells are an exciting prospect currently available only in Crohn's disease, but indications are likely to expand.

MANAGEMENT OF THE RECURRENT FISTULA

Failure of sphincter-preserving methods and persistent symptoms may make lay-open the most sensible option and the patient's goals and appetite for risk may evolve during their journey. Some patients may prefer to live with a long-term loose seton, and others favour further attempts with SPPs, whilst a few require defunctioning ostomy formation due to intractable and severe symptoms.

After fistulotomy, many patients are able to lead normal lives. However, some may request sphincter repair. MRI is a useful way of making sure that there is no covert pathology before embarking on repair. Over a 3-year period at St Mark's Hospital, 20 patients underwent sphincteroplasty for incontinence after previous surgery for idiopathic fistulas. A good outcome (Parks' grade 1 or 2 continence score) was obtained in 13 (65%).[85]

It is important to consider the possibility of an extra-sphincteric fistula arising from pelvic or abdominal disease or from a pre-sacral dermoid cyst when a high 'blind' tract is encountered. Failure to image (usually with MRI) is a major reason for delayed diagnosis. If a tract is truly high and blind, this might be because the internal opening has closed, or because surgery has dealt with the primary tract and recurrence is because of an overlooked secondary extension. In such cases, the component of the tract outside the sphincters should be laid open and curetted. As the resulting wound may be large, it is often wise to make a circular rather than radial incision to avoid sphincter damage. Following granulation tissue with curette and probe must be done extremely carefully if false tracts and iatrogenic openings are to be avoided. If the tract peters out before reaching the inter-sphincteric space, it is safest to stop and come back another day. If the tract enters the inter-sphincteric space but no internal opening can be identified, it is reasonable to assume that the opening has healed or is extremely small; internal sphincterectomy of that quadrant is then justified to try to prevent recurrence.

Key points

- A fistula has a primary tract and may have secondary extensions – complete eradication of both will lead to cure.
- All lay-open procedures divide some of the internal sphincter, so patients should be warned of a one in three chance of inadvertent passage of wind and 'skid marks' in the underwear; 'incontinence' is an unhelpful word.
- Lay-open is the most certain treatment where it is feasible and when the risks have been properly explained and accepted.
- Anterior fistulas in women should only rarely be laid open, as the risk of impaired continence is high.
- Sphincter preserving procedures carry limited success rates but are generally safe and require a particular fistula morphology.
- Newer techniques appear regularly. Promising early results need long-term evaluation or MRI confirmation of healing.
- STIR sequence MRI is the gold standard for imaging but several newer techniques are under investigation.
- A permanent, comfortable, loose seton will preserve continence and prevent much (although not all) future abscess formation, but continual discharge means patients need careful counselling, and a minority find it unacceptable in the long term.
- In the balance between minor soiling with almost certain cure or potential recurrence with a less than certain technique, many patients allowed the choice will choose the former, but preferences vary between patients and within an individual patient's journey.

RECOMMENDED VIDEOS

- Documentary exploring the management of fistula-in-ano – https://tinyurl.com/yd26552u
- Delormes advancement flap for ano-vaginal fistula – https://tinyurl.com/ycbfcy66
- Rectal advancement flap – https://www.youtube.com/watch?v=d-qVauLWgZ5k
- LIFT –https://www.youtube.com/watch?v=7YXOJzIrKFM
- FiLaC – https://www.youtube.com/watch?v=8cT4CV1gkAA
- OTSC – https://www.youtube.com/watch?v=ZqPfWvCGL1g

KEY REFERENCES

[16] Quah HM, Tang CL, Eu KW, et al. Meta-analysis of randomized clinical trials comparing drainage alone vs primary sphincter-cutting procedures for anorectal abscess-fistula. Int J Colorectal Dis 2006;21(6):602–9. PMID: 16317550.

[17] Malik AI, Nelson RL, Tou S. Incision and drainage of perianal abscess with or without treatment of anal fistula. Cochrane Database Syst Rev 2010;7:CD006827. PMID: 20614450.

Meta-analyses showing that fistulotomy in setting of acute sepsis resulted in reduction in risk of recurrence at final follow-up without a higher risk of flatus incontinence and soiling.

[59] Stellingwerf ME, van Praag EM, Tozer PJ, Bemelman WA, Buskens CJ. Systematic review and meta-analysis of endorectal advancement flap and ligation of the intersphincteric fistula tract for cryptoglandular and Crohn's high perianal fistulas. BJS Open 2019;3(3):231–41. https://doi.org/10.1002/bjs5.50129. Erratum in: BJS Open. 2020;4(1):166–241. PMID: 31183438; PMCID: PMC6551488.

A systematic review including almost 500 patients suggests a success rate for LIFT of 65–70% with a new continence impairment rate of 1.6%.

[74] Jayne DG, Scholefield J, Tolan D, FIAT Trial Collaborative Group, et al. A multicenter randomized controlled trial comparing safety, efficacy, and cost-effectiveness of the surgisis anal fistula plug versus surgeon's preference for transsphincteric fistula-in-ano: the FIAT Trial. Ann Surg 2021;273(3):433–41. https://doi.org/10.1097/SLA.0000000000003981. PMID: 32516229.

Randomised controlled trial of about 300 patients showed a success rate at 12 months of around 50% for plug, similar to the surgeon's preference group.

References available at http://ebooks.health.elsevier.com/

Pasquale Giordano | Gaetano Gallo

HAEMORRHOIDS

ANATOMY AND PHYSIOLOGY

Haemorrhoids are vascular arteriovenous plexuses that form two sets of anal cushions in the normal rectal anatomy. These plexuses are located in the upper anal canal above the dentate line (internal haemorrhoidal plexus), and at the anal verge (external haemorrhoidal plexus). The internal haemorrhoidal plexus or internal haemorrhoids, also known as *anal cushions*, lie above the dentate line and are covered by columnar epithelial cells that have visceral innervations. Anal cushions or internal haemorrhoids are classically described as being in the right anterior, right posterior and left lateral aspect of the anal canal ('4-7-11 o'clock' in the lithotomy position).[1,2] Newer technologies investigating the rectal and anal canal vasculature as a potential target for the treatment of haemorrhoidal disease have established an average of six haemorrhoidal arteries originating from the superior rectal artery and reaching the haemorrhoidal zone (range 1–8).[3] The internal haemorrhoidal plexus drains via the middle rectal veins into the internal iliac vessels. The internal haemorrhoids complement anal sphincter function in normal physiology by providing fine control over the continence of liquid and gas, however, their abnormal enlargement produces haemorrhoidal disease, corresponding to the common complaints experienced by patients and treated by colorectal surgeons. It has been demonstrated that the anal cushions can contribute to up 20% of the resting anal pressure.[4] The external haemorrhoidal plexus also known as *external haemorrhoids*, lie below the dentate line in the subcutaneous tissue at the anal verge and drain via the inferior rectal veins into the pudendal vessels and then into the internal iliac vein. These haemorrhoids are not normally visible and do not really contribute to the physiology of the anal canal. These vessels are covered by anoderm that is comprised of modified squamous epithelium containing pain fibres, thus affecting the way they present and are treated.

The words 'haemorrhoids' and 'haemorrhoidal disease' are not synonymous and should be used specifically to name either the presence of normal arteriovenous plexuses or the disease produced by their engorgement, respectively.

AETIOLOGY AND PATHOGENESIS

Haemorrhoidal disease affecting the internal haemorrhoids develops when tissues supporting the anal cushions deteriorate and allow them to slide down into the anal canal,[2] which in turn leads to impaired venous drainage, progressive venous engorgement, local stasis and transudation of fluid. The anal cushions function normally when they are fixed to their proper sites within the anal canal by fibromuscular ligaments, which are the anal remnants of the longitudinal layer of the muscularis propria from the rectum (Treitz's ligaments). When these submucosal fibres fragment, the anal cushions are no longer restrained from engorging excessively with blood and may result in bleeding and prolapse. These fibres may be fragmented by prolonged and repeated downward stress related to straining during defaecation. Veins that traverse the anal sphincter are blocked whereas arterial inflow continues, leading to increasing haemorrhoidal congestion. Once prolapse occurs, further engorgement of these vascular cushions leads to pain, and anal spasm then prevents reduction, leading to a vicious cycle of prolapse and congestion of the vascular cushions. Risk factors for this condition are those, which directly or indirectly are associated with excessive straining and/or increased intra-abdominal pressures (i.e., constipation, hard stools, pregnancy).[5] The progressive descent of the internal cushions produces various degrees of prolapse (see later), one the main symptoms of haemorrhoidal disease, while external haemorrhoidal disease manifests directly with venous engorgement. Defaecation in the squatting position may also aggravate the tendency to prolapse as it increases perineal descent and pressure. The anatomical alterations modify the vascular haemodynamics by decreasing venous reflux (especially in the erect position) and increasing the intravascular venous pressure. Microtrauma elicited during defaecation of hard solid stools produces small lacerations of the vessel wall and, consequently, another important symptom – bleeding. The venous hypertension of the diseased anal cushions augments the filtration of fluid through the vessel wall (transudate) producing what has been referred to 'soiling' (although its pathogenesis is not because of anal incontinence) and local itching. Local blood stasis also promotes venous thrombosis, and the sudden onset of venous hypertension stretches the mucosa overlying the cushion and causes the typical severe perianal pain during the attack (thrombosed haemorrhoidal disease). The external haemorrhoidal plexus also known as *external haemorrhoids*, lie in the subcutaneous tissue at the anal verge, are not normally visible and only cause symptoms when acutely thrombosed causing localised swelling and severe acute pain.

CLASSIFICATION

The classic staging of haemorrhoidal disease refers to the internal plexus prolapse and is classified into four degrees (Goligher's classification): grade 1 – the anal cushions bleed but do not prolapse; grade 2 – the anal cushions prolapse through the anus on straining but reduce spontaneously; grade 3 – the anal cushions prolapse through the anus on straining or exertion and require manual replacement into the anal canal; and grade 4 – the anal cushions are constantly prolapsed. This classification is therefore a clinical classification based on the actual symptoms rather than size or appearance of haemorrhoids.

SYMPTOMS AND DIAGNOSIS

The most frequent symptom of haemorrhoidal disease is bleeding, normally reported as bright red.[6] Bleeding is usually self-limiting, although in patients on anticoagulation or with predisposing bleeding diathesis can be more abundant. Other symptoms include prolapse (Fig. 17.1), mucous discharge, itching and feeling of a lump. Thrombosed haemorrhoid from the internal plexus normally presents as a very large and painful prolapsed pile. This non-reducible haemorrhoid should not be described as 'external haemorrhoids'. Thrombosis of external haemorrhoids is also responsible for acute anal pain irrespective of bowel movements.[6] In contrast to thrombosed haemorrhoids from the

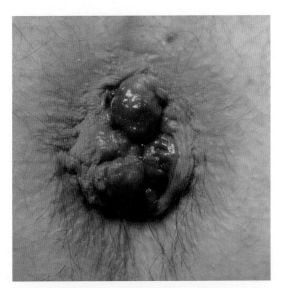

Figure 17.1 Prolapsed haemorrhoids.

internal plexus, thrombosed haemorrhoids from the external plexus will present as a relatively small and well-defined nodule at the anal verge. This very painful condition is also known as *perianal haematoma*. External haemorrhoids should not be confused with anal skin tags that are always present and not normally painful.

Haemorrhoidal disease can be diagnosed by history, examination (including inspection of the anal canal). Fresh bleeding not associated with any other anal symptoms and without any other colorectal alarm symptoms (i.e., change in bowel habit, abdominal pain) or without family history of colorectal neoplasia should still be investigated with a flexible sigmoidoscopy. Positive faecal occult blood, anaemia or right-sided abdominal pain/palpable mass should be evaluated by a complete colonic examination (either a colonoscopy or computed tomography [CT] virtual colonography).

MANAGEMENT

Therapeutic strategies normally depend on the severity of symptoms and the amount of haemorrhoidal tissue prolapsing beyond the anal verge (Goligher classification; see Table 17.1 later).[7]

FIRST DEGREE

Dietary changes

If the piles are not prolapsing, non-operative methods should be attempted first. The primary problems of constipation and straining at stool need to be addressed. In some patients, improving bowel action with laxatives in the form of fibres may help to control the symptoms, especially bleeding.[8–10]

Phlebotonics

Phlebotonics consist of plant extracts (i.e., flavonoids) and synthetic compounds (i.e., calcium dobesilate), which improve venous tone, stabilise capillary permeability and increase lymphatic drainage.[11] There are several available phlebotonics but Daflon 500® (Les Laboratoires Servier, France) is by far the best evaluated in the medical literature, and is widely used in Europe and the Far East.[12] Its

Table 17.1 Level of evidence for the treatment of haemorrhoids according to the severity of prolapse

| | Level of evidence | | | |
	I	II	III	IV
First degree		Dietary changes and flavonoids	Rubber-band banding Sclerotherapy Infrared coagulation	
Second degree	Rubber-band ligation	HAL*/THD**	Stapled haemorrhoidopexy	
Third degree	Stapled haemorrhoidopexy	Haemorrhoidectomy	HAL*/THD** Rubber band ligation	
Fourth degree		Haemorrhoidectomy	Stapled haemorrhoidopexy, THD/HAL with haemorrhoidopexy	
Single external cushion			Haemorrhoidectomy (Ultracision, Ligasure)	

*HAL, Haemorrhoidal arterial ligation.
**THD, Transanal hemorrhoidal de-arterialisation.

pharmacological properties include noradrenalin-mediated venous contraction, reduction in blood extravasation from capillaries and inhibition of prostaglandin (PGE_2, PGF_2)-mediated inflammatory response.[13] Phlebotonics, although currently not available in the UK, improve pain, bleeding, leakage and pruritus in meta-analyses of randomised controlled trials (RCTs)[11,14] and have been introduced in national guidelines.[10]

Other forms of treatment that can give more immediate symptomatic relief include rubber-band ligation (RBL), injection sclerotherapy, infrared coagulation. Only cases refractory to non-operative methods should undergo these more invasive treatments.[7,10] Topical applications are popular with many patients, who testify relief from bleeding and pain. There are, however, no clinical trials to demonstrate any benefit from such applications.

✓ Dietary changes, fibres and phlebotonics help control symptoms in first degree haemorrhoidal disease. Invasive treatments should be reserved for refractory cases.[10]

SECOND DEGREE
Rubber-band ligation

RBL is the technique of choice for second-degree haemorrhoidal disease,[7,10] for which it is effective in 68% of patients at 5 years follow-up with a 2–5% risk of secondary haemorrhage. Rubber bands are applied in an outpatient clinic or at the end of an endoscopic examination, at the apex of the haemorrhoidal tissues just above the dentate line, taking care to avoid catching the dentate line. The strangulated tissue then becomes necrotic and sloughs off in a few days, after which the wound fibroses, resulting in fixation of the mucosa akin to forming new suspensory ligaments for the anal cushions. The haemorrhoidal tissue is thus prevented from engorging and prolapsing.

✓ RBL is the treatment of choice for second-degree haemorrhoidal disease when compared with excisional haemorrhoidectomy. In this group, it achieved similar results without the side effects of surgery. Surgery should be reserved for recurrent or third-degree haemorrhoids.[15]

Anal pain, although uncommon, is a well-known sequela of RBL, however, the procedure is relatively painless if correctly performed above the dentate line. The use of local anaesthetic infiltration before the RBL decreases the amount of post-procedure pain experienced.[16] Bleeding can occur up to 14 days after the ligation and can be important especially on patients receiving anticoagulants, therefore RBL should be used with caution in these cases and following careful discussion about the necessity to suspend anticoagulants for 2 weeks following the procedure.[17] Some patients may still experience tenesmus for a day or two that is partially relieved by oral analgesia. Up to three haemorrhoids can be banded on the same occasion although at the expenses of greater discomfort. RBL can easily be repeated and is often offered as a course rather than one-off treatment; and approximately 4 weeks is usually waited between each session.[7] More severe complications

have rarely been reported such as severe local and systemic sepsis and death.[10]

Sclerotherapy

Injection sclerotherapy is an alternative technique used for the treatment of second-degree haemorrhoids, providing at least some temporary symptomatic relief in 69% of patients.[7,10] Sclerosant agents used include phenol (5%) in almond oil or sodium tetradecyl sulphate. These are injected into the submucosa around the pedicle of the pile, at the level of the anorectal ring, and cause local inflammation leading to reduced blood flow into the haemorrhoids. The sclerosant also causes fibrosis, which draws minor prolapse back into the anal canal.

✓ Inadvertently deep injections can cause perirectal fibrosis, prostatitis, infection and urethral irritation. Rare but major complications as impotence, fatal necrotising fasciitis and abdominal compartment syndrome following sclerotherapy have been reported.[7,10]

Other treatments

Various other methods have been used less or completely abandoned over the years. Infrared photocoagulation produced less pain compared to RBL and sclerotherapy, but requires an additional device.[10,18] Cryotherapy results in unpleasant and foul smelling discharge and, if not performed properly, can destroy the internal anal sphincter producing anal stenosis and incontinence. Anal stretch, based on the belief that haemorrhoidal disease derives from a narrowing of the lower canal, is not performed anymore due to the concerns of damage to the internal anal sphincter and subsequent impairment to anal sphincter function.

THIRD DEGREE

Traditionally, third-degree haemorrhoidal disease was removed by excisional haemorrhoidectomy.[10] Haemorrhoidectomy as first described by Milligan and Morgan consists of the excision of the diseased anal cushions. Since then, numerous variations to the technique have been described. It can be conducted under local or general anaesthesia; excision of haemorrhoidal cushions can be conducted with scissors,[19] diathermy, laser, vessel-sealing technology (Ligasure), ultrasonic technology (Harmonic Scalpel)[20] or radiofrequency devices;[21] mucosal wounds can be closed (Ferguson, Parks) or left open (Milligan-Morgan). Open and closed haemorrhoidectomies produced similar results for post-operative pain, complications and hospital stay.[22] However, according to a more recent meta-analysis[23] of 11 RCTs and 1326 patients comparing OH and CH, the Ferguson procedure was associated with reduced post-operative pain, faster wound healing, lesser risk of post-operative bleeding, and longer procedure time. The comparison of Ligasure versus diathermy haemorrhoidectomy also showed lower post-operative pain and urinary retention rate, shorter operative time, hospital stay and return to work for Ligasure haemorrhoidectomy.[24–26] Similar advantages were found for Harmonic Scalpel versus conventional haemorrhoidectomy with regard to post-operative pain and return to work.[27]

Nowadays, two new procedures have been added to the surgical armamentarium for the treatment of symptomatic haemorrhoids, namely stapled haemorrhoidopexy and haemorrhoidal arterial ligation also known as *transanal haemorrhoidal de-arterialisation* (HAL/THD).[10]

Stapled haemorrhoidopexy

Conventional haemorrhoidectomy deals with the symptoms alone by excising the anal cushions once they bleed or are painful. It does not act on the pathophysiological mechanism that produced the haemorrhoidal disease, the descent of the mucosal anal cushions. In 1998 a transanal circular stapling instrument was used to treat haemorrhoidal disease. The technique consisted of a circumferential mucosectomy and mucosal lifting (haemorrhoidopexy), aimed not to excise the 'diseased' haemorrhoidal cushions but rather to reconstitute the normal anatomy and physiology of the haemorrhoidal plexus.[28] Once reduced, the engorged haemorrhoidal tissue will decongest and shrink. It is thought that the stapling device restores the normal anatomy of the anal canal and enables the haemorrhoidal cushions to perform their role in continence, as opposed to haemorrhoidectomy techniques that only excise abundant tissues.

Since its introduction, numerous studies have assessed the short- and long-term efficacy of stapled haemorrhoidopexy, and thus far this technique has produced the largest amount of evidence-based analyses comparing it to classic and modern haemorrhoidectomies. Stapled haemorrhoidopexy produced better results compared to traditional haemorrhoidectomies with regard to early post-operative outcomes such as post-operative pain, bleeding and length of hospital stay,[29–32] but produced similar results to Ligasure haemorrhoidectomy for post-operative pain, bleeding, urinary retention, difficulty in defaecation, anal fissure, return to normal activities, and hospital stay.[33–38]

✔ Short-term outcomes are significant improved in stapled haemorrhoidopexy compared to techniques of traditional haemorrhoidectomy[26–29] but are similar to those achieved by Ligasure haemorrhoidectomy.[33–38]

Although the rates of anal stenoses are lower compared to traditional open haemorrhoidectomy, faecal incontinence rates and tenesmus are higher.[39,40] Furthermore, stapled haemorrhoidopexy is associated with increase recurrence of haemorrhoidal prolapse and anal skin tags, worse quality of life and is less cost-effective when compared to classic haemorrhoidectomy on long-term follow-up.[28,31,32,40–42]

✔ Stapled haemorrhoidopexy loses its early advantages compared to classic haemorrhoidectomy when considering faecal incontinence, tenesmus, recurrence rates and quality of life at long-term follow-up.[28,39,40]

An additional feature of stapled haemorrhoidopexy is the potential to produce significant and sometimes serious morbidity and even mortality in the immediate post-operative period. These complications, albeit rare and reported mostly as case reports, seriously endanger patients' lives for what is the treatment of an otherwise benign disease and are often heralded by abdominal pain, urinary retention and fever.[43–45] It is believed that such complications derive from a full-thickness (or near full-thickness) staple line and resulting anastomotic leakage. Furthermore, distressing new

symptoms such as tenesmus are probably related to the mucosal stimulation of the staples and sometimes require a second operation for their removal.[46]

Haemorrhoidal arterial ligation/transanal haemorrhoidal de-arterialisation

This non-excisional technique is based on the occlusion of the haemorrhoidal arterial flow that feeds the haemorrhoidal plexus, by Doppler-guided identification and ligation of the terminal branches of the superior rectal artery using a specially designed proctoscope. The reduction in blood flow to the haemorrhoids leads to shrinkage of the anal cushions. Although the sensitive anoderm below the dentate line is avoided to minimise post-operative pain, this is still present in 18.5% of patients.[3] Anal stenoses are less frequent compared to traditional haemorrhoidectomy, but recurrence rates are higher.[39] After 1 year follow-up, recurrence was present in 4.8% for third-degree and 26.7% for fourth-degree haemorrhoidal disease, although the addition of a mucosal plication (mucopexy) further decreased such occurrence in fourth-degree patients.[3,47]

✔ HAL/THD produced less post-operative pain and anal stenosis but results in higher recurrence rates compared to traditional haemorrhoidectomy.[39,48] The addition of a mucopexy to HAL/THD lowers the long-term recurrence rates to levels similar to traditional haemorrhoidectomy.[47]

In recent years numerous meta-analyses compared results of HAL/THD to stapled haemorrhoidopexy.[49–51] Based on the one including the largest number of studies, stapled haemorrhoidopexy produced higher post-operative bleeding and no significant difference in terms of operating time, post-operative pain, hospital time and return-to-work time. However, the total recurrence rate was higher in the HAL/THD group than in the stapled haemorrhoidopexy group.[49]

More recently, the HubBle trial compared HAL/THD to RBL for the treatment of second- and third-degree haemorrhoids.[52] The study showed that 1-year post-procedure, 49% of patients in the RBL group and 30% of patients in the HAL group had haemorrhoid recurrence (adjusted odds ratio [aOR] 2.23, 95% confidence interval [CI], 1.42–3.51; $P = 0.0005$).[52] In a post-hoc analysis comparing a subgroup of patients who underwent an outpatient course of RBL treatment consisting of multiple procedures to patients who received one HAL procedure, the difference in recurrence rate was 37% for RBL and 30% for HAL (aOR, 1.35; 95% CI, 0.85–2.15; $P = 0.20$).[52] However, these post-hoc analysis results have to be interpreted very cautiously because of the definition adopted for recurrence and different follow-up length between the two groups.[53]

FOURTH DEGREE

Haemorrhoidectomy is the main treatment for fourth-degree haemorrhoids (grade 2 evidence) with a recurrence rate of 2–8%.[10] Closed haemorrhoidectomy has reduced post-operative pain, faster wound healing and a lesser risk of post-operative bleeding compared to open procedures.[23] Some authors have suggested that THD may have a role for the treatment of advanced haemorrhoidal disease.[10,54–56] In general, newer technologies significantly reduce post-operative pain and speed up post-operative recovery and return to work at the expense of increased costs due to the disposable devices and increased recurrence rate.

POST-OPERATIVE PROBLEMS

Common but transient problems that occur after haemorrhoidectomy include urinary retention, transient incontinence to flatus and faecal impaction. Post-operative pain, bleeding, anal stenosis and fissures also occur and must be mentioned to patients.[10] Permanent anal incontinence is present in up to 6% of patients.[10]

Post-operative pain

Despite the numerous treatments that over the decades have been proposed for the surgical treatment of haemorrhoids, the essential problems encountered remain similar. Whichever technique is used, pain may still be significant in some patients in the post-operative period. Some authors have described post-haemorrhoidectomy pain as being akin to passing glass fragments, such that many patients would rather suffer the discomfort of large prolapsing haemorrhoids for years than submit to surgery. Pain is multifactorial, spasm of the internal sphincter as well as the actual skin wound with its exposed nerves being the most significant factors.

Numerous meta-analyses have evaluated the effects of various adjuncts to oral analgesics (non-steroidal anti-inflammatory drugs, paracetamol and opiates) to control post-operative pain. Local anaesthetic infiltration (pudendal nerve block) has been shown to significantly improve immediate post-operative pain.[57] The effects of oral and topical metronidazole on post-operative pain have been assessed in numerous comparative studies with contrasting results,[58–63] and unfortunately no meta-analysis is currently available on this topic. All treatments acting on the internal anal sphincter have an effect on post-operative pain. Glyceryl trinitrate (GTN) is thought to decrease muscle spasm and increase anodermal blood flow; in the first 2 post-operative weeks following haemorrhoidectomy it improves pain, healing and resumption of daily activities at the expense of an increased incidence of headaches.[64] Similar results were also achieved with local calcium-channel blockers and botulinum toxin A.[65,66] Concomitant lateral internal sphincterotomy at the time of haemorrhoidectomy significantly reduces post-operative pain at the expense of an increase in faecal incontinence rates (1.8% vs. 6.6%).[67]

✔ Local anaesthetics, GTN, calcium-channel blockers and botulinum toxin are useful post-operative adjuncts for post-operative pain. Lateral internal sphincterotomy decreases pain at the expense of an increase in faecal incontinence.

Post-operative haemorrhage

A less frequent problem is post-operative haemorrhage. Bleeding in the immediate post-operative period is usually because of inadequate intra-operative haemostasis. Submucosal adrenaline (epinephrine) injection has been shown to be effective for addressing bleeding after excisional haemorrhoidectomy.[68] Secondary bleeding is more often as a result of post-operative infection and it affects approximately 5% of patients undergoing haemorrhoidectomy. The advocated treatment is antibiotics. Following stapled

haemorrhoidectomy, bleeding may follow the rare staple-line dehiscence.

Anal stenosis

Post-haemorrhoidectomy anal stricture is an uncommon occurrence seen in only 3.7% of haemorrhoidectomies,[69] and represents a technical failure to leave sufficient mucocutaneous skin bridges. The stricture usually presents 6 weeks post-operatively and is treated with anal dilatation and stool softeners.

Thrombosed haemorrhoids

Prolapsed thrombosed internal haemorrhoids (Fig. 17.2) and perianal haematoma are best managed conservatively. The course of these conditions is self-limiting and normally symptoms resolve within a couple of weeks. Laxatives, stool softeners, sitz baths, ice packs, oral and topical analgesia are often helpful. Perianal haematomas presenting very early may be considered for surgical excision or drainage. Very rarely prolapsed thrombosed internal haemorrhoids with gangrenous component may also require excision (Fig. 17.3).

ANAL FISSURE

INTRODUCTION

An anal fissure is an ulceration of the squamous epithelium of the anal canal distal to the dentate line. It is a common complaint in the colorectal clinic. Medical treatment is simple but is frequently not adhered to and is not successful in a significant number of cases. Surgical management has become less frequently used due to the application of botulinum toxin.

AETIOLOGY

Two main factors contribute to the formation of posterior anal fissures. First, hard faeces contribute by increasing the local trauma on the anal mucosa, although 25% of fissures present in patients without constipation.[70] Second, affected patients frequently present with internal anal sphincter hypertonia, which in turn, enhances the traumatic effects of the hard faeces and provokes a relative tissue ischemia with decreased blood supply to the anal mucosa. The internal anal sphincter alone appears to be responsible for the hypertonia.[71] Hypertonia of the internal anal sphincter is caused by the decreased production of nitric oxide by the internal sphincter, a substance that normally relaxes muscle contraction. This produces the high mean resting anal pressures frequently seen in affected patients.

After the initial tear, a vicious cycle of non-healing and repeated trauma leads to development of chronic deep fissures. In this cycle, local pain increases sphincter reflex contraction, which in turn worsens the effect of hard stools and local tissue ischaemia. This mechanism can explain the achievement of high healing rates with therapies, which reduce the sphincter tone and improve the local blood flow.[72]

Although this mechanism is valid for most patients, other factors have to be considered in elderly patients or post-partum patients where anal fissures have been reported in

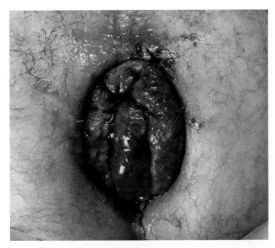

Figure 17.2   Thrombosed prolapsed internal haemorrhoids.

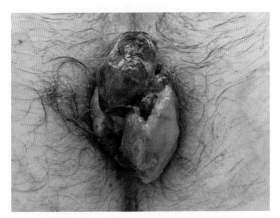

Figure 17.3   Gangrenous haemorrhoids.

the presence of normal or hypotonic internal sphincters *(see anterior anal fissures later)*.[73]

CLASSIFICATION

Anal fissures are classified according to their duration into acute or chronic, their morphological appearance into 'superficial' or 'deep' fissures, and according to their location into posterior (80–90%), anterior (2.5–10%), or in unusual positions. Furthermore, primary anal fissures are not caused by underlying chronic disease whereas secondary anal fissures are associated with other diseases such as chronic inflammatory bowel disease, human immunodeficiency virus, tuberculosis, syphilis, and some neoplasms.[73] Secondary fissures are usually multiple or located in unusual positions.

Anal fissures are considered to be acute if they have been present for less than 6 weeks, are superficial, and have well-demarcated edges. They are considered chronic if they have been present for more than 6 weeks and have keratinous edges, if there is a sentinel tag and hypertrophied anal papilla and if the fibres of the internal anal sphincter are visible in the base of the fissure (Fig. 17.4).[73]

Superficial fissures, as the name implies, involve only the superficial mucocutaneous layers of the anal canal, presenting with a superficial separation of the anoderm with sharp edges. The base of the fissure does not reach the internal

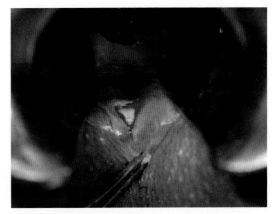

Figure 17.4   Chronic anal fissure with visible fibres of the internal anal sphincter and sentinel skin tag.

anal sphincter. The vast majority of superficial fissures will heal spontaneously within days or within a few weeks of appropriate conservative treatment. Deep anal fissures are recognised by the characteristic deep, wide pear-shaped ulcer, often with visible fibres of the internal anal sphincter and minimal granulation tissue at the base. Other features of a chronic anal fissure include the distinctive triad of indurated ulcer edges, a distal skin tag (sentinel pile) and a proximal hypertrophic anal papilla. Deep fissures often persist and either tend not to heal without intervention or recur regularly.

Posterior anal fissure presents in the posterior triangular space, also called *space of Brick* or *triangle of Minor.* The space is formed by the peculiar architectural arrangement of the sphincter mechanism on the posterior midline, where there is a 'Y'-shaped deficiency of the fibres of the external sphincter.[74] This space is an area where traumatic factors act most and where there are high-resting anal pressures and reduced local perfusion. Furthermore, branches of the inferior rectal artery at the posterior commissure are less dense in the sub-anodermal space and within the internal anal sphincter in the posterior midline.[75] In contrast, anterior anal fissures are more frequent in women and usually associated with occult external anal sphincter injuries and impaired sphincter function. Such pathogenetic mechanisms have important implications and exclude treatments such as lateral sphincterotomies or Botulinum toxin injection.[76]

✔ Anterior fissures have aetiopathogenetic mechanisms different from those located posteriorly. High sphincter pressures seem less responsible for these fissures and therefore treatments not acting on the anal pressures, such as anal flaps, should be preferred.

SYMPTOMS AND DIAGNOSIS

Pain is usually the predominant symptom in anal fissures with or without the presence of fresh bleeding. The pain classically presents during defaecation and is described as excruciating and sharp, like 'a knife cutting', which last for several minutes or the entire day. Anal fissures can be visualised by gentle parting the buttocks with eversion of the anal verge. Intra-anal examinations should not be attempted in the clinic due to the severe pain. If the clinical suspicion of a secondary pathology is high, digital rectal and proctoscopic examinations should be performed under regional or general anaesthesia.

Differential diagnoses include all causes of secondary fissures, anal cancers and inter-sphincteric abscesses. Where there is doubt, biopsy and appropriate histological examination and/or cultures are indispensable.

MANAGEMENT

The current treatment of anal fissures in the UK is summarised into the recommendations of the Association of Coloproctology of Great Britain and Ireland (ACPGBI) statement. This relies on a stepwise approach from conservative to progressively more invasive treatments, taking into consideration particular cases such as women following vaginal deliveries or men with previous proctological surgery.[70]

INITIAL TREATMENT – CONSERVATIVE MEASURES

When managing anal fissures, the logical strategy is to treat factors that influence the persistence of the fissure. Any abnormal pattern of defaecation (hard constipated stools) needs to be addressed by appropriate dietary advice and medication (increasing liquid intake, stool softeners and topical analgesics). Patients with relatively normal bowel function but excessive straining at defaecation might benefit from anorectal biofeedback. All these treatments are non-specific, aim at softening the stools and facilitate regular bowel movements; these alone result in healing anal fissures in almost 50% of cases.[77]

Glyceryl trinitrate

If non-specific conservative treatment fails, specific medical treatments can be offered to reversibly decrease the hypertonic sphincter spasm and improve local tissue ischaemia. These are used with a stepwise approach, from the least to the most invasive. GTN and diltiazem are two local creams most commonly used that help to relax the internal anal sphincter. Botulinum toxin, recently introduced, acts by blocking the release of the acetylcholine neurotransmitter. These approaches, also called '*chemical sphincterotomy*' (as opposed to the surgical sphincterotomy), are effective when associated with modification of the predisposing factors (hard stools, constipation, straining).

✓✓ GTN is better than placebo in healing anal fissure. Diltiazem and botulinum toxin are equivalent to GTN in efficacy with fewer adverse events. Medical therapy is not as effective as surgical sphincterotomy, however, is not associated with the risk of incontinence in any of the RCTs reported.[78]

GTN acts by relaxing the internal anal sphincter musculature through the local donation of nitric oxide. It has been shown to produce fissure healing in 68% of patients after 8 weeks of treatment, but late recurrence is in the range of 50% of those initially cured.[78] However, almost half of these could be successfully treated by a second topical course.

The National Institute for Health and Care Excellence (NICE) guideline: topical 0.4% GTN cream (Rectogesic 4 mg/g rectal ointment) is licensed in the UK for the relief of pain associated with chronic anal fissure in adults for a maximum of 8 weeks, generally applied twice daily. This is the first drug to be used in patients with anal fissure that require medical treatment.

No cases of permanent faecal incontinence have been described. The major drawback to the use of GTN local cream is the occurrence of significant headaches, which has been reported in 25% of patients.[69] This can be sufficient to reduce compliance to the treatment including definitive withdraw from it in 3% of cases.[79]

Diltiazem

Diltiazem is a calcium-channel blocker and vasodilator, which increases blood flow to smooth muscles and relaxes muscle tone.

✓✓ In a recent meta-analysis that compared diltiazem to GTN, the former was equally effective but was associated with a lower incidence of side effects, headache and recurrence.[80] No cases of permanent incontinence were reported. Although the ACPGBI recommends topical diltiazem as first-line treatment in the management of anal fissure (twice daily for 8 weeks), according to the NICE guidelines this product is not licensed in the UK for treating chronic anal fissure.

Botulinum toxin

Botulinum toxin normally binds to presynaptic cholinergic nerve terminals and inhibits the release of acetylcholine at the neuromuscular junction. This leads to relaxation of the anal sphincter for 2–3 months, an effect that appears to be independent of the technique, site of injection or the dose used (median 23 Units, range 10–100 U).[68]

In a meta-analysis of six RCTs, botulinum toxin was as effective as GTN for the management of chronic fissures (healing rates 76%), produces lower rates of headaches but higher rates of transient anal incontinence (5–10% of cases).[81,82] The main drawback is related to its higher costs (£200 for 100 U), not including costs of administration (often general or regional anaesthesia in a hospital operating theatre), which limit its use to refractory cases.[70] To decrease costs, patients can be grouped on the same list and one vial can be used for four patients.[70]

SURGICAL TREATMENTS

ANAL DILATATION

Anal dilatation was first described in 1838 by Lord in the treatment of haemorrhoids. Lord's original eight-finger dilatation was abandoned in favour of a more gentle four-finger stretch for four minutes and more recently, a standardised dilatation procedure using a Parks' retractor opened to 4.8 cm. Although anal dilatation resulted in successful healing of anal fissures comparable to lateral internal sphincterotomy, both the internal and external sphincters can be irregularly disrupted with a higher risk of incontinence than sphincterotomy. This treatment has therefore only an historical role and is definitely abandoned in modern practice.[83]

LATERAL ANAL SPHINCTEROTOMY

Lateral sphincterotomy involves the division of the internal anal sphincter to restore a normal anal sphincter tone from the initial hypertonia. It can be performed either as an open or closed procedure with little difference in terms of fissure persistence or risk of incontinence.[78] The optimal amount of sphincter to be divided is a matter of discussion, and additional factors have to be considered such as age of the patient, sex, previous vaginal deliveries or operations involving the anal canal. Theoretically, 30% of the sphincter muscle fibres should be divided, which does not correspond anatomically to 30% of the sphincter length. As a rule of thumb, in a tailored sphincterotomy, the internal sphincter is divided up to the highest point of the fissure only (in the past sphincterotomy was done with division of the internal sphincter up to the level of the dentate line). This more conservative approach seems to decrease the impairment of continence. Healing rates are in the range of 85%.[70] In a pooled analysis of 4512 patients, flatus incontinence was present in 9%, soiling in 6% and incontinence to solid stool in 0.83%.[84]

Compared to all other treatments for anal fissure, lateral sphincterotomy produces the highest healing rates but also a significant risk of incontinence.[85]

FISSURECTOMY

Surgical removal of the fissure (fissurectomy) has shown promising results. Fissurectomy includes excision of the fibrotic edge of the fissure, curettage of its base and excision of the sentinel tag and/or anal papilla if present.[70] Success rates have been reported in 67% of patients when associated with botulinum toxin injections,[86] 100% when associated with advancement flap anoplasty, with 0–7% de-novo incontinence.[87] Recurrence after fissurectomy was 11.6% at 5 years follow-up,[88] and nil when associated with other treatments (isosorbide dinitrate, botulinum toxin injections, skin flap anoplasty).[86,87,89,90]

ANAL ADVANCEMENT FLAP

Anal fissures without anal hypertonia (low pressure sphincter) pose a peculiar challenge for the colorectal surgeon.[76] Common therapies that decrease the sphincter tone cannot be used in this situation because they would not resolve the fissure and actually produce or exacerbate incontinence. Patients with low resting sphincter pressures may be helped by anal cutaneous advancement flaps (anoplasty),[91] with or without fissurectomy.[92] Similarly, patients with recurrence after lateral sphincterotomy necessitate anal manometry and ultrasound to identify those with low resting anal pressures from patients with persistently raised resting pressures, therefore guiding treatment towards a repeat lateral sphincterotomy in the opposite lateral quadrant or an advancement flap anoplasty. More recently, indications have further expanded and flaps have been used with good results for the treatment of all chronic fissures (not just low-pressure ones) because of their ability to decrease local pain and therefore help in the relaxation of the hypertonic sphincter complex.[93,94]

The literature on this matter is quite mixed as various types of flaps exist (island, V-Y, rotational) and are frequently associated with other procedures (botulinum toxin, fissurectomy).[93,95] In a recent meta-analysis ,advancement flaps have shown less incontinence rates but similar healing rates compared to lateral internal sphincterotomy.[96]

PRURITUS ANI

Pruritus ani is a frequent symptom, sometimes managed by dermatologists, however, it is not uncommon for the colorectal surgeon to also be referred these patients. The surgical assessment is mostly based on excluding associated and sometimes more sinister causes, which might require an operation.

AETIOLOGY AND PATHOGENESIS

There are numerous direct causes of perianal itch (Box 17.1). Clinically, however, idiopathic pruritus ani is most usually associated with a minor degree of faecal incontinence. The object of history taking and examination is to find the likely cause of faecal leakage. This may be due to local pathology permitting stool to leak to the outside or to difficulty with thorough anal cleansing, or to anal sphincteric dysfunction or other contributory causes such as irritative foods and, importantly, a high-fibre diet. In addition, applications of inappropriate topical creams and even excessive cleansing may further aggravate the situation.

DIAGNOSIS

The diagnosis of causes of minor anal leakage is most often revealed by good history taking and physical examination. Physical examination should include any evidence of skin

---

Box 17.1 Secondary causes of pruritis ani

Neoplasia
- Rectal adenoma
- Rectal adenocarcinoma
- Anal squamous cell carcinoma
- Malignant melanoma
- Bowen's disease
- Extra-mammary Paget's disease

Benign anorectal conditions
- Haemorrhoids
- Fistula-in-ano
- Anal fissure
- Rectal prolapse
- Anal sphincter injury or dysfunction
- Faecal incontinence
- Radiation proctitis
- Ulcerative colitis

Infections
- Condyloma acuminatum
- Herpes simplex virus
- Threadworm
- *Candida albicans*
- Syphilis
- *Lymphogranuloma venereum*

Dermatological
- Neurogenic dermatitis
- Contact dermatitis
- Lichen simplex
- Lichen planus
- Lichen atrophicus

disease elsewhere. The perineum and underclothes should be carefully inspected for any reason for soiling.

Digital rectal examination may reveal anal sphincteric dysfunction or other reasons for the pruritus. Wiping with moist gauze may confirm staining and thus anal leakage. Repeat examination after straining may be required to reveal a rectal prolapse. Endoscopy may be required in certain cases. Skin lesions may need to be biopsied and examined for fungus or other dermatological problems.

Another cause of pruritus ani is *Enterobius* or threadworm. Placing a piece of adhesive tape to the anus and then transferring to a microscopy slide may reveal these. The presence of ova is indicative of infection.

TREATMENT

Treatment is dependent on the primary pathology. Advice should be cautious before any surgical intervention, as cure is not certain. In primary pruritus ani, the aims of treatment are the reduction of leakage, maintenance of good personal hygiene and the prevention of further injury to the perianal skin. Reducing flatulence by lowering dietary fibre and adding probiotics may decrease soiling. Loose stools may also be solidified with anti-motility medications. Small amounts of loose stool trapped within the anus may leak out and cause irritation later in the day long after the perineum had been cleaned.

Cleansing of the perineum using water with drying by gentle dabbing is preferred to vigorous rubbing with toilet paper. An anti-itch powder and the use of anti-histamine medication may be useful to break the vicious cycle of itching and scratching. Loose underwear made of non-allergenic material may decrease the chance of contact dermatitis.

The desire to scratch may be due to fresh leakage and immediate flushing with water may obviate the desire to scratch, which otherwise may be well nigh irresistible. Short-term use of a hydrocortisone cream may help to break the cycle, but steroid use should not be prolonged.

In a study by Lysy et al.,[82] topical capsaicin has been shown to be effective for idiopathic pruritus ani; 44 patients were randomised to topical capsaicin 0.006% or placebo (menthol 1%) and crossover was carried out after 4 weeks. Of these patients, 31 experienced relief with capsaicin but none with menthol.

In patients with refractory pruritus ani, anal tattooing with methylene blue destroys the nerve endings around the anus, leading to hypo-aesthesia of perianal skin and relief from the annoying itch.

PILONIDAL SINUS

The word 'pilonidal' is derived from the Latin words *pilus* meaning hair and *nidus* meaning nest, because of trapped hair found within the sinus. It usually affects hirsute young adults, males twice as often as females.[97]

AETIOLOGY

Pilonidal sinus is an acquired disease with the traditional theory suggesting it results from a foreign body reaction to extruded hair in the skin. Keratin plugs and other debris

may contribute further to the inflammation. This theory arose from the observation of pilonidal sinus appearing in the hands of a barber.[98] Bascom postulated that the disease arose from infection of hair follicles in the natal cleft, which may have been occluded by keratin.[99] The infected hair follicle theory is supported by epidemiological findings that the age of presentation starts after puberty, affecting young adults. Obesity is another risk factor. Hormonal changes at puberty and obesity are closely linked to an increased incidence of infected pilosebaceous glands. Whether the cause is exclusive to either theory or a combination of both is unclear.

However, most authors agree that propagation of the inflammation to a chronic sinus is related to a foreign body reaction from a non-healing abscess. Loose hairs from the region tend to gather toward the natal cleft due to the anatomy and suction of the buttocks on movement. These hairs migrate into the sinus, tip first, and get trapped, aggravating the inflammatory process.[100]

CLINICAL MANIFESTATION

An asymptomatic pilonidal disease does not require treatment; however, it often presents as an acute abscess in the midline of the sacrococcygeal region. Following incision and drainage, many patients still develop a pilonidal sinus with a primary tract epithelialised and forming a small pit in the midline of the natal cleft. Some patients also develop secondary tracts, which persist as discharging sinuses lined by granulation tissue.

Hence, patients often present either in the acute abscess stage or with an off-midline discharging sinus. When they present with a chronic pilonidal sinus, it is common to note midline pits in the natal cleft that correspond to the healed primary tracts. In such cases, the pilonidal sinus will be situated slightly cephalad to the primary pit, 1–3 cm lateral to the midline, over the underlying sacrum.

If no primary pits are seen or if the sinus drains either lateral to the sacrum or appears caudal to the primary pits, other diagnoses should be considered. It is very unusual to find multiple sinuses that open into both buttocks simultaneously. In such a case, the differential diagnosis would include hydradenitis suppurativa, complex anal fistula, osteomyelitis with draining sinuses to the skin, as well as infective conditions, such as tuberculosis or actinomycosis.

TREATMENT

PILONIDAL ABSCESS

Simple incision and drainage is the treatment for pilonidal abscesses when diagnosed, with up to 58% of patients having complete healing.[101] Meticulous skin care and good hygiene, avoiding skin maceration and regular hair shaving prevents hair from penetrating the healing scar. Such diligent wound care may further lower recurrence rates. As such, whichever surgical technique is used, careful attention to skin hygiene and hair exfoliation is often recommended.

CHRONIC PILONIDAL SINUS

A chronic pilonidal sinus is a pilonidal sinus appearing after treatment of an acute pilonidal abscess. The term is also used for patients who have a discharging sinus at first presentation with or without an abscess. The surgical management of a chronic pilonidal sinus aims to obliterate the epithelialised sinus tract and heal the wound.

OUTPATIENT OPTIONS

Simple outpatient options include phenol injection and excision and lay-open of the chronic tract. Phenol destroys the epithelium in the tract and sterilises the wound. An injection of 1–2 mL of 80% phenol is given into the tract, with great care taken to protect the surrounding skin with paraffin or other ointments. The surrounding hair is shaved off and wound dressing performed daily. The phenol injection can be repeated every 4–6 weeks till the wound has healed. This simple technique has the advantage of minimal time away from work, with a variable healing rate of 59–95%. However, the side effects include skin necrosis and abscess formation in up to 22% of patients. Some authors have advocated a reduced strength of 40% phenol, with a reduced complication rate of 12% and a healing rate of 77%.[102]

Alternatively, the sinus tract can be laid open under local anaesthesia and dressed in the outpatient setting. Some authors have advocated using fibrin sealant or regular wound brushing to reduce the wound healing time or recurrence rate. However, whatever modifications are used, the recurrence rate is generally low, from 10–18%, with the added advantage of minimal complications or time away from work.

INPATIENT OPTIONS

Once a surgeon decides to perform a more complex procedure, the options increase but the best method remains debatable. The principles of the operation are to eradicate the sinus tract, ensure complete healing of the overlying skin and prevent recurrence. The options include laying the wound open to heal by secondary intention or primary closure of the surgical wound. The techniques with primary closure are further categorised into midline closure or off-midline closure.

Lay-open methods include simple excision of subcutaneous tract (sinectomy), wide excision down to sacral periostium and marsupialisation of the wound.

Lay-open methods involving wide radical excisions are associated with long healing times, limited excisions with shorter times (sinusotomy/sinectomy).[103]

Conversely, many have adopted primary closure techniques because the time to wound healing and return to work is shorter.

Theoretically, off-midline closure should be favoured over midline techniques, there being fewer recurrences with off-midline closure (1.4% vs. 10.3% for midline closure) and wound infections (6.3% vs. 10.4% for midline closure).[104]

One theory behind off-midline techniques is that the natal cleft is an anatomical trough, which loose hairs tend to gravitate toward. Negative pressure in the natal cleft produced by movement of the buttocks on sitting and walking also creates a suction effect attracting the tips of loose hair towards the natal cleft. Any wound in the midline will

preferentially gather loose hairs in the wound, predisposing midline wounds to recurrence. Techniques of off-midline closure change the natal cleft contour and disperse suction pressure over a wider area, thereby reducing the likelihood of loose hair implanting in the healing wound. The Karydakis flap and the Limberg flap are most thoroughly analysed off-midline procedures.

A meta-analysis confirmed that recurrence rates are lower but healing times slower after open healing compared to primary closure techniques. For primary closure recurrence are lower and healing times faster after off-midline compared to midline closure techniques.[104]

Drainage following primary closure seems to have no role in the prevention of post-operative infections or recurrences.[105] Furthermore, administration of a gentamicin collagen sponge after surgical excision of sacrococcygeal pilonidal sinus disease showed no influence on wound healing and recurrence rate, but a trend towards a reduced incidence of surgical site infections was noted.[106]

Various techniques of closures have been proposed over the years for the treatment of pilonidal sinus. In the Bascom operation, an incision is made lateral to the midline to curette the deep cavity free of loose hairs and granulation tissue, together with excision of the primary midline pits using small stab incisions of about 7 mm. The midline incisions are closed primarily and the lateral wound left to heal by secondary intention.[99] Some authors close the lateral wound over a drain to reduce the healing time, with good results. Another popular technique is the Karydakis flap procedure where a 'semilateral' 'D-shaped' incision is made incorporating the sinus tract down to the presacral fascia:[107] the defect is convex on one side and straight on the other (next to the midline) (Fig. 17.5a). The flap of tissue on the straight wound side is mobilised down to the fascia to allow the flap to be brought over to the convex wound edge and sutured down in layers (Fig. 17.5b). Karydakis reported a recurrence rate of only 1%, with 8.5% wound complication rate.[99] Other flaps (Z-plasty, modified Z-plasty, gluteus maximus myocutaneous flap, V-Y fasciocutaneous flap and rhomboid fasciocutaneous flap – Limberg/Dufourmentel) have also been used for closure of primary and recurrent sinuses, the most frequent being the advancement Limberg flap (Fig. 17.6). Overall, flaps reduce the risk of recurrence, have a shorter duration of incapacity to work, a lower risk of wound infections, a lower risk of skin wound complications, and a shorter duration of hospitalisation versus direct closure, and a shorter time to complete wound healing versus the laying open technique.

Based on these data, flaps are currently the most reliable and effective method for treating both primary and recurrent pilonidal sinuses.[108]

Off-midline closures are superior compared to midline closures.[109] The Karidakis flap is usually preferred for primary pilonidal sinus because simpler to perform, while more complex flaps (i.e., Limberg) are chosen for recurrent disease in view of the significant amount of scarring already present.[109] Limberg flap is superior to Karydakis procedure in terms of infection rates and wound dehiscences[110,111] but not for recurrence rates.[112]

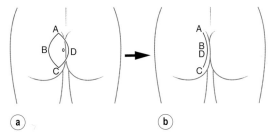

Figure 17.5 Asymmetric elliptical excision with closure of the cavity with Karydakis flap. **(a)** Asymmetric elliptical incision and excision. **(b)** Longitudinal closure of the wound after creation of the flap.

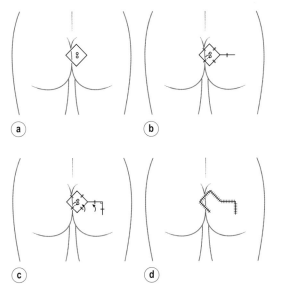

Figure 17.6 Modified Limberg flap for recurrent pilonidal sinus showing: (a) off-midline rhomboid-shaped incision incorporating sinus tracts; (b) lateral extension of incision of length equal to the side of the rhomboid incision; (c) caudal extension perpendicular to lateral incision; and (d) securing rotated flap with sutures.

More recently, a procedure called *endoscopic pilonidal sinus treatment (EPSiT)* has been proposed. The procedure involves removal of hairs and debris under vision of a miniendoscope (fistuloscope) introduced through the pits. Subsequently, a monopolar electrode is used to treat the pilonidal tissue from the inside, finally a 'curettage' of the fistula tract is performed and again haemostasis with the monopolar electrode.[113] Complete healing is generally achieved in 33 days with a failure rate of 6.3%.[114] EPSiT for recurrent disease demonstrated complete wound healing in 95% of the patient, with a mean complete wound healing time of 29 ± 12 days and 5.1% recurrences.[115] The use of ultraportable negative pressure wound therapy may further improve wound management after EPSiT, facilitating a quicker recovery and possibly improving overall patient satisfaction.[116]

ANAL STENOSIS

Anal stenosis is an abnormal narrowing of the anal canal with physical obstruction at that level. This is in contrast to anal canal spasm secondary to painful lesions or functional abnormalities where examination shows a supple and fully compliant anus.

AETIOLOGY

The commonest cause is surgery with excessive mucocutaneous excision, usually but not only following haemorrhoidectomy. Other causes are listed in Box 17.2. Recurrent anal fissures, perianal abscesses with repeated surgical procedures and excessive excision of perianal skin in Bowen's or Paget's disease may present with anal canal stenosis.

CLINICAL PRESENTATION

A history of constipation, decreasing stool calibre, difficulty in voiding with the need to strain excessively and tenesmus are usually the first symptoms of anal stenosis. Bleeding may occur from traumatic defaecation or digitation. Scarring from previous anal surgery may be obvious, if digitation is possible, the stenosis may be mild to moderate and the level of the stenosis relative to the dentate line as well as the length of the stenosis must be noted. Anatomical findings may not correlate well with the magnitude of the obstructive symptoms.

TREATMENT

A biopsy may be essential if there is no history of previous surgery or anal trauma. Treatment of anal stenosis depends on the severity and level of stenosis within the anal

---

Box 17.2 Aetiology of anal stenosis

Congenital
- Imperforate anus
- Anal atresia

Acquired
- Irradiation
- Lacerations
- Following surgery of anal canal/low rectum (commonly anastomotic failure)

Neoplastic
- Perianal or anal cancers
- Leukaemia
- Bowen's disease
- Paget's disease

Inflammatory
- Crohn's disease
- Tuberculosis
- Amoebiasis
- *Lymphogranuloma venereum*
- Actinomycosis

Other
- Chronic anal fissure
- Ischaemic

canal, as well as when it has arisen in relation to any prior anal operation. Anal stenosis below the dentate line is often related to previous anal surgery, such as excisional haemorrhoidectomy, or to inflammatory conditions, such as Crohn's disease. Anal stenosis above the dentate line may be secondary to stapled haemorrhoidectomy or low anterior resection because of partial staple-line dehiscence or infection.

PREVENTION

The key to treatment lies in its prevention with good surgical judgment. Excessive removal of the anoderm during haemorrhoidectomy is often the cause of significant anal stenosis. Preserving a 'mucocutaneous skin bridge' of anoderm at least 1-cm wide between wounds and limiting the distal extent of tissue resection to the anal verge may minimise anal stenosis. However, preserving anodermal 'bridges' is crucial to all anal surgery and not haemorrhoidectomy alone.

ANAL DILATATION

Mild stenosis (tight anal canal but permitting the passage of the index finger) may be treated occasionally with bulk laxatives, but the recurrence rate is high. After initial manual dilatation, many surgeons have recommended regular dilatation with the patient's own finger or an appropriately sized anal dilator (e.g., St Mark's anal dilator or Hagar dilator) to maintain the anal diameter. Good functional results may be achieved in this manner for mild cases, particularly if a post-surgical stenosis is caught early. The patient should be guided to pass the dilator beyond the anal stricture twice daily for 2 months, but regular anal dilatation may not work if the scarring has already matured at the time of diagnosis. Further forceful dilatation at this stage may worsen the fibrosis and lead to more serious stenosis.

✔ Four-finger manual dilatation performed under anaesthesia should never be performed and is always unnecessary. The uncontrolled manner of anal tearing can lead to excessive anal sphincter damage and subsequent faecal incontinence.

A very scarred and stenotic anus, or one associated with Crohn's disease, may occasionally be self-maintained using Hagar dilators after initial Hagar graded dilatation under general anaesthesia if the patient is not keen on more complicated surgery. However, a worsening of scarring with time is inevitable. The principles of surgical treatment are outlined in Box 17.3.

SPHINCTEROTOMY

In the past, some surgeons believed that a hypertrophied internal anal sphincter could cause anal stenosis and hence recommended anal sphincterotomy. However, there are no studies to verify this. These patients with so-called 'anal stenosis' actually have anismus or dyssynergic defaecation. Anecdotal experience of sphincterotomy showing benefit is likely because of reduction of anal pressure in the short term. In the longer term, it could theoretically lead to faecal

> **Box 17.3 Principles of surgical treatment for anal stenosis**
>
> - Stool bulking
> - Anal dilatation
> - Examination under anaesthesia with graded Hagar's dilator followed by post-operative self-maintenance
> - Removal of cutaneous scarring
> - Stricturoplasty for anal stenosis proximal to dentate line (worst cases may need an abdominal pull-through operation)
> - Skin advancement (inwards)
> - Mucosal advancement (outwards)
> - Colostomy in desperate cases

incontinence, though this is yet unproven. These patients are better treated with biofeedback, a form of re-training of the various muscles involved to provide an appropriate coordination of defaecation. Injection of botulin toxin may also help.

STRICTUROPLASTY

Severe anal stenosis, with inability to pass the index finger through the stenosis, will usually require surgical intervention. In cases of anal stenosis proximal to the dentate line, as in stapled haemorrhoidopexy, stricturoplasty has proved to be a simple and reliable method of treatment. The stricture along the anastomosis is palpated and two to four vertical incisions are made over the scar with a narrow proctoscope. This incision is deepened until the entire thickness of the scar is incised without cutting the muscle layer of the rectal wall. The mucosa is approximated transversely with sutures and not left to heal by secondary intention. Two (anterior and posterior midline) or four (at 3, 6, 9, 12 o'clock positions) incisions across the stenosis can be performed based on the degree of stenosis. Special care must be taken not to cause full-thickness perforation to prevent septic and bleeding consequences. Adequacy of stricturoplasty is assessed by digital examination showing a supple and distensible anorectal wall at the level of the previous stenosis.

FLAP PROCEDURES

Mucosal advancement flap (above down)

This involves the advancement of anal mucosa into the stenotic area by way of a vertical incision made in the stenotic area perpendicular to the dentate line in the lateral position. An excision of the scar tissue allows widening of the stenosis. The incision is then undermined for about 2 cm and closed in a transverse manner, stitching the mucosal edge down onto the skin edge of the anoderm.

Y-V advancement flap (outside in)

Originally described by Penn in 1948, a Y incision is made, with the vertical limb of the Y in the anal canal above the proximal level of the stenosis. The 'V' of the Y is drawn on the lateral perianal skin. The skin is incised, and a V-shaped flap is raised; the length-to-breadth ratio must be less than three. After excision of the underlying scar tissue in the anal canal the flap can be mobilised into the anal canal and stitched into place. This may be done bilaterally with good results and provides relief in 85–92% of cases. Tip necrosis occurs in 10–25% of cases and stenosis may recur.[117]

V-Y advancement flap (outside in)

Unlike the Y-V advancement flap, the V-Y flap has the advantage of bringing a wider piece of skin into the stenosis to keep it open. The V is drawn with the wide base parallel to the dentate line about 2 cm long. A similar length-to-base ratio as in the Y-V flap should be maintained. Marking the skin flap is followed by its mobilisation such that it may move without tension into the anal canal. Sufficient subcutaneous tissue must be mobilised with the flap, which derives its blood supply from the perforating vessels arising within the fat. The skin is then closed behind the flap to produce the limb of the Y. A treatment success rate of 96% has been reported with this flap.

Island advancement flap (outside in)

First described in 1986, the island flap may be constructed in various shapes (e.g., diamond, house or U-shaped).[118] The flap is mobilised from its lateral margins together with the subcutaneous fat after the scar tissue in the stenotic area has been excised. A lateral sphincterotomy may or may not be performed. A broad skin flap (up to 50% of the circumference) may be brought into the entire length of the anal canal and simultaneously allow for closure of the donor site. Improvement of symptoms may be as high as 91% at 3 years of follow-up; 18–50% suffer minor wound separation.[119]

SEXUALLY TRANSMITTED INFECTIONS

Sexually transmitted infections (STIs) often present to colorectal surgeons. Signs and symptoms include diarrhoea, rectal bleeding, tenesmus and ulcerative or fistulous lesions of the rectum, anus and perineum. All healthcare providers should be aware that high-risk behaviours, including unprotected sex, multiple partners and illicit drug use, can increase transmission of STIs as well as human immunodeficiency virus (HIV).[99] The presence of more than one infecting organism is not uncommon.

The commonest organisms causing STIs of the anorectum present in three symptom categories: suppurative, ulcerative and fistulous disease (Table 17.2). The diseases presented in Table 17.3 are categorised by aetiological agent. Medications are suggested, but clinicians should consult full prescribing information and request specialist advice before using them.

HUMAN PAPILLOMAVIRUS AND ANAL WARTS

This is covered in Chapter 8 on Anal Neoplasia.

OTHER SEXUALLY TRANSMITTED INFECTIONS AFFECTING THE ANORECTUM

Herpes simplex (HSV) is a deoxyribonucleic acid (DNA) virus of the Herpesviridae family that includes varicella zoster, Epstein–Barr and cytomegalovirus. HSV-1 is usually associated with oral, labial or ocular lesions, but with increasing oral–genital contact the rate of HSV-1 genital infections has increased and accounts for up to 13% of anorectal herpes infections. HSV-2 is more typically responsible for anogenital infections from direct anogenital contact, accounting for almost 90% of such infections.

Molluscum contagiosum is caused by a virus of the pox virus family and transmitted by direct contact. It presents with painless discrete 2–6 mm skin-coloured papules with central umbilication. Multiple lesions are common; however, immunocompromised patients can develop a severe form with hundreds of skin lesions. While it is generally a self-limiting disease, treatment can be used to prevent spread and for cosmetic purposes. Treatments include curettage, cryotherapy, trichloracetic acid and electrocautery but none have proven superior in trials.

Chlamydia trachomatis is the most frequently reported bacterial STI in western countries. It is an obligate intracellular

---

Table 17.2   Anorectal sexually transmitted infections (STIs) categorised by predominant presentation

STIs with proctitis	STIs with ulcers	STIs with fistulas

• Gonorrhoea
• *Chlamydia*
• Herpes simplex virus
• Syphilis
• AIDS-associated anal ulcers
  • *Lymphogranuloma venereum*
  • Primary syphilis – chancre
  • Chancroid
  • Granuloma inguinale
  • Herpes simplex virus
• *Lymphogranuloma venereum*
  • Complex Bushke–Lowenstein tumours		

Table 17.3 Sexually transmitted organisms that affect the anorectum

Organism	Symptoms	Anoscopy/proctoscopy	Laboratory	Treatment
Viral				
HIV	Pain unrelated to defaecation	Broad-based ulcers proximal to dentate line	Serology	HAART, debridement, unroofing cavities, intra-lesional steroid injection
Herpes simplex virus (HSV)	Anorectal pain, pruritus, rectal bleeding	Perianal erythema, vesicles, ulcers, diffusely inflamed and friable rectal mucosa (Fig. 17.7)	Cytological examination of scrapings or viral culture of vesicle fluid PCR	Acyclovir or Famciclovir or Valaciclovir
Human papillomavirus (condylomata acuminatum)	Pruritus, bleeding, discharge, pain	Perianal warts (Fig. 17.8)	Excisional biopsy to determine serotype	Topical agents. Excision or destruction
Molluscum contagiosum	Painless skin lesions	Flattened, round, umbilicated lesion	Excisional biopsy and staining for molluscum bodies	Expectant, excision or destruction
Bacterial				
Chlamydia trachomatis	Tenesmus, perianal pain	Friable, often ulcerated mucosa	Tissue culture, nucleic acid amplification, serological antibody titres	Azithromycin or Doxycycline
Lymphogranuloma venereum (LGV)	Systemic symptoms, inguinal adenopathy, anogenital ulceration	Friable ulcerated rectal mucosa	LGV serotyping with nucleic acid amplification, confirmation at specialty laboratories	Doxycycline or Erythromycin
Haemophilus ducreyi (chancroid)	Anal pain	Anorectal abscesses and ulcers	Culture, Gram stain with 'school of fish' pattern, PCR	Azithromycin or Ceftriaxone or Ciprofloxacin or Erythromycin
Neisseria gonorrhoeae (gonorrhoea)	Rectal discharge	Proctitis, mucopurulent discharge	Culture of discharge on Thayer–Martin or Modified New York City agar	Ceftriaxone PLUS Treatment for *Chlamydia* if chlamydial infection is not ruled out Alternative regimen Spectinomycin
Calymmatobacterium granulomatis (granuloma inguinale)	Perianal mass, ulceration	Hard, shiny perianal masses	Smear or biopsy of mass or ulceration	Doxycycline or Azithromycin or Ciprofloxicin or Erythromycin or Trimethoprim-Sulfamethoxazole, or until all lesions have healed
Treponema pallidum (syphilis)	Primary syphilis Painful anal chancre, inguinal lymphadenopathy, lesions infected with spirochetes Secondary syphilis Condyloma lata, foul discharge, lesions infected with spirochetes Tertiary syphilis Rectal gumma, tabes dorsalis, severe perianal pain, paralysis of anal sphincters	See text	Dark-field microscopy of ulcer scrapings, immunostaining from biopsy, serology	Benzathine penicillin G

HAART, Highly active anti-retroviral therapy; *HIV*, human immunodeficiency virus; *PCR*, polymerase-chain-reaction.

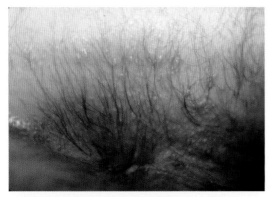

Figure 17.7 Herpetic vesicles. (Courtesy of L. Gottesman, MD.)

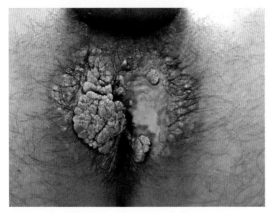

Figure 17.8 Anal warts. On the patient's left side is an area from previous surgical excision.

bacterium that is sexually transmitted and can cause infections that resemble gonorrhoea. Anorectal transmission occurs primarily through anoreceptive intercourse. Clinical syndromes resulting from chlamydial infection include cervicitis, pelvic inflammatory disease, urethritis and proctitis. Small vesicles that become ulcerated are the initial signs of infection at the site of inoculation. Areas of necrosis occur within the lymph nodes, which can then form abscesses, or a large matted mass with overlying erythema, mimicking syphilis. After resolution of these an anogenitorectal syndrome occurs, with signs of systemic infection (fevers, myalgia) and a more aggressive infection involving the perianal, anal and rectal areas resulting in ulceration, rectal pain, discharge, bleeding and severe proctitis. On sigmoidoscopy, there is a severe, non-specific granular proctitis with mucosal erythema, friability and ulceration. Biopsies of the mucosa are consistent with infectious proctitis, including crypt abscesses, infectious granulomas and giant cells, and can be difficult to distinguish from Crohn's disease.[106] Diagnosis is by culture, microimmunofluorescent antibody titres or polymerase chain reaction.

Long-term chronic inflammation from lymphogranuloma venereum results in stricture, fistulas, lymphoedema and in women can lead to the development of rectovaginal fistulas. Sexual contacts from the past 60 days should be treated, and patients should refrain from sexual activity for 7 days after completion of treatment (doxycycline).

Chancroid, caused by *Haemophilus ducreyi* is a gram-negative coccobacillus that is a frequent cause of painful anogenital ulcerations in underdeveloped countries, but is uncommon in the USA and Western Europe.

Neisseria gonorrhoeae is a gram-negative intracellular diplococcus. Symptoms of anorectal involvement include pruritus ani, bloody or mucoid discharge, tenesmus and anorectal pain. Mucopurulent discharge in combination with proctitis is the characteristic physical finding in gonococcal proctitis. On anoscopy, there is a thick, yellow mucopurulent discharge that can be expressed from anal crypts when pressure is applied. Even when the anal canal is spared, one may still see perianal erythema. A single intra-muscular dose of ceftriaxone plus treatment for chlamydia (i.e., azithromycin or doxycycline) are first-line therapy.

Syphilis is a mucocutaneous STI caused by the spirochete *Treponema pallidum*. It can present in one of several progressive stages: primary (chancre or proctitis), secondary (condyloma lata) or tertiary (with involvement of the nervous and vascular systems). Anal syphilis occurs during anoreceptive intercourse. The primary stage begins within 2–10 weeks of exposure with the appearance of an anal ulcer called a *chancre*. This is a raised, 1–2 cm lesion that begins as a small papule, which progresses into an indurated, clean-based ulcer without exudate. Anal ulcers are frequently painful (in contrast to genital ulcers), may be single or multiple, and can be located on the perianal skin, in the anal canal or in the distal rectum. Differentiation from idiopathic anal fissure may be difficult, however, chancres are usually eccentrically located (off the midline), multiple and, if opposite each other, are known as '*kissing ulcers*'. Painless but prominent lymphadenopathy is also common. If secondary bacterial infection occurs, patients can experience worsening anorectal pain. Rectal mucosal involvement results in tenesmus, rectal discharge or bleeding, though proctitis may occur with or without chancres.[107] Untreated lesions usually heal in 2–4 weeks. If primary syphilis is untreated, haematogenous spread occurs 4–10 weeks after the primary lesions and leads to secondary syphilis. This presents with systemic symptoms including fever, malaise, arthralgia, weight loss, sore throat and headache, and as a non-pruritic macular rash on the trunk, limbs, palms and/or soles. Condyloma lata, a grey or whitish wart-like lesion teeming with spirochetes, may be found near the initial chancre. These lesions are smoother and more moist than anal condyloma from HPV, are pruritic and have a foul discharge. Mucosal patches or ulcerations may appear in the rectum.[108] Tertiary syphilis is rare and presents with classic neurological and vascular symptoms.

Treponema pallidum cannot be cultured. Serology, specific immunofluorescent staining or dark-field microscopy of scrapings from chancres or lymph nodes help with the diagnosis. Treatment is with Benzathine penicillin G.

Key points

- Haemorrhoidal disease is common but other more significant diseases must be excluded, before ascribing symptoms to haemorrhoids. Treatment by RBL is appropriate in early stages. Consideration should be given either to transanal haemorrhoidal artery ligation, stapled haemorrhoidopexy or excisional haemorrhoidectomy for more severe degrees of prolapsing piles, depending on the degree present and the expertise available.
- Most anal fissures derive from an increased anal sphincter tone and treatment is based on a stepwise approach from non-invasive approaches to lateral sphincterotomy in refractory cases. Low-pressure fissures may need flap closure to control pain and achieve remission.
- Pruritus ani may result from many anorectal or dermatological conditions and remains a difficult problem to manage and treat. Reduction of anal leakage, reduction in fibre consumption and good personal hygiene remain important aspects of treatment.
- Treatment of pilonidal sinus depends upon presentation as well as patient preferences in terms of healing time, time off work and recurrence rates. Incision and drainage are the preferred treatment for acute presentation. Open wound surgery is associated with less recurrence but longer healing time compared to wound closures. Off-midline wound closure is preferred to midline if primary wound closure is performed. Flap techniques of reconstruction may be required in recurrent cases due to the significant scarring.
- Anal stenosis has many aetiologies but the commonest is a result of anal surgery. Treatments range from anal dilatation to flap procedures.
- Although STI are managed by an STI service, a high index of suspicion and knowledge of the most common lesions is required because they might present to the colorectal surgeon. An appropriate sexual history of patients and physical examination are important because these diseases are usually associated and present with other infections such as Hepatitis and HIV. Patients and partners should be involved in the process.

▶ RECOMMENDED VIDEOS

- LIFT procedure https://www.youtube.com/watch?v=zHSYutaulK4
- THD https://youtu.be/GfJbTk9Sut8
- Stapled Haemorrhoidopexy https://www.youtube.com/watch?v=X-v2y8XtGCCY

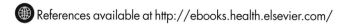 References available at http://ebooks.health.elsevier.com/

Index